A Practical Guide to Management of Femoral Head Fracture-Dislocation

Ramesh Kumar Sen • Sujit Kumar Tripathy
Editors

A Practical Guide to Management of Femoral Head Fracture-Dislocation

Springer

Editors
Ramesh Kumar Sen
Institute of Orthopedic Surgery
Max Super Speciality Hospital
Mohali, Punjab, India

Sujit Kumar Tripathy
Department of Orthopedics
All India Institute of Medical Sciences
Bhubaneswar, Odisha, India

ISBN 978-981-96-9851-6 ISBN 978-981-96-9852-3 (eBook)
https://doi.org/10.1007/978-981-96-9852-3

This Springer imprint is published by the registered company Springer Nature Singapore Pte Ltd.
The registered company address is: 152 Beach Road, #21-01/04 Gateway East, Singapore 189721, Singapore

By Dr. Ramesh Kumar Sen

To my beloved family, who stood by me through countless late nights, whose patience never wavered, and whose love provided the foundation for everything I've been able to accomplish.

And to my patients, who trusted me with their care, who taught me more about healing and humanity than any textbook ever could. Your stories are woven into the fabric of these pages. This book exists because you do.

By Dr. Sujit Kumar Tripathy

To my beloved wife—your unwavering support, love, and quiet strength have been my greatest inspiration.

To my two adorable little kids—your laughter and wonder remind me of life's purest joys.

And to all the patients who graciously offered their time, stories, and trust—thank you for granting me the opportunity to reflect, learn, and write.

This book is for you all.

Foreword

Fracture-dislocations of the femoral head are among the most challenging injuries in orthopaedic trauma. It was Pipkin who in 1957 first drew attention to fractures of these lesions with a series not larger than 26 patients. A collective of 62 patients was published in 1962 by Epstein. The authors of this comprehensive book published in 2021 their series of 138 patients, treated over a period of 22 years. These numbers impressively underline the rarity of this injury. Pipkin fractures occupy a unique space due to their anatomical complexity, demanding surgical management, and significant risk of long-term complications if not addressed with precision. Despite their clinical importance, there has been a noticeable lack of comprehensive, focused literature dedicated to this topic.

Professor Ramesh Kumar Sen and **Professor Sujit Kumar Tripathy** have shown a lifelong interest in this specific entity of orthopaedic trauma by treating the highest number of patients, and registering the characteristics and long-term outcome of each of their patients. Both esteemed orthopaedic surgeons and academicians offer an authoritative exploration of Pipkin fracture-dislocations in this seminal textbook. The book is subdivided into the milestones of management: trauma mechanism, diagnostic challenges, classification systems, treatment algorithms, complications, and outcome. Each chapter has been meticulously authored by globally recognised experts in the field, enriched with personal insights and case-based wisdom drawn from years of clinical experience.

Despite advances in diagnostic modalities and surgical techniques since its initial description, the management of Pipkin fractures continues to pose significant challenges. This volume overlooks the full management spectrum, focusing on the role and limitations of different surgical approaches, from traditional open techniques to modern minimally invasive procedures, from diagnostic dilemmas to evidence-based decision-making. The evolving roles of advanced imaging, hip arthroscopy, and orthobiologics are thoughtfully incorporated, making this book a true reflection of the contemporary state of care. The progression from foundational principles to cutting-edge interventions makes this textbook unique and indispensable for trauma surgeons and arthroplasty specialists.

This exceptional book connects theoretical knowledge with practical application. Thanks to the large experience of the contributing authors, academic in-depth analysis is combined with real-world surgical decision-making. Topics such as classification controversies, intraoperative strategies, and long-term outcome optimisation are discussed clearly and deeply, elements often underrepresented in standard texts.

I congratulate Professors Sen and Sujit for the realisation of this masterpiece. With this work, they contribute much to the understanding of a seldom and complex injury. This book reflects the relentless dedication of the editors to orthopaedic education, innovation, and mentorship. Their commitment to academic excellence and clinical relevance and the choice of the renowned chapter contributors ensure that this volume will serve as a definitive guide for residents, fellows, and practising surgeons.

I strongly recommend this excellent theoretical and practical book to every orthopaedic training institute, departmental library, and personal collection. It nicely reflects the evolving science and enduring art of managing femoral head fracture-dislocations.

It is both an honour and a privilege to write this foreword for my friends Ramesh and Sujit, and to endorse their significant contribution to orthopaedic scholarship.

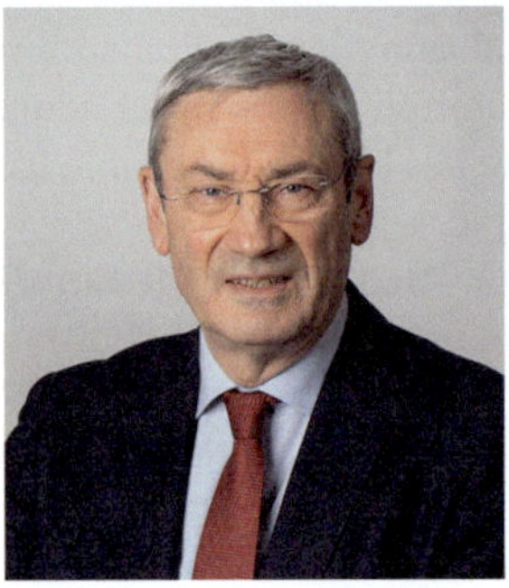

Pol M. Rommens

University Medical Centre
Johannes Gutenberg-University
Mainz, Germany

Preface

Fracture-dislocations of the femoral head, particularly Pipkin injuries, represent some of the most complex and technically demanding challenges in orthopaedic trauma. Their rarity, combined with the intricate anatomy of the hip joint, the critical importance of preserving femoral head vascularity, and the high risk of complications, demands a high level of surgical expertise and clinical acumen. Yet, despite their clinical significance, Pipkin fractures remain underrepresented in orthopaedic literature—often relegated to subsections within broader trauma texts.

This book was conceived from a deep academic curiosity and a clear clinical necessity. Over the years, the management of these injuries—in all their varied presentations, from acute dislocations and delayed diagnoses to avascular necrosis and post-traumatic arthritis—has shaped our understanding and highlighted the need for a focused, evidence-based, and experience-driven resource.

The literature on femoral head fracture-dislocations is notably scarce. Much of what we know stems from small case series and isolated case reports. High-quality, large-scale studies remain elusive, largely due to the rarity, heterogeneity, and surgical complexity of these injuries. Consequently, there exists a pressing need for a consolidated, expert-driven reference that provides clarity, guidance, and practical insights into this often-misunderstood condition.

What this book offers is a comprehensive exploration of Pipkin fracture-dislocations—from historical perspectives and evolving classifications to diagnostic challenges, surgical decision-making, emerging imaging modalities, hip arthroscopy, orthobiologics, rehabilitation, and long-term outcomes. Each chapter is authored by globally renowned experts who bring not only academic authority but also invaluable personal experience, bridging the gap between theoretical understanding and real-world surgical practice. We are deeply honoured that a distinguished leader in orthopaedics has agreed to write the foreword, lending his voice and endorsement to this endeavour.

This book is not merely a compendium of knowledge. It is a reflection of years of clinical dedication, scholarly rigour, and, above all, a commitment to improving outcomes for patients with one of the most challenging injuries in orthopaedic trauma. We hope it serves as a valuable companion for residents, fellows, trauma and arthroplasty surgeons, and all those striving to master the management of Pipkin fractures.

Mohali, Punjab, India — Ramesh Kumar Sen
Bhubaneswar, Odisha, India — Sujit Kumar Tripathy

About the Book

A Practical Guide to Management of Femoral Head Fracture-Dislocation is the first comprehensive monograph dedicated exclusively to one of the most complex and underexplored injuries in orthopaedic trauma. Fracture-dislocations of the femoral head—especially Pipkin variants—are rare but devastating injuries that demand precision in diagnosis, surgical expertise, and long-term clinical foresight.

This book offers an in-depth analysis of every aspect of Pipkin fractures, from foundational principles to the latest surgical innovations. Authored and edited by **Prof. Ramesh Kumar Sen** and **Prof. Sujit Kumar Tripathy**, two internationally recognised orthopaedic surgeons, and contributed to by a distinguished panel of global experts, the text combines academic rigour with real-world surgical insight.

Key highlights include:

- **Historical evolution and classification systems**, with a critical appraisal of their clinical relevance
- **Advanced imaging modalities** and their role in preoperative planning
- **Detailed surgical approaches**—open, minimally invasive, arthroscopic—including step-by-step techniques and tips from masters
- **Complications, pitfalls, and long-term management strategies**
- **Rehabilitation protocols** tailored to injury patterns and surgical interventions
- **Emerging roles of orthobiologics and hip preservation techniques**

Enriched with case illustrations, clinical pearls, high-quality imaging, and intraoperative photographs, this book fills a critical gap in orthopaedic literature. It is designed to be a practical, go-to reference for orthopaedic residents, trauma surgeons, arthroplasty specialists, and hip preservation experts.

Whether you're managing your first Pipkin case or seeking nuanced insights into complex presentations, this book provides the clarity, confidence, and evidence you need at every step of care.

Contents

Surgical Anatomy of the Femoral Head

1

Sujit Kumar Tripathy, Shahnawaz Khan, and Ankit Bhagat

1.1 Introduction

The hip joint is a complex joint of the pelvic girdle. It is a ball and socket joint comprising two articular surfaces: the femoral head and the acetabular socket. This joint is essential for a wide range of movements, including flexion, extension, abduction, adduction, rotation, and circumduction, enabling activities such as walking, running, sitting, and squatting. The femoral head is a vital component of this joint, and any pathology in it can affect a person's normal gait, affecting the quality of life. Understanding the femoral head anatomy is of paramount importance to address such pathologies. Moreover, a good understanding of the anatomy can enable a surgeon to perform various surgical procedures like arthroplasty, hip arthroscopy, and fracture fixations. In this chapter, we will discuss the anatomy of the femoral head.

1.2 Osseous Anatomy

With the exception of the fovea, a tiny, medially positioned depression posteroinferior to its center, the femoral head, also known as the caput femoris, is spherical and entirely covered with hyaline cartilage. This depression provides attachment to the ligament of the head of the femur (ligamentum capitis femoris) that connects the head of the femur to the acetabulum. The femoral head is seated deep in the acetabulum. At any position, the acetabulum covers only 40% of the acetabulum [1]. This necessitates additional structures like the acetabular labrum and capsuloligamentous complex to increase the depth and aid in the coverage of the head. This further

S. K. Tripathy (✉) · S. Khan · A. Bhagat
Department of Orthopaedics, All India Institute of Medical Sciences, Bhubaneswar, Odisha, India
e-mail: ortho_sujit@aiimsbhubaneswar.edu.in

R. K. Sen, S. K. Tripathy (eds.), *A Practical Guide to Management of Femoral Head Fracture-Dislocation*, https://doi.org/10.1007/978-981-96-9852-3_1

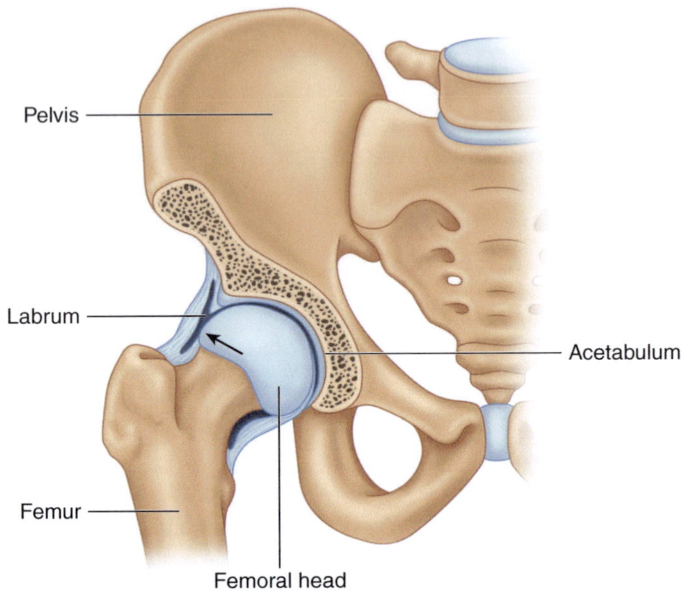

Fig. 1.1 Anatomy of femur head. The blue arrow indicates the area of the head that remains uncovered despite the acetabular labrum

increases the depth by another 33% [1]. Despite the reinforcements, 23% of the femoral head remains uncovered (Fig. 1.1). The iliofemoral, pubofemoral, and ischiofemoral ligaments make up the majority of the thick longitudinal fibers that encircle the capsular ligaments, which run in a spiral pattern to limit hip extension and offer extra support in the lateral plane [2]. The capsule is thinner posteroinferiorly and thicker anterosuperiorly, where most weight-bearing forces occur.

The femoral neck, which connects the femur head to the rest of the femur, gives it its anteversion and inclination. The spatial arrangement of the femur head and proximal femur creates leverage for the hip muscles and influences weight distribution across the hip joint.

1.3 Vascular Anatomy

A surgeon must know the blood supply to the femoral head and how it flows. The blood flow to the femoral head depends on two major arterial systems: the femoral arterial system and the obturator artery system. The amount of flow from these sources varies according to the age.

The primary blood supply to the femoral head comes from the circumflex femoral arteries, namely, the medial circumflex femoral artery (MCFA) and the lateral circumflex femoral artery (LCFA). Out of the two, the medial circumflex femoral artery forms the significant blood supply to the femoral head (Fig. 1.2).

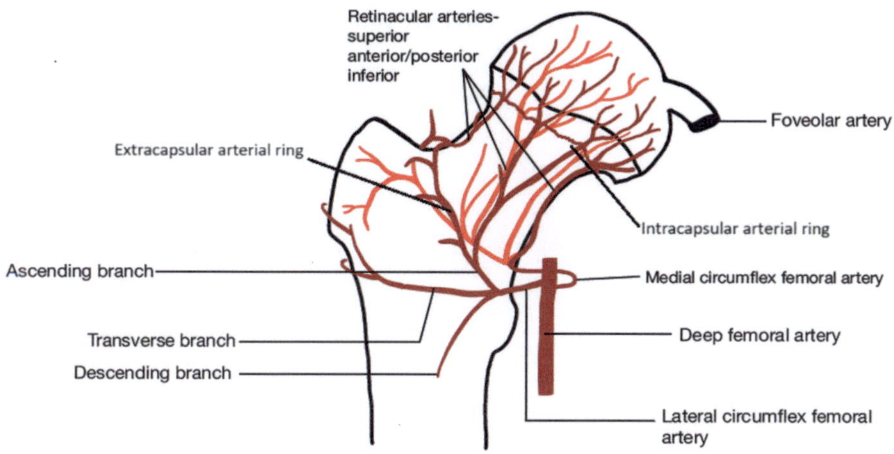

Fig. 1.2 Blood supply to the femoral head

Medial Circumflex Femoral Artery There are differences in the source of the circumflex femoral arteries. In about 50% of patients, the MCFA as well the LCFA originate from the profunda femoris artery [3]. Adachi first described this in 1928 as "truncus profundocircumflexus perfectus" [4]. In 31% of patients, the "truncus profundocircumflexus lateralis" type of division was found where the common or superficial femoral artery is the source of MCFA and the LCFA originates from the profunda femoris. In 15%, the "truncus profundocircumflexus medialis" was found where the common or superficial femoral artery is the source of the LCFA, while the deep femoral artery is the source of the MCFA [3]. In rare cases, both the MCFA and the LCFA branch off from the common femoral artery, while in some cases, either of them is absent [3, 5]. A classification for the origin of MCFA in the year 2016 made the understanding even simpler (Fig. 1.3) (Table 1.1) [6].

In a normal individual, the MCFA originates posteromedially from the profunda femoris artery approximately 50–53 mm below the mid-inguinal point [6]. It then passes along the posterior aspect of the femur between the pectineus and the iliopsoas and then between the adductor brevis and the obturator externus (Fig. 1.4). Near the upper border of the adductor brevis, it branches off into five divisions: an ascending branch, a descending branch, an acetabular branch, a superficial branch, and a deep branch [7].

The inferior gluteal artery, LCFA, and the first of the perforating arteries of the deep femoral artery establish an anastomosis with the superficial branch of the medial circumflex femoral artery, which is situated between the quadratus femoris and the upper border of the adductor magnus. The acetabular branch enters the acetabulum and supplies the acetabular fat.

The deep branch ascends obliquely between the quadratus femoris and obturator externus tendon toward the trochanteric fossa. Here, it is joined by the smaller anterior branches of the lateral circumflex femoral artery to form the extracapsular arterial ring at the base of the femoral neck. The artery pierces the joint capsule between

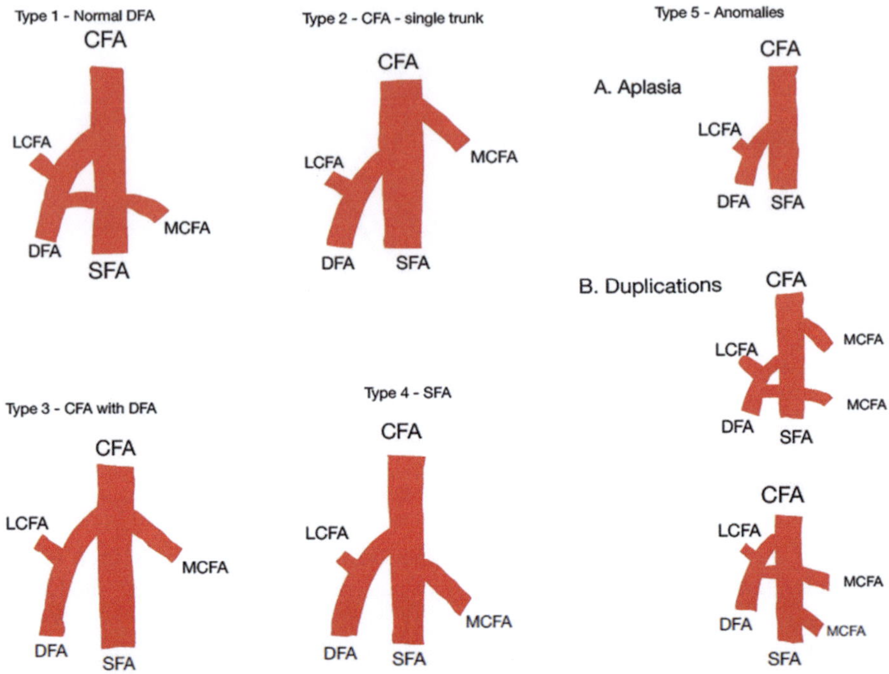

Fig. 1.3 Anatomic variations in the origin of MCFA

Table 1.1 Classification of MCFA origin

Type 1 (normal)	MCFA branching from the DFA
Type 2	MCFA branching from the CFA as a single trunk
Type 3	MCFA branching from the CFA with the DFA
Type 4	MCFA branching from the SFA
Type 5	Anomalies
Type 5A	MCFA aplasia
Type 5B	MCFA duplications

Abbreviations: *MCFA* medial circumflex femoral artery, *DFA* deep femoral artery, *SFA* superficial femoral artery, *CFA* common femoral artery

the triceps coxae (superior and the inferior gemelli and the obturator internus) and the piriformis.

The extracapsular ring gives rise to the following vessels:

- A lateral branch that supplies the greater trochanter.
- Ascending cervical branches: Travel outside the capsule.
- Retinacular vessels: Travel inside the capsule. There are three retinacular vessels, namely, superior, inferior and posterior.

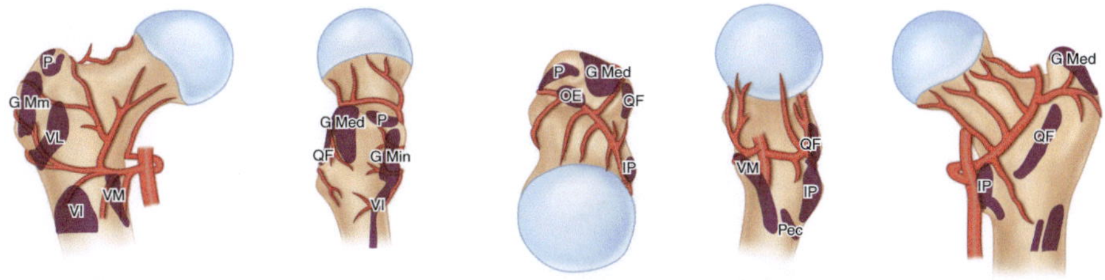

Fig. 1.4 Relation of vasculature with muscle *VI* vastus intermedius, *VL* vastus laterallis, *VM* vastus medialis, *G min* gluteus minimus, *P* pyriformis, *G med* gluteus medius, *OE* obturator externus, *QF* quadratus femoris, *IP* ilio-psoas, *Pec* pectineus

The retinacular vessels (superior, inferior, and posterior) travel just beneath the capsule in synovial folds to the femoral head's base, forming another anastomosis called the sub-synovial arterial ring of Chung. The epiphyseal arteries emerge from this anastomosis and supply the intra-osseous segment of the caput femoris. The lateral epiphyseal artery is the most important, supplying the major part of the femoral head.

1.3.1 Sites of MCFA Injury

This artery may get injured while performing a posterior approach to the acetabulum, like the Kocher-Langenbeck approach, or the safe surgical dislocation to fix Pipkin's fracture. Since the artery lies just below the insertion of the piriformis, it may get injured if the tendon is released entirely from its insertion. At least 1 cm of tendon is left from the lateral end to avoid this complication.

Furthermore, the MCFA may get injured just before piercing the joint capsule during trochanteric digastric osteotomy owing to its close presence to the piriformis tendon. To avoid this injury, the segment of the trochanter that will stay on the shaft should have a 5 mm cuff of the posterior border of the gluteus medius attached to it at the proximal end of the trochanteric flip osteotomy (Fig. 1.5). An intact obturator externus further prevents the kinking of MCFA during the safe surgical dislocation.

The artery may also get kinked in hip dislocations, jeopardizing the blood flow to the femoral head. The retinacular branches are prone to kinking or compression by hematoma in the neck of femur fractures. The sub-capital neck of the femur fracture disrupts the end arterial supply at the femur head's base, increasing the chances of avascular necrosis.

Lateral Circumflex Femoral Artery It has a less prominent role in the blood supply of the femoral head. It arises from the profunda femoris artery anteriorly and ascends along the intertrochanteric crest and the greater trochanter under the sartorius and rectus femoris. This vessel may get injured while performing the Smith-Peterson approach.

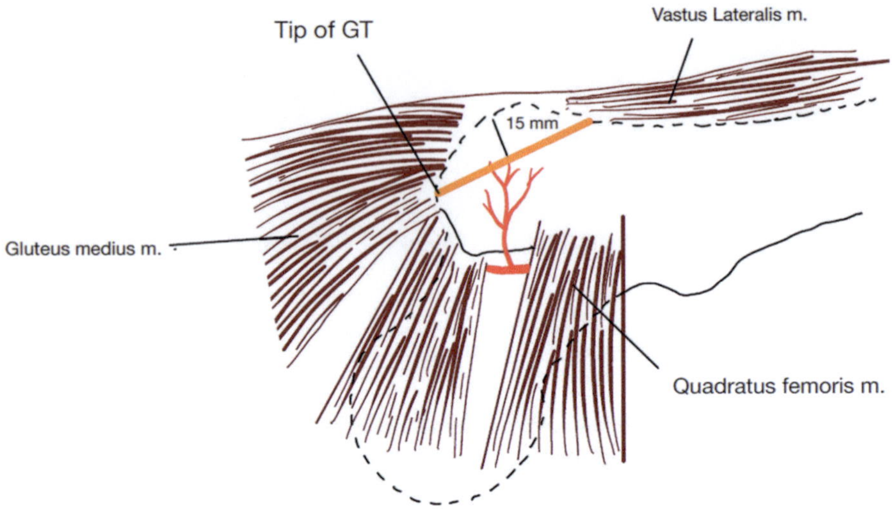

Fig. 1.5 Correct site for trochanteric flip osteotomy. Some gluteus medius fibers must remain attached to the greater trochanter

Obturator Artery The femur head also gets its supply from the obturator artery. The obturator vessel supplies the region near the fovea centralis through the foveal artery. This artery provides a significant amount of blood supply in children [8].

1.4 Nutrient Foramina Distribution

The majority of nutritional foramen are located in the spaces between the muscle attachment sites and along the vascular route. These can be found in the central part of the fovea capitis femoris, subcapital and basicervical areas of the femoral neck, and muscle attachment gaps of the femoral trochanter [9]. The superior and posterior aspects of the femoral neck have a denser distribution of nutritional foramina than the anterior aspect (Fig. 1.6). During hip surgery, the terminal branch of the nutrition arteries that enter the nutrient foramina may sustain iatrogenic injury, particularly when there are close bone exposures. Hence, the anterior approaches carry a lesser risk of development of avascular necrosis. This fact needs to be kept in mind while performing osteotomies of neck and femoral head surgeries.

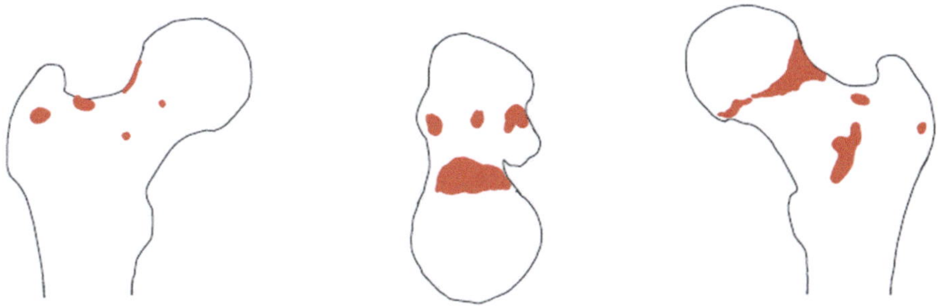

Fig. 1.6 Location of nutrient foramina

1.5 Superior Gluteal Vessels

The internal iliac artery gives rise to the superior gluteal artery. It passes through the upper part of the greater sciatic notch and travels along the lateral ilium, closely adhering to the periosteum. Here, it is associated with the superior gluteal nerve [10]. The artery is also accompanied by vena comitantes. The nerve lies caudal to the artery. The superior gluteal artery divides into a superficial and a deep branch. The gluteus maximus is supplied by the superficial branch, while the gluteus medius and minimus are supplied by the deep branch. The deep branch further divides into a superior and an inferior branch. The artery joins the lateral femoral circumflex artery and the deep circumflex iliac artery, forming the "trochanteric anastomosis," which also supplies the femoral head.

This artery is also injured in traumatic pelvis injury and acetabular posterior-column injuries. The deep inferior branch of this artery is frequently injured in the Kocher-Langenbeck approach [10, 11]. This can be minimized by carefully splitting the gluteus maximus till the vascular pedicle is encountered. Many surgeons opt for a digastric osteotomy of the greater trochanter to avoid this injury.

1.6 Neural Anatomy

There are no nearby nerves that are connected to the femur head. However, the knowledge of nerves around the hip is crucial because the femur head exposure requires a tremendous amount of soft tissue dissection.

The important nerves we will discuss comprise the lateral circumflex femoral and sciatic nerve.

The femur head fractures are typically approached either through a posterior approach by safe surgical dislocation of the hip joint or through an anterior approach.

1.7 Sciatic Nerve

The posterior approach is either a Kocher-Langenbeck approach or a Gibson's approach, the latter more preferred for isolated femoral head fractures. These approaches put the sciatic nerve at risk. In around 9–15% of cases involving posterior approaches to surgery, sciatic nerve damage has been documented [12, 13]. The sciatic nerve comprises the tibial and common peroneal nerves, with the latter being more superficial and injury-prone.

1.7.1 Relation of Sciatic Nerve to the Hip Joint

The formation of the sciatic nerve comes from the anterior and the posterior rami of the L4 to S3 nerve roots. Through the greater sciatic foramen, the sciatic nerve then descends posteriorly and exits the pelvis. Together with the posterior femoral cutaneous nerve, posterior gluteal nerve, inferior gluteal artery and vein, posterior femoral cutaneous nerve, posterior pudendal nerve, and internal pudendal artery and vein, it runs inferior to the piriformis muscle. The nerve then passes into the posterior thigh, where it traverses between the long head of the biceps femoris and the adductor magnus. The nerve can be injured due to posterior dislocation of the hip or posterior wall and column fractures of the acetabulum [14]. Also, iatrogenic injuries have been reported in this region due to the placement of the retractors or an improper dissection while performing posterior approaches to the hip or acetabulum. A large hematoma can also compress the sciatic nerve in this location, leading to postoperative weakness.

DeLee et al. opined that keeping the hip extended and the knee flexed relaxes the sciatic nerve and takes it away from the operative field.

1.7.2 Anatomical Variations at Sciatic Nerve Origin

There are six anatomical variants of the sciatic nerve with respect to the piriformis muscle in the gluteal region, with type 1 being the most commonly encountered variations as described by Beaton and Anson [15, 16] (Table 1.2). The anatomic variants of the sciatic nerve must be kept in mind while performing a posterior approach to avoid inadvertent damage to the nerve (Fig. 1.7).

Table 1.2 Beaton and Anson's classification of variation in sciatic nerve

Type	Description
Type 1	Undivided nerve below undivided muscle
Type 2	Divisions of the nerve between and below the undivided muscle
Type 3	Divisions above and below undivided muscle
Type 4	Undivided nerve between heads
Type 5	Divisions between and above heads
Type 6	The undivided nerve above the undivided muscle

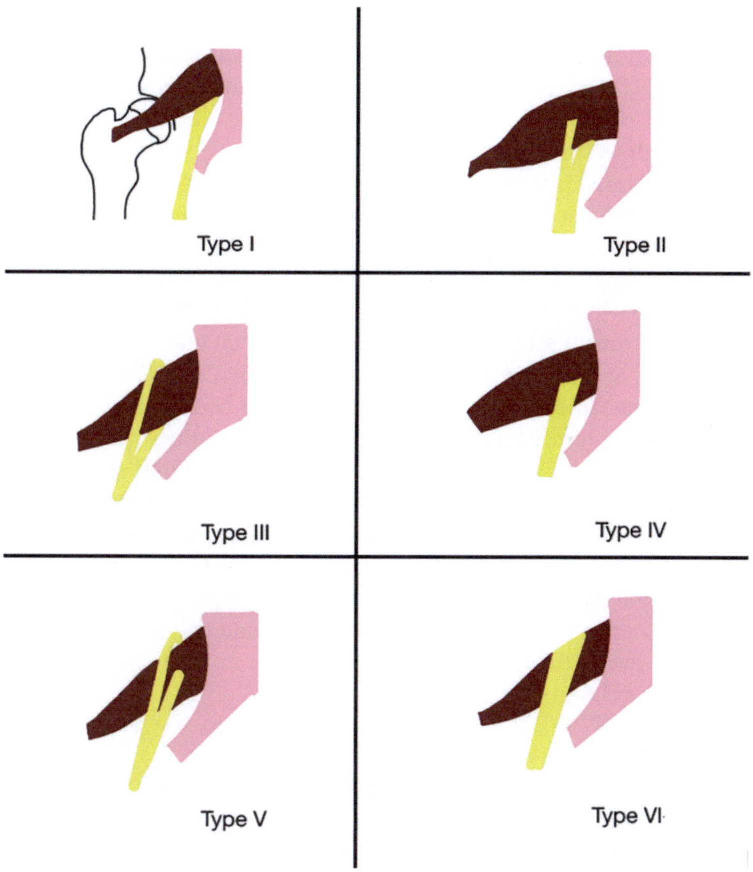

Fig. 1.7 Variation in sciatic nerve with respect to the piriformis muscle

1.8 Superior Gluteal Nerve

This nerve lies in close relation to the deep part of the superior gluteal artery and supplies the gluteus medius and the minimus [11]. It can be injured with the superior gluteal artery during trauma and surgery. Weakness of hip abductors, which manifests as Trendelenburg gait, is caused by injury to this nerve.

1.9 Lateral Femoral Cutaneous Nerve (LFCN)

LFCN requires special mention as it is exposed during the Smith-Peterson approach. The frequency of this nerve damage in anterior approaches may vary from 0.1% to 81% [17–20]. LFCN arises from the anterior rami of the L1 and L2 nerves. It supplies the parietal peritoneum in the iliac fossa and the skin over the anterolateral aspect of the thigh as far as the knee.

The nerve is divided into four segments: lumbar, iliac, inguinal, and femoral. The LFCN's lumbar segment passes between the psoas major muscle's deep and superficial regions. This is followed by the iliac segment, where the nerve passes through two layers of fascia on the iliacus muscle after emerging from the lateral border of the psoas major muscle and descending obliquely around the pelvis. The inguinal part of the LFCN runs through the "aponeurotico-fascial tunnel" with the iliopubic tract on one side and the inguinal canal on the other [21]. The LFCN normally enters the thigh beneath the inguinal ligament and can be found anywhere between 6.5 cm medial and 6 cm lateral to the anterior superior iliac spine [22, 23]. The LFCN splits into anterior and posterior branches in the femoral segment. The skin of the lateral and anterior thighs is supplied by the anterior branch. The anterior branch, on the other hand, pierces the fascia lata lower than the posterior branch. The posterior branch supplies the skin from the greater trochanter to around mid-thigh on the lateral side.

The femoral segment is prone to injury during the anterior approaches. The nerve may be injured due to direct surgical trauma or due to traction-induced ischemia leading to perineural fibrosis [24].

1.9.1 Variations in the Course of LFCN

Numerous variations are reported along the course of LFCN [25, 26]. However, we discuss only the variations in the inguinal and the iliac parts. The nerve may pass through a slit-like opening in the inguinal ligament. Additionally, the nerve may pass medially, under, through, or across the tendinous part of the sartorius muscle. It may cross the iliac crest just behind the ASIS, rarely [25]. Due to limited mobility and tethering, the nerve may be prone to traction injury if it passes through the inguinal ligament or the sartorius. Variations are also noted in the femoral part of the nerve. There are three categories for the thigh's LFCN branching pattern [27]:

- Sartorius type: The lateral border of the sartorius has a dominating anterior branch, and the anterior part of the thigh has additional branches.
- Posterior type: The thickness of the posterior branch is either the same as or greater than that of the anterior branch in this type. Distal to the anterosuperior iliac spine, it extends laterally and passes over the medial border of the tensor fascia lata muscle.
- Fan-shaped: On the anterolateral side of the proximal aspect of the thigh, there are several nerve branches of equal thickness that cross the lateral border of the sartorius and the tensor fascia lata.

Sugano demonstrated that all anterior variants of the LFCN were safe because none of its sartorius or fan-shaped branches passed over the main longitudinal skin incision. On the other hand, 68% of the posterior-type LFCN was spanned by the skin incision and is prone to injury in the Hueter or Smith-Peterson approach [28].

1.10 Summary

Given the intricacy and difficulties of its approach, surgeons must have a thorough understanding of the femoral head's surgical anatomy. Femoral head fractures are often linked to posterior hip dislocations, which may result in sciatic nerve paralysis, which may cause foot drop, or avascular necrosis due to vascular disruption.

The vascular supply of the femoral head, the sciatic nerve, and the superior gluteal arteries are all at risk of harm with posterior-based techniques like the Kocher-Langenbeck approach, especially if exposure reaches the sciatic notch. On the other hand, one of the safest methods for fixing femur head fractures is the safe surgical dislocation of the hip, which protects the piriformis tendon and posterior structures while successfully preserving the femoral head's blood supply.

Anterior-based approaches, while offering alternative access, involve the risk of injury to the **lateral femoral cutaneous nerve**, which can result in **meralgia paresthetica**. Understanding these anatomical considerations is essential to minimize complications and optimize outcomes in surgical management.

References

1. Glenister R, Sharma S. Anatomy, bony pelvis and lower limb, hip. In: StatPearls. Treasure Island: StatPearls Publishing; 2024.
2. D'Ambrosi R, Ursino N, Messina C, Della Rocca F, Hirschmann MT. The role of the iliofemoral ligament as a stabilizer of the hip joint. EFORT Open Rev. 2021;6:545–55. https://doi.org/10.1302/2058-5241.6.200112.
3. Zlotorowicz M, Czubak-Wrzosek M, Wrzosek P, Czubak J. The origin of the medial femoral circumflex artery, lateral femoral circumflex artery and obturator artery. Surg Radiol Anat. 2018;40:515–20. https://doi.org/10.1007/s00276-018-2012-6.
4. Adachi B (1928) Das Arteriensystem der Japaner. Band 0

5. Massoud TF, Fletcher EW. Anatomical variants of the profunda femoris artery: an angiographic study. Surg Radiol Anat SRA. 1997;19:99–103. https://doi.org/10.1007/BF01628133.
6. Tomaszewski KA, Henry BM, Vikse J, Roy J, Pękala PA, Svensen M, Guay DL, Saganiak K, Walocha JA. The origin of the medial circumflex femoral artery: a meta-analysis and proposal of a new classification system. PeerJ. 2016;4:e1726. https://doi.org/10.7717/peerj.1726.
7. Gautier E, Ganz K, Krügel N, Gill T, Ganz R. Anatomy of the medial femoral circumflex artery and its surgical implications. J Bone Joint Surg Br. 2000;82:679–83. https://doi.org/10.1302/0301-620x.82b5.10426.
8. Gold M, Munjal A, Varacallo M. Anatomy, bony pelvis and lower limb, hip joint. In: StatPearls. Treasure Island: StatPearls Publishing; 2024.
9. Wu S, Quan K, Wang W, Zhang Y, Mei J. 3D mapping of bone channel of blood supply to femoral head in proximal femur. Front Surg. 2022;9:852653. https://doi.org/10.3389/fsurg.2022.852653.
10. Collinge CA, Ziran NM, Coons DA. Relationship between the superior gluteal vessels and nerve at the greater sciatic notch. Orthopedics. 2015;38:e929–33. https://doi.org/10.3928/01477447-20151002-62.
11. Ebraheim NA, Olexa TA, Xu R, Georgiadis G, Yeasting RA. The quantitative anatomy of the superior gluteal artery and its location. Am J Orthop (Belle Mead NJ). 1998;27:427–31.
12. Staresinic M, Lindtner RA, Krappinger D, Gänsslen A. Posterior approaches to the acetabulum. Arch Orthop Trauma Surg. 2024;144:4633–40. https://doi.org/10.1007/s00402-024-05583-0.
13. Negrin LL, Benson CD, Seligson D. Prone or lateral? Use of the Kocher-Langenbeck approach to treat acetabular fractures. J Trauma. 2010;69:137–41. https://doi.org/10.1097/TA.0b013e3181b28ba6.
14. Cornwall R, Radomisli TE. Nerve injury in traumatic dislocation of the hip. Clin Orthop Rel Res. 2000;377:84–91. https://doi.org/10.1097/00003086-200008000-00012.
15. Beaton LE, Anson BJ. The relation of the sciatic nerve and of its subdivisions to the piriformis muscle. Anat Rec. 1937;70:1–5. https://doi.org/10.1002/ar.1090700102.
16. Beaton LE, Anson BJ. The sciatic nerve and the piriformis muscle: their interrelation a possible cause of coccygodynia. JBJS. 1938;20:686.
17. Restrepo C, Parvizi J, Pour AE, Hozack WJ. Prospective randomized study of two surgical approaches for total hip arthroplasty. J Arthroplast. 2010;25:671–679.e1. https://doi.org/10.1016/j.arth.2010.02.002.
18. Kennon RE, Keggi JM, Wetmore RS, Zatorski LE, Huo MH, Keggi KJ. Total hip arthroplasty through a minimally invasive anterior surgical approach. J Bone Joint Surg Am. 2003;85-A(Suppl 4):39–48. https://doi.org/10.2106/00004623-200300004-00005.
19. Goulding K, Beaulé PE, Kim PR, Fazekas A. Incidence of lateral femoral cutaneous nerve neuropraxia after anterior approach hip arthroplasty. Clin Orthop. 2010;468:2397–404. https://doi.org/10.1007/s11999-010-1406-5.
20. Homma Y, Baba T, Sano K, Ochi H, Matsumoto M, Kobayashi H, Yuasa T, Maruyama Y, Kaneko K. Lateral femoral cutaneous nerve injury with the direct anterior approach for total hip arthroplasty. Int Orthop. 2016;40:1587–93. https://doi.org/10.1007/s00264-015-2942-0.
21. Witkin LR, Gulati A, Zhang T, Karl HW. Lateral femoral cutaneous nerve entrapment. In: Peripheral nerve entrapments: clinical diagnosis and management; 2016. p. 667–81.
22. Hanna AS. Lateral femoral cutaneous nerve transposition: renaissance of an old concept in the light of new anatomy. Clin Anat. 2017;30:409–12. https://doi.org/10.1002/ca.22849.
23. Hanna A. The lateral femoral cutaneous nerve canal. J Neurosurg. 2017;126:972–8. https://doi.org/10.3171/2016.1.JNS152262.
24. Kiyama T, Naito M, Shiramizu K, Shinoda T, Maeyama A. Ischemia of the lateral femoral cutaneous nerve during periacetabular osteotomy using Smith-Petersen approach. J Orthop Traumatol. 2009;10:123–6. https://doi.org/10.1007/s10195-009-0055-5.
25. de Ridder VA, de Lange S, Popta J. Anatomical variations of the lateral femoral cutaneous nerve and the consequences for surgery. J Orthop Trauma. 1999;13:207.
26. Haładaj R, Wysiadecki G, Macchi V, de Caro R, Wojdyn M, Polguj M, Topol M. Anatomic variations of the lateral femoral cutaneous nerve: remnants of atypical nerve growth pathways

revisited by intraneural fascicular dissection and a proposed classification. World Neurosurg. 2018;118:e687–98. https://doi.org/10.1016/j.wneu.2018.07.021.

27. Rudin D, Manestar M, Ullrich O, Erhardt J, Grob K. The anatomical course of the lateral femoral cutaneous nerve with special attention to the anterior approach to the hip joint. J Bone Joint Surg Am. 2016;98:561–7. https://doi.org/10.2106/JBJS.15.01022.
28. Sugano M, Nakamura J, Hagiwara S, Suzuki T, Nakajima T, Orita S, Akazawa T, Eguchi Y, Kawasaki Y, Ohtori S. Anatomical course of the lateral femoral cutaneous nerve with special reference to the direct anterior approach to total hip arthroplasty. Mod Rheumatol. 2020;30:752–7. https://doi.org/10.1080/14397595.2019.1637992.

2 Mechanism of Injury and Various Fracture Classifications

Sujit Kumar Tripathy, Shahnawaz Khan, Ankit Bhagat, and Ramesh Kumar Sen

2.1 Introduction

Femoral head fractures are relatively rare injuries, accounting for approximately 5–15% of cases associated with posterior hip dislocations [1–3]. The incidence of these injuries has risen in recent years, likely attributable to the increasing prevalence of road traffic accidents [2, 3]. These fractures have garnered significant attention in the orthopedic community due to their high complication rates and notable rates of reoperation [4–6].

Accurate diagnosis can be challenging, as femoral head fractures may be easily overlooked without meticulous evaluation of radiographic imaging [7]. Furthermore, analyzing the injury mechanism and classifying the fracture based on imaging findings can be complex, especially in the high-pressure environment of a busy trauma bay. The existence of multiple classification systems often adds to the confusion, making it difficult for clinicians to select and apply the most appropriate system in real-time clinical practice.

This chapter explores the various mechanisms underlying femoral head fractures and provides a detailed discussion of their classification systems. The rationale for each system and its clinical significance will be emphasized to aid in the systematic evaluation and management of these challenging injuries.

S. K. Tripathy (✉) · S. Khan · A. Bhagat
Department of Orthopaedics, All India Institute of Medical Sciences, Bhubaneswar, Odisha, India
e-mail: ortho_sujit@aiimsbhubaneswar.edu.in

R. K. Sen
Institute of Orthopaedic Surgery, Max Super Speciality Hospital, Mohali, Punjab, India
e-mail: rameshkumar.sen@maxhealthcare.com

R. K. Sen, S. K. Tripathy (eds.), *A Practical Guide to Management of Femoral Head Fracture-Dislocation*, https://doi.org/10.1007/978-981-96-9852-3_2

2.2 History of Femoral Head Fracture-Dislocation

The first documented case of a femoral head fracture was reported in 1869 by the English surgeon John Birkett (1815–1904), a prominent figure in surgery known for his contributions to breast disease management and advocacy for the integration of histology into medical diagnostics [8]. During the autopsy of a 35-year-old woman who sustained fatal injuries from a fall, Birkett identified a hip dislocation with an associated femoral head fracture. Notably, the avulsed fragment of the femoral head, including the ligamentum teres (ligamentum capitis femoris) attachment, was located within the acetabulum.

In 1872, Walter Moxon (1836–1886) described another case during an autopsy of a man struck by a train [9]. The findings included a compound iliac dislocation of the hip with partial avulsion of the femoral head. Subsequently, in 1885, Bernhard Moritz Carl Ludwig Riedel (1846–1916) became the first to diagnose and surgically manage a femoral head fracture in a living patient [10]. The case involved a 15-year-old boy presenting with a 3-month history of hip injury, iliac dislocation, and persistent crepitation. Riedel discovered a femoral head fracture, with both fragments dislocated outside the acetabulum, and a posterior rim impression on the acetabulum. A loose fragment was excised, and the femoral head was reduced. Although the fracture healed, the patient developed hip ankylosis and 2 cm of limb shortening.

In subsequent years, additional cases were reported, including by Braun (1891), Crile (1891), and Robert (1896) [11–13]. In 1904, Durand was among the first to utilize radiographic imaging to diagnose femoral head fractures, identifying the injury in three cases [14].

In 1926, Frederick Christopher (1889–1967) advanced the understanding of femoral head fractures through a comprehensive review of 14 cases documented in the literature, to which he added a case of his own from 1924 [15]. His patient, a woman with a posterior hip dislocation and avulsion of the inferior femoral head, was successfully treated with closed reduction under general anesthesia. The patient recovered with an excellent functional outcome, experiencing only transient peroneal nerve palsy caused by the hip dislocation. Christopher categorized the cases into two groups: nine involving posterior hip dislocations and six without dislocation.

Further contributions to the literature culminated in 1957 when Garrett Pipkin analyzed 25 cases, including those from his practice and colleagues, with follow-ups extending up to 18 years [16]. From this analysis, Pipkin proposed a classification system that has since been widely adopted, and the injury became known as the "Pipkin fracture-dislocation."

2.3 Mechanism of Injury

Isolated femoral head fractures are rare occurrences [17]. These injuries are typically associated with concurrent acetabular fractures or posterior hip dislocations and are the result of high-energy trauma, such as dashboard injuries in motor vehicle accidents or falls from height. The primary mechanisms leading to femoral head fractures are (1) impaction of the femoral head into the acetabulum, (2) shearing of the femoral head against the acetabular wall, and (3) avulsion of the ligamentum teres femoris [18].

These fractures most commonly occur when the hip is in a flexed position. The coronal plane alignment of the lower limb during flexion plays a critical role in determining the size and nature of the fracture fragment (Fig. 2.1). When the hip is abducted, forces are dissipated through the posterior acetabular wall, sparing the femoral head and resulting in a posterior wall fracture with or without hip dislocation. Conversely, when the hip is fully adducted, compression forces on the femur align parallel to the posterior acetabular wall, leading to posterior hip dislocation. In such cases, shearing forces may produce small osteochondral fractures of the femoral head, which are often radiographically occult and necessitate advanced imaging, such as CT scans, for accurate diagnosis [19].

With the hip flexed and the limb in a neutral or mild adduction position, compression forces on the femur become perpendicular to the posterior acetabular wall. This alignment increases the likelihood of posterior wall fractures. If the posterior wall withstands the force, the shearing stress on the medial aspect of the femoral head can cause supra-foveal fractures, with the fracture fragment

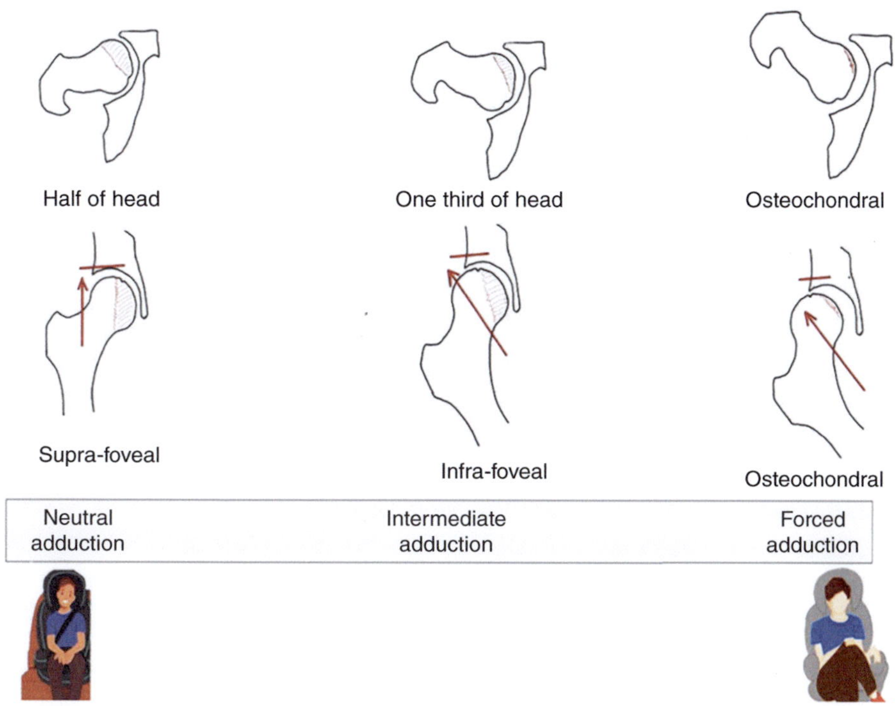

Fig. 2.1 Injury mechanisms of femoral head fracture-dislocation

typically displaced inferiorly within the joint. Under greater force, the femoral neck may fail, resulting in a concurrent femoral neck fracture (Pipkin type III) (Fig. 2.1).

As the limb transitions from full adduction to a neutral position, the contact surface area between the femoral head and the posterior acetabular wall increases. Consequently, the size of the fracture fragment enlarges as adduction decreases (Fig. 2.1). Individuals with reduced femoral anteversion (greater internal rotation) are more susceptible to isolated hip dislocations due to altered rotational alignment of the femoral head [20–22]. Conversely, femoral head fractures are more likely to occur in individuals with greater anteversion or reduced internal rotation, as these conditions predispose to the application of higher forces during dislocation events (Table 2.1).

Anterior hip dislocations, although less common than posterior dislocations, occur when the hip is abducted and externally rotated. Flexion or extension of the hip in this position results in inferior obturator dislocations or superior pubic dislocations, respectively (Fig. 2.2). Anterior dislocations are often accompanied by impaction or indentation fractures of the femoral head. These fractures carry a particularly poor prognosis when the indentation exceeds 4 mm.

Femoral head fractures can also occur in the absence of total hip dislocation, typically in the context of subluxation. This mechanism involves an impacting force transferred through the femoral head and neck against the acetabulum, creating a "hammer-and-anvil" effect [16, 23].

Low-velocity injuries can lead to pathological or insufficiency fractures of the femoral head in individuals with osteopenic or osteoporotic bone, caused by subchondral impaction. Similar fractures may also occur as stress injuries, commonly seen in military personnel and athletes. These fatigue fractures often necessitate magnetic resonance imaging (MRI) for accurate diagnosis.

Table 2.1 Hip position and fracture pattern in femoral head fracture-dislocation

Hip position	Resulting injury
Extreme flexion, adduction, and internal rotation (FADIR)	Dislocation of the hip joint posteriorly, typically without any associated fracture
Moderate flexion with slight adduction or abduction	Posterior hip dislocation accompanied by fractures in either the acetabulum or the femoral head due to shear forces
Flexion, abduction, and external rotation (FABER)	Anterior-inferior hip dislocation, often referred to as an obturator dislocation
Extension, abduction, and external rotation (EABER)	Anterior-superior dislocation of the hip, classified as iliac or pubic based on its location

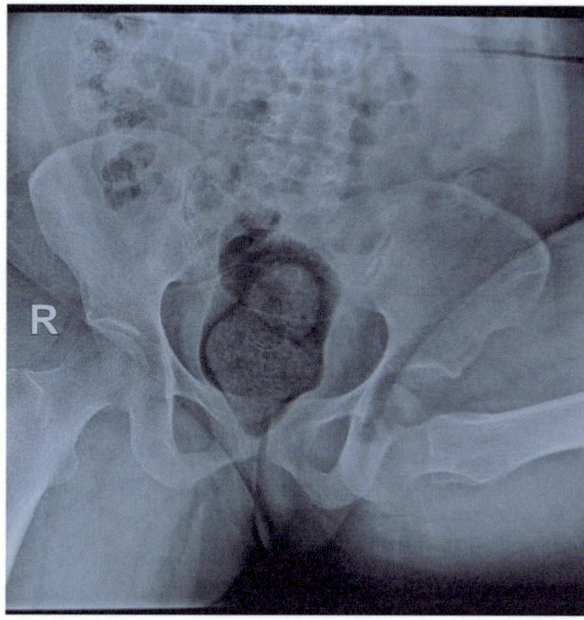

Fig. 2.2 Injury mechanism (flexion-abduction-external rotation) of anteroinferior hip dislocation (obturator) along with femoral head fracture

2.4 Classification

Numerous classification systems have been developed to describe femoral head fractures, particularly since the 1950s. Among the earliest systems were those proposed by Thompson and Epstein and Stewart and Milford [20].

Thompson and Epstein devised a classification system primarily focused on posterior hip dislocations, with type V representing posterior hip dislocations accompanied by femoral head fractures. However, this system did not account for cases involving fractures of the femoral neck. Conversely, Stewart and Milford (1954) included fractures of the femoral head or neck in their classification, categorizing such injuries as grade IV [20].

Due to the shared mechanisms of injury, subsequent classification systems have often categorized femoral head fractures as subtypes of hip dislocations. This concept was further refined in 1957 by Pipkin, who introduced a more detailed classification to enhance understanding of these fractures' management and outcomes [16]. Pipkin's system is based on the location of the fracture line relative to the fovea centralis (Fig. 2.3), as follows:

Type I: The fracture line is inferior to the fovea centralis and does not involve the weight-bearing region of the femoral head.

Type II: The fracture line passes superior to the fovea centralis, involving the weight-bearing region. In these injuries, the ligamentum teres femoris often

Fig. 2.3 Pipkin's classification of femoral head fracture-dislocation

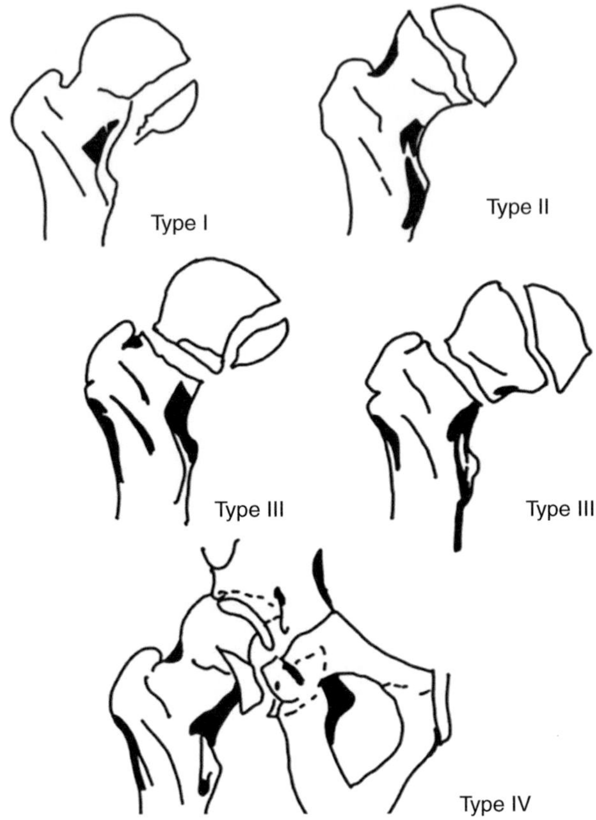

remains attached to the fractured femoral head fragment, contributing to its rotation.

Type III: Femoral head fractures is accompanied by a concomitant femoral neck fracture.

Type IV: Femoral head fractures are associated with a concomitant acetabular fracture.

The Pipkin classification remains the most widely used system for femoral head fractures due to its simplicity and clinical relevance. However, the prognosis of these injuries worsens as their complexity increases [23]. By providing a standardized framework, the Pipkin classification has significantly contributed to the understanding and management of femoral head fractures.

Brumback et al. (1987) described a more comprehensive classification of femur head fractures wherein the direction of the dislocating force, joint stability, and severity of acetabular fracture were taken into account (Table 2.2) [24]. A significant fracture of acetabular rim leads to a dislocation. This classification system also

Table 2.2 Brumback classification of femur head fracture

Fracture type	Description
Type 1A	Infero-medial fracture with minimal or no acetabular rim fracture with a stable hip joint
Type 1B	Type 1A fracture with significant acetabular rim fracture resulting in an unstable hip joint
Type 2A	Supero-medial head fracture with minimal or no acetabular rim fracture with a stable hip joint
Type 2B	Type 2A with significant acetabular rim fracture with an unstable hip joint
Type 3A	Anterior or posterior hip dislocation with a femoral neck fractures
Type 3B	Type 3A with a femur head fracture
Type 4A	Anterior hip dislocation with an indentation type of femur head fracture
Type 4B	Anterior hip dislocation with a transchondral type of femoral head fracture
Type 5	Central hip dislocation with a femoral head and acetabulum fracture

takes into account the indentation fractures and chondral injuries of the femoral head (Fig. 2.4). This system also has a prognostic value with type 2B fractures having the best prognosis and the type 3B and type 5 having the worst prognosis [25, 26].

Yoon et al. (2001) proposed a classification system exclusively for femoral head fracture which could guide the treatment (Fig. 2.5) [27]. They divided the fracture into four types (Table 2.3). However, the lack of validation of this classification system limits its use in daily practice. Moreover, this classification system also does not include the smaller osteochondral fractures and the associated ipsilateral neck of femur and acetabulum fractures.

The AO/OTA classification simplifies the previously existing classification systems [28]. The femoral head fractures are classified by AO/OTA as 31C (Fig. 2.6). This is further divided into two groups:

1. Split fractures (31C1)
2. Depressed fractures (31C2)

The split fractures are further classified into three types:

(i) Avulsion of ligamentum teres (31C1.1)
(ii) Infra-foveal split fracture (31C1.2)
(iii) Supra-foveal split fracture (31C1.3)

The depressed fractures are further classified into three types:

(i) Depression of the cartilage/chondral lesion (31C2.1)
(ii) Depression impaction fracture (31C2.2)
(iii) Split depression fracture (31C2.3)

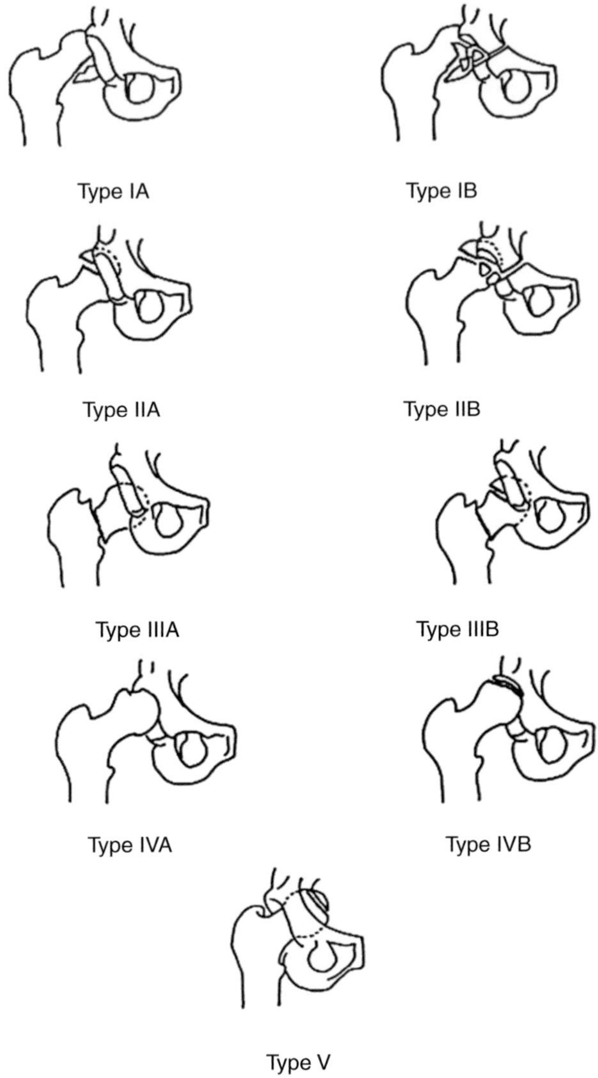

Fig. 2.4 Brumback classification of femoral head fracture-dislocation

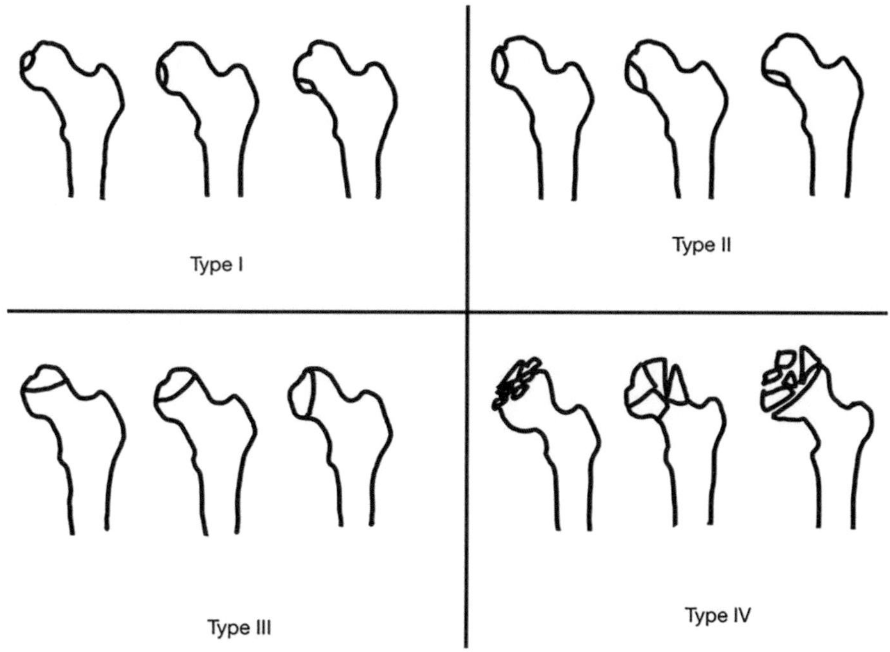

Fig. 2.5 Yoon's classification of femoral head fracture dislocation

Table 2.3 Yoon's classification of femoral head fractures

Type	Description	Treatment
Type I	Fracture fragment distal to fovea too small or fragmented to be fixed by screws	Excision
Type II	Large head fragment distal to fovea	Open reduction and internal fixation
Type III	Large head fragment proximal to fovea centralis	
Type IV	Comminuted fracture of head of femur	Arthroplasty

However, this classification system does not describe the exact location of fracture. Moreover, the osteochondral fragments and the associated injuries are also overlooked by this system.

Chiron's classification (2013, CT based) is the latest classification system which takes into account the shortcomings of all other classifications [18, 29]. It is a comprehensive classification which includes the size of the fragment along with the

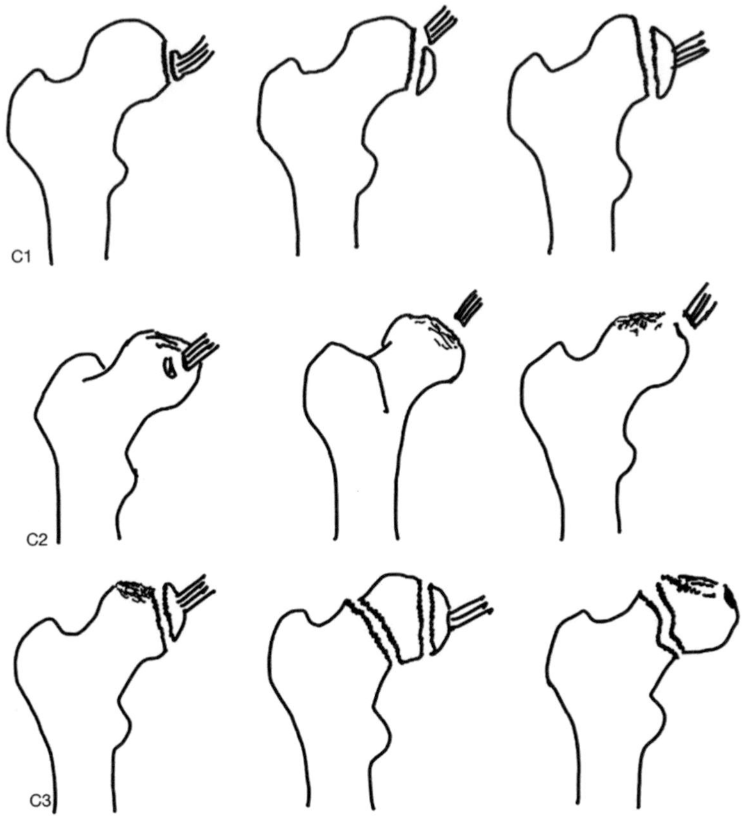

Fig. 2.6 AO classification of femoral head fracture-dislocation

associated injuries (Fig. 2.7). The fracture is classified into four types depending upon the size of the head fragment (Table 2.4). Each type is further divided into three types depending upon the associated injury as follows:

A: Isolated head fracture
B: Associated with acetabulum fracture
C: Associated with femur neck fracture

Though it is a descriptive classification, it fails to give much information regarding the associated joint instability, direction of dislocation, etc. Types I and II are managed by arthroscopic removal of the fragment. Type III and IV fractures are fixed. Types IV and V in individuals older than 60 years should be managed by primary total hip arthroplasty.

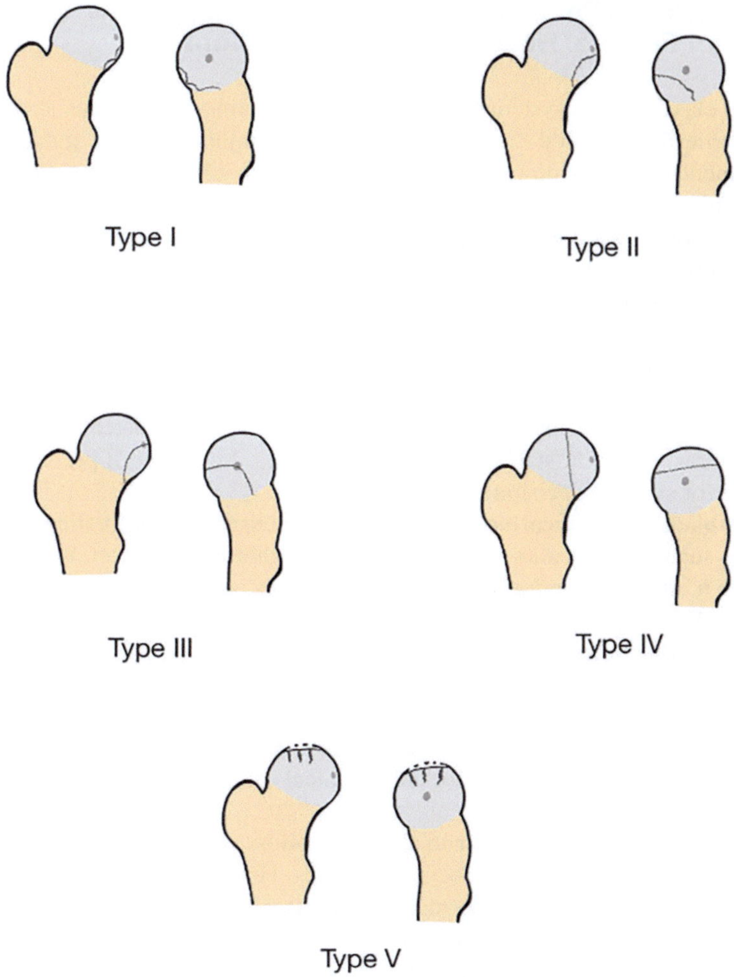

Fig. 2.7 Chiron's classification of femoral head fracture dislocation

Table 2.4 Chiron's classification of femur head fracture

Type	Size of the fracture fragment
Type I	Osteochondral fragments
Type II	1/4th of the head fragment
Type III	1/3rd of the head fragment
Type IV	1/2 of the head fragment
Type V	Superior collapse

2.5 Author's Perspective on Classification Systems for Femoral Head Fracture-Dislocations

An ideal classification system for femoral head fracture-dislocations should fulfil several criteria: it should encompass all possible injury patterns, guide surgical management, and provide reliable prognostic information. However, the rarity of these injuries and the limited number of case series have impeded the development and validation of such a system. Among the existing classification systems, none fully meet these criteria.

Pipkin's classification remains the most widely utilized system due to its simplicity. While it is helpful for communication and offers some prognostic insights, particularly with **type I** and **type II** injuries generally showing better outcomes than **type III** and **type IV**, the system has significant limitations. It fails to account for critical factors such as fragment comminution, the size of associated head or acetabular fractures, and joint stability in **type IV** injuries. Moreover, it provides limited guidance for surgical decision-making.

Brumback's classification is more comprehensive, incorporating additional variables such as dislocation direction and joint stability. However, its complexity can make it cumbersome for clinical use, and it does not clearly delineate treatment pathways. From a prognostic perspective, **type 3B** and **type 5** injuries are associated with poorer outcomes, whereas **type 2B** fractures tend to have more favorable results.

The **AO classification** system, while widely known, lacks comprehensiveness and practical utility in guiding treatment. Conversely, **Yoon's classification** is more treatment-oriented and practical for daily clinical use, making it particularly useful in operative planning.

The most recent system, **Chiron's classification**, provides a detailed CT-based description that incorporates associated injuries. However, it is primarily descriptive, offering limited information regarding critical aspects such as joint instability and dislocation direction, which are important for clinical decision-making.

In practice, **Pipkin's classification** continues to be favored for its simplicity and ease of communication. However, for complex cases where Pipkin's system proves inadequate, **Brumback's classification** may be employed as a more detailed alternative. Despite the availability of multiple classification systems, the field still lacks a universally accepted system that addresses all clinical and prognostic considerations effectively.

References

1. Sahin V, Karakaş ES, Aksu S, Atlihan D, Turk CY, Halici M. Traumatic dislocation and fracture-dislocation of the hip: a long-term follow-up study. J Trauma. 2003;54:520–9. https://doi.org/10.1097/01.TA.0000020394.32496.52.
2. Enocson A, Wolf O. Pipkin fractures: epidemiology and outcome. Eur J Trauma Emerg Surg. 2022;48:4113–8. https://doi.org/10.1007/s00068-022-01951-w.

3. Droll KP, Broekhuyse H, O'Brien P. Fracture of the femoral head. J Am Acad Orthop Surg. 2007;15:716–27. https://doi.org/10.5435/00124635-200712000-00005.
4. Bettinelli G, Placella G, Moharamzadeh D, Belluati A, Salini V. Articular femoral head fracture management: a meta-analysis of literature. Indian J Orthop. 2021;55:304–13. https://doi.org/10.1007/s43465-021-00431-4.
5. Engel JL, Johnsen P, Patel NK, Satpathy J, Mounasamy V. Pipkin type IV femoral head fractures: a case series and review of literature. Eur J Orthop Surg Traumatol Orthop Traumatol. 2021;31:791–5. https://doi.org/10.1007/s00590-020-02838-5.
6. Wang J, Cai L, Xie L, Chen H, Guo X, Yu K. 3D printing-based Ganz approach for treatment of femoral head fractures: a prospective analysis. J Orthop Surg. 2019;14:338. https://doi.org/10.1186/s13018-019-1383-7.
7. Lubovsky O, Liebergall M, Mattan Y, Weil Y, Mosheiff R. Early diagnosis of occult hip fractures: MRI versus CT scan. Injury. 2005;36:788–92. https://doi.org/10.1016/j.injury.2005.01.024.
8. Birkett J. Description of a dislocation of the head of the femur, complicated with its fracture; with remarks. Medico-Chir Trans. 1869;52:133–8.
9. Moxon W. Compound dislocation of hip-joint, the bone thrust through skin. 1872.
10. Reider B. Längsfraktur von Schenkelkopf und –Hals. Bericht über die Verh Dtsch Ges Chir XIV. 1885.
11. Braun H. Seltenere Fracture des Oberschenkels. Arch Klin Chir. 1891;42:107–11.
12. Crile GW. VII. Report of three fractures with fatal termination. Ann Surg. 1891;13:373–7. https://doi.org/10.1097/00000658-189101000-00074.
13. Roberts JB. Iliac dislocation complicated with fracture of the head and neck of the femur and of the edge of the acetabulum; arthrotomy. Ann Surg. 1896;23:207–12.
14. Durand D. Les fractures de la tête fémorale. Bul Soc Chir Lyon. 1903;6:376–82.
15. Christopher F. Fractures of the head of the femur. Arch Surg. 1924;12:1049–61.
16. Pipkin G. Treatment of grade IV fracture-dislocation of the hip. J Bone Joint Surg Am. 1957;39-A:1027–1042 passim.
17. Menger MM, Braun BJ, Herath SC, Küper MA, Rollmann MF, Histing T. Fractures of the femoral head: a narrative review. EFORT Open Rev. 2021;6:1122–31. https://doi.org/10.1302/2058-5241.6.210034.
18. Chiron P, Lafontan V, Reina N. Fracture-dislocations of the femoral head. Orthop Traumatol Surg Res. 2013;99:S53–66. https://doi.org/10.1016/j.otsr.2012.11.007.
19. Calisir C, Fishman EK, Carrino JA, Fayad LM. Fracture-dislocation of the hip: what does volumetric computed tomography add to detection, characterization, and planning treatment? J Comput Assist Tomogr. 2010;34:615–20. https://doi.org/10.1097/RCT.0b013e3181d344fb.
20. Stewart MJ, Milford LW. Fracture-dislocation of the hip; an end-result study. J Bone Joint Surg Am. 1954;36:315–42.
21. Scorcelletti M, Reeves ND, Rittweger J, Ireland A. Femoral anteversion: significance and measurement. J Anat. 2020;237:811–26. https://doi.org/10.1111/joa.13249.
22. Klim SM, Reinbacher P, Smolle MA, Hecker A, Maier M, Friesenbichler J, Leithner A, Leitner L, Draschl A, Lewis J, Brunnader K, Maurer-Ertl W. Femoral anteversion in total hip arthroplasty: retrospective comparison of short- and straight-stem models using CT scans. J Clin Med. 2023;12:2391. https://doi.org/10.3390/jcm12062391.
23. Marchetti ME, Steinberg GG, Coumas JM. Intermediate-term experience of Pipkin fracture-dislocations of the hip. J Orthop Trauma. 1996;10:455–61. https://doi.org/10.1097/00005131-199610000-00002.
24. Brumback RJ, Kenzora JE, Levitt LE, Burgess AR, Poka A. Fractures of the femoral head. Hip. 1987;1987:181–206.
25. Stannard JP, Harris HW, Volgas DA, Alonso JE. Functional outcome of patients with femoral head fractures associated with hip dislocations. Clin Orthop Relat Res. 2000;377:44–56. https://doi.org/10.1097/00003086-200008000-00008.
26. Romeo NM, Firoozabadi R. Classifications in brief: the Pipkin classification of femoral head fractures. Clin Orthop. 2018;476:1114–9. https://doi.org/10.1007/s11999.0000000000000045.

27. Yoon TR, Rowe SM, Chung JY, Song EK, Jung ST, Anwar IB. Clinical and radiographic outcome of femoral head fractures: 30 patients followed for 3–10 years. Acta Orthop Scand. 2001;72:348–53. https://doi.org/10.1080/000164701753541998.
28. Marsh JL, Slongo TF, Agel J, Broderick JS, Creevey W, DeCoster TA, Prokuski L, Sirkin MS, Ziran B, Henley B, Audigé L. Fracture and dislocation classification compendium – 2007: orthopaedic trauma association classification, database and outcomes committee. J Orthop Trauma. 2007;21:S1–133. https://doi.org/10.1097/00005131-200711101-00001.
29. Tonetti J, Ruatti S, Lafontan V, Loubignac F, Chiron P, Sari-Ali H, Bonnevialle P. Is femoral head fracture-dislocation management improvable: a retrospective study in 110 cases. Orthop Traumatol Surg Res. 2010;96:623–31. https://doi.org/10.1016/j.otsr.2010.03.020.

Emergency Care in Patients Having Femur Head Fractures

3

Sameer Aggarwal, Vishal Kumar, and Ansh Gupta

3.1 Introduction

Since the hip is an inherently stable joint, femoral head fractures are usually due to high-velocity trauma; however, subchondral fractures may occur without trauma in patients with osteoporosis and acetabular dysplasia [1]. The femoral head fractures are usually associated with posterior hip dislocation and may have additional systemic injuries such as abdominal injury, head injury, and chest injury. Hence, a standard systemic evaluation in the emergency should be performed.

Suraci et al. reported that up to 95% of patients have injuries which require hospitalization independent of their fracture dislocation [2]. Commonly seen skeletal injuries include pelvic ring and femoral shaft fractures, spine injuries, and ligament injuries around the knee. Knee injuries occur in approximately 25% of the cases and can occur along with patella fracture in cases of dashboard injuries [3]. Craniofacial and neck injuries may occur in 21%, head injury in 24%, thoracic injury in 21%, and abdominal injuries in 15% of the cases [4]. Direct injury due to the dislocation may lead to sciatic nerve palsy in 10% of the cases, usually with posterior dislocations and acetabular wall fractures. Femoral artery injury has also been reported in a few case reports [5].

S. Aggarwal (✉) · V. Kumar · A. Gupta
Department of Orthopedics, Postgraduate Institute of Medical Education and Research, Chandigarh, India

R. K. Sen, S. K. Tripathy (eds.), *A Practical Guide to Management of Femoral Head Fracture-Dislocation*, https://doi.org/10.1007/978-981-96-9852-3_3

Outcomes of femoral head fractures depend on the timing and precision of reduction with the aim being to perform an emergent reduction to achieve a congruent and stable hip. The most important factor for the development of secondary osteoarthritis is avascular necrosis of the femoral head. The risk of avascular necrosis increases as the duration between injury and reduction increases [6]. Therefore, emergency care plays a vital role in the management of these patients.

3.2 Clinical Assessment

These patients should be managed in line with the Advanced Trauma Life Support (ATLS) guidelines by the American College of Surgeons when they present in the emergency [7]. Following a brief history of the age, gender, and mechanism of injury, a rapid assessment of the airway, breathing, and circulation should be conducted. Very often, the hip trauma may be detected early in the assessment but should not distract the hospital care from more important life-saving measures [4, 8]. Since femoral head fractures and hip dislocations are markers of extreme injury, proceeding to secondary surgery and detailed clinical assessment should only begin after adequate resuscitation of the patient [9].

A detailed history can help in understanding the mechanism of injury and possible associated injuries. It may not be possible to always take the history from the patients who are drowsy, unconscious, or uncooperative. Additional information can be obtained from the first responders who provided primary care and other accompanying personnel. It is important to assess if the patient was under the influence of alcohol or other drugs since they may need to be managed appropriately.

A through physical examination of the affected torso and limbs should be conducted. Any open wound should be adequately lavaged with copious amounts of prewarmed saline and covered with sterile dressing. At the same time, it is important to look for other physical signs of injury, including bruises, skin discoloration, abrasions, and penetrating wounds. Bruising on the anterolateral thigh could occur due to internal degloving leading to the formation of a Morel-Lavallée lesion [10]. Identification of this is important since it can interfere with surgical incisions and therefore operative planning.

The attitude of both the limbs should be noted. This not only provides information about the possible dislocation but also suggests the pattern of injury to the femoral head. Posterior hip dislocations usually lie in adduction and internal rotation, are more commonly associated with head split fractures, and have a poorer prognosis [11]. Superior anterior hip dislocations lie in extension and external rotation; inferior anterior dislocations lie in abduction and external rotation and tend to be associated with femoral head osteochondral impaction [12, 13]. Patients may also have other associated injuries including fractures of the acetabulum, femoral neck, femoral shaft, patella, proximal tibia, and knee dislocations as often seen in dashboard injuries. Soft tissue injuries to the acetabular labrum and the cartilage of the hip joint may also occur. These injuries may change the clinical presentation such as a patient may not have an attitude of internal rotation if there is an associated femoral shaft fracture [14, 15]. It is vital to document the neurovascular status at presentation. Injury to the sciatic nerve may occur in posterior dislocations but should be checked for in all cases. It is more often incomplete and involves the peroneal division due to the higher sensitivity of the L5 nerve root in comparison to the S1 nerve root [11, 14]. The neurological deficit can occur due to stretch at the level of the lumbosacral plexus, the main trunk as it passes through the greater sciatic foramen, at the level of the external rotators adjacent to the posterior wall of acetabulum, or distally at the level of the knee due to associated injuries. Therefore, a detailed sensory motor mapping should be done, which may be difficult due to the pain [16]. Injury to the femoral nerve has also been documented in some cases [12]. Albeit rare, injury to the femoral artery can occur in anterior dislocations, and therefore distal pulses at the knee and ankle should always be checked and compared with the opposite side.

3.3 Radiographic Assessment

A plain anterior-posterior radiograph of the pelvis with bilateral hips performed during the secondary survey is the first X-ray to be done in all cases. While a fracture dislocation is fairly obvious by the incongruency of the femoral head with the acetabulum and a break in the Shenton line, the X-ray should be systematically reviewed to compare the femoral heads, joint lines, rotation of proximal femur, and associated fractures of the femoral neck, proximal shaft, acetabulum, and pelvis [17].

On the AP view, the femoral head appears smaller in size in cases of posterior dislocation (90% of the cases), with the lesser trochanter being poorly visualized due to the internal rotation. The opposite occurs in cases of anterior dislocations (10% of the cases). The variation in the size occurs due to the change in magnification as the proximity of the femoral head to the film changes [8]. The fracture in the femoral head may not be visible until the beam is in plane with the fracture line. Femoral neck fractures should be ruled out. All further radiology should ideally be undertaken after emergent reduction of the hip unless femoral neck fracture cannot be ruled out or there is a clinical suspicion of an ipsilateral lower limb injury which may interfere with the ability to perform a closed reduction.

After reduction of the hip joint, all standard views of the pelvis should be obtained which are AP, inlet, outlet, and the two Judet oblique views focusing on the center of the pelvis to compare both hips. After a successful reduction, there should be no loss of parallelism between the acetabular sourcil and femoral head. The joint spaces should be comparable.

A non-contrast computed tomogram (NCCT) should be performed in all cases after reduction of the hip. The CT scan provides vital information about the femoral head fracture, the displacement of the fragments, intraarticular loose bodies, condition and congruency of the joint, and other missed fractures. Thin axial slices of 1–2 mm should be evaluated such that smaller osteochondral fragments which may become free-floating loose bodies are not missed [14, 17, 18].

Differences as less as 0.5 mm may indicate hip subluxation. Impaction injuries and femoral head fracture are better visualized on post-reduction CT scans. CT scan also helps in planning the surgery, by identifying the location and size of the fragments in a communited fracture. The direction of the fracture line can be used take specific angled oblique pelvic radiographs which have a higher accuracy when compared with conventional radiographs for determining fracture displacement and joint congruency as described by Moed and Maxey. Post-operative follow-up radiographs taken along this angle can be useful to access healing in cases treated nonoperatively [19].

However, a CT scan may be conducted before reduction if an occult fracture of the femur neck is suspected on the basis of the X-ray or the patient needs a CT scan for a head or thoraco-abdominal injury. In that case, thicker slices of 3 mm may be used to decrease radiation exposure and scan duration. The CT scan helps identify the femur fracture line and classify it. A concomitant femur neck fracture will require fixation before the hip can be reduced. If closed reduction cannot be achieved in the ER, and the patient is being shifted to OT, then a CT scan can be done before shifting to help in planning the surgical fixation simultaneously.

There is no role of magnetic resonance imaging in emergency management of femoral head fractures [20]. However, in the acute setting, it is useful to check for occult injuries such as subchondral bony contusions, superficial cartilaginous abrasions, chondral fragments, and the status of acetabular labrum, iliofemoral, and ilioinguinal ligaments [16]. MRI has a higher sensitivity in detecting small intraarticular loose fragments over a CT scan especially if hemarthrosis is present. It can help prognosticate nerve recovery in cases of neuropraxia based on edema around the sciatic nerve and risk of AVN based on the status of the obturator externus tendon. Tannast et al. suggested that rupture of the tendon is an indirect indicator of damage to the medial circumflex femoral artery which is the major source of blood supply to the femoral head [21]. In short-term follow-up (6–8 weeks), MRI can be useful to check for development of avascular necrosis of the femoral head [22]. Most cases develop AVN within the first 2 years post trauma (Figs. 3.1, 3.2, 3.3 and 3.4).

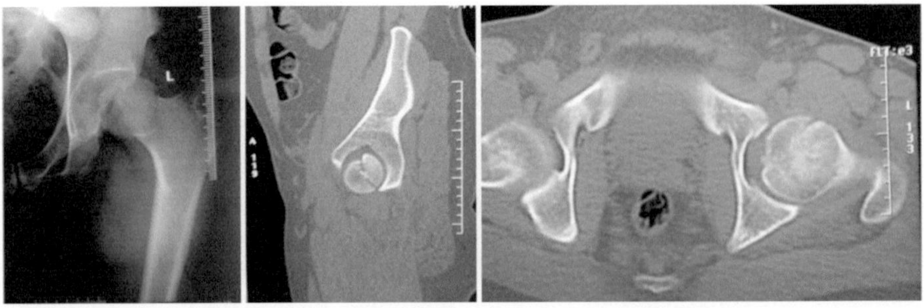

Fig. 3.1 X-rays and CT scan of a case of femoral head fracture dislocation. Note: CT scan done after achieving closed reduction of the hip joint

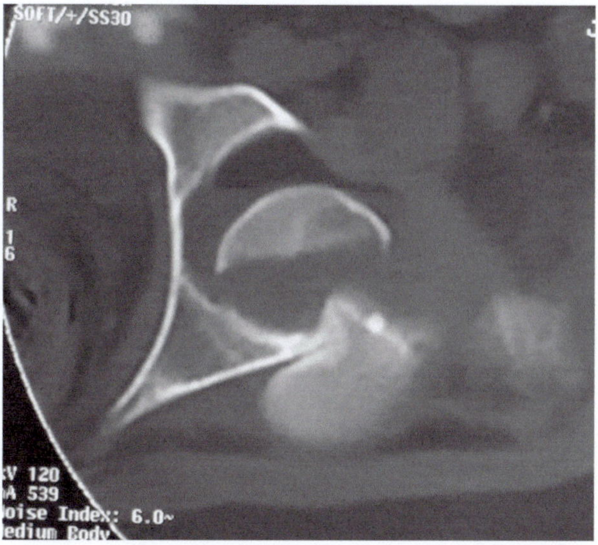

Fig. 3.2 CT scan of an irreducible femoral head fracture dislocation due to the fractured femoral head fragment being incarcerated in the acetabular socket

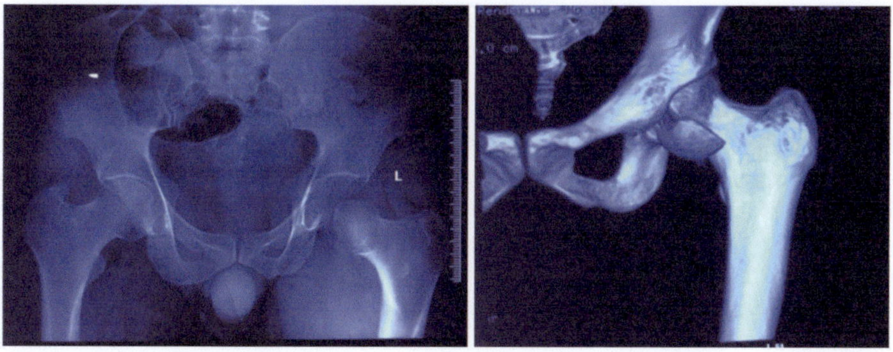

Fig. 3.3 X-ray of what appears to be an isolated hip dislocation but reveals a femoral head fracture after closed reduction

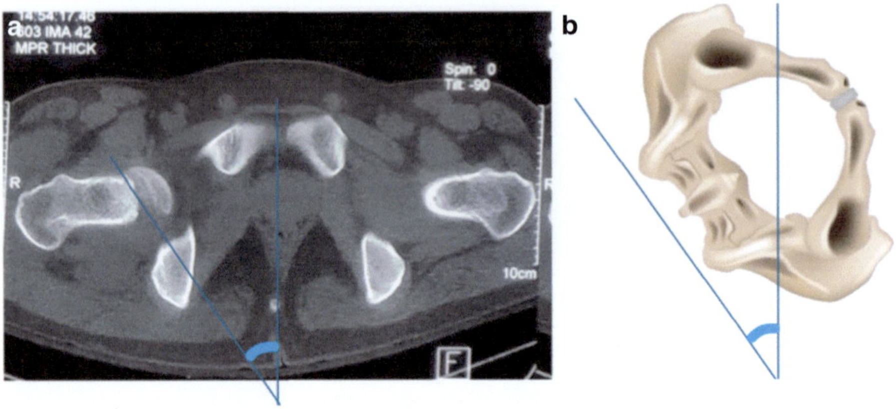

Fig. 3.4 (**a**) CT determination of the angle of the femoral head fracture relative to the sagittal plane and (**b**) patient positioning to obtain a radiograph with the fracture being parallel to the beam as described by Moed and Maxey

3.4 Emergency Management

Femoral head fracture dislocation is an orthopedic emergency. Immediate attempt must be made to reduce the joint to reduce the risk of avascular necrosis, preferably within 6 h, irrespective of the femoral head fracture [6, 23]. Delay in reduction to more than 12 h is associated with a fivefold increase in the risk of AVN [24]. Early reduction helps to restore blood supply which may be disrupted due to kinked vessels.

Closed reduction can be attempted under sedation in the emergency room using intravenous opiates and benzodiazepines. A maximum of two attempts should be made in the emergency department [25]. Multiple attempts can lead to cartilage damage and may also cause an iatrogenic fracture. Combination of fentanyl and midazolam has often been used since they have a fast onset, but there is an associated risk of prolonged sedation, respiratory depression, and severe hypotension [26]. They should be used with caution, especially in elderly patients. Etomidate has a lower risk of hypotension but can lead to myoclonus [27]. All sedation procedures should be performed under a one-to-one care and monitoring. However, sedatives do not provide adequate muscle relaxation. Inadequate analgesia may lead to more pain and make the procedure difficult to perform. General anesthesia is preferred since it provides analgesia, amnesia, and muscle relaxation. Various methods have been described for closed reduction of the dislocated hip, with the earliest literature dating back to 1870 [28]. The principle however remains constant; reduction can be achieved by traction, flexion, internal rotation, and adduction followed by extension and abduction. The commonly used methods are as follows.

Allis Method [29] With the patient in supine position, the leg is grasped and lifted such that hip and knee are flexed to 90°. With the assistant stabilizing the pelvis by applying pressure on the anterior superior iliac spines, inline traction is applied while further flexing the hip. As the hip reduces, the hip is extended and externally rotated to permit the femoral head to enter the acetabulum (Fig. 3.5).

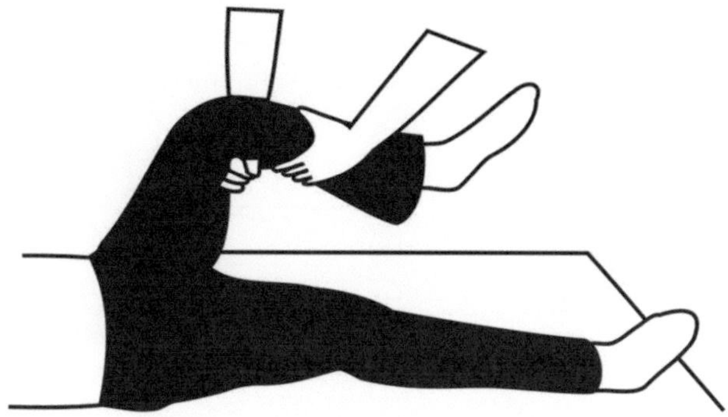

Fig. 3.5 Allis method

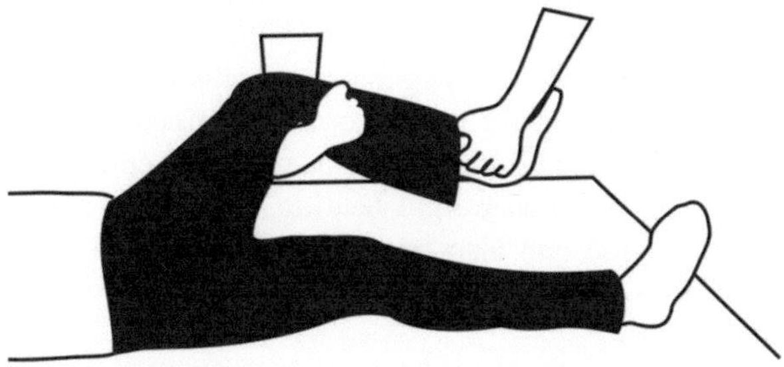

Fig. 3.6 Bigelow method

Bigelow Method [28] With the patient in supine position and the surgeon by the side, the affected limb is grasped at the knee with the forearm and at the ankle by the hand. It is flexed, adducted, and internally rotated while the pelvis is being stabilized by the assistant. Inline traction followed by abduction external rotation and extension should reduce the hip (Fig. 3.6).

Lefkowitz Method [30] The patient is laid supine, and the affected limb is placed over the surgeon's thigh as he kneels close to the affected hip. Flexion of the knee with stabilization of anterior thigh provides inline traction, and the leg can be used to maneuver the rotation (Fig. 3.7).

Other methods have also been described such as those by Captain Morgan, the East Baltimore Lift maneuver, lateral traction, and gravity method but are however less commonly used [31].

A successful reduction can be indicated by a "pop sound," regaining similar limb lengths and attitude, and a reduction in the patients' pain. This should be followed by fresh radiographs to confirm the reduction. The reduced hip should be flexed to 90° to check for stability. If unstable, the patient requires skeletal traction. Else the patient can be given a gentle skin traction. This helps to decrease the pain, immobilize the limb, and prevent cartilage damage due to the femoral head fracture. Neurovascular status should be reassessed after reduction.

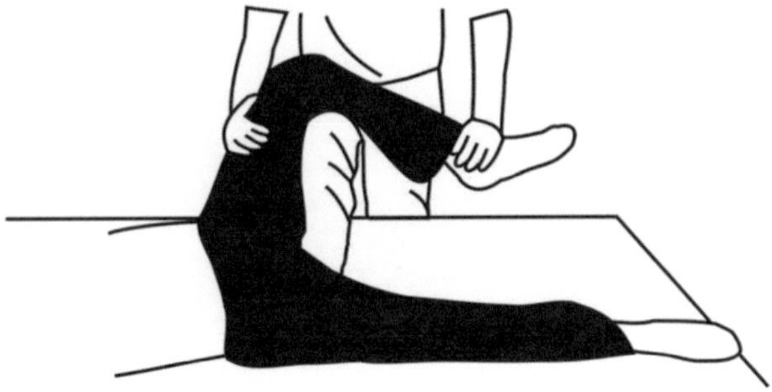

Fig. 3.7 Lefkowitz method

A thin-sliced CT scan should then be obtained to assess the femora head and check for the congruity of the hip joint. Any bony fragments should be noted. An incongruous reduction suggests incarcerated soft tissue which could lead to arthrosis. The final plan for the femoral head fracture is now decided based on the CT scan. Undisplaced fractures can be managed conservatively with traction and keeping the patient non-weight-bearing. Type I fractures not involving the weight-bearing region can also be managed conservatively. Displaced and communited fractures involving the weight-bearing region will need open reduction and internal fixation.

Closed reduction should not be attempted in cases with a femoral neck or shaft fractures or in patients who are hemodynamically unstable. Attempt at closed reduction in cases with undisplaced femoral neck fractures can lead to displacement of the fracture and further increase in the risk of AVN. These cases should undergo emergency fixation of the neck fracture before reduction.

Closed reduction may not be possible due to entrapped soft tissue structures. This could include the labrum, the capsule, pulvinar and synovium, the ligamentum teres, or the iliopsoas tendon. The femoral head fracture fragments could also block the reduction. These cases require open reduction. The hip may re-dislocate due to inadequate support from a fractured acetabulum [12]. Such cases may warrant a heavier skeletal traction after reduction.

Direct open reduction should be planned as early as possible in cases having a non-concentric reduction; associated fractures of the acetabulum, femoral head, and femoral neck; and for dislocations which are not reducible by closed techniques. Approach for reduction is usually posterior (Kocher-Langenbeck), and the femoral head can be fixed directly or via a trochanteric flip osteotomy. All cases should get a CT scan post reduction (Fig. 3.8).

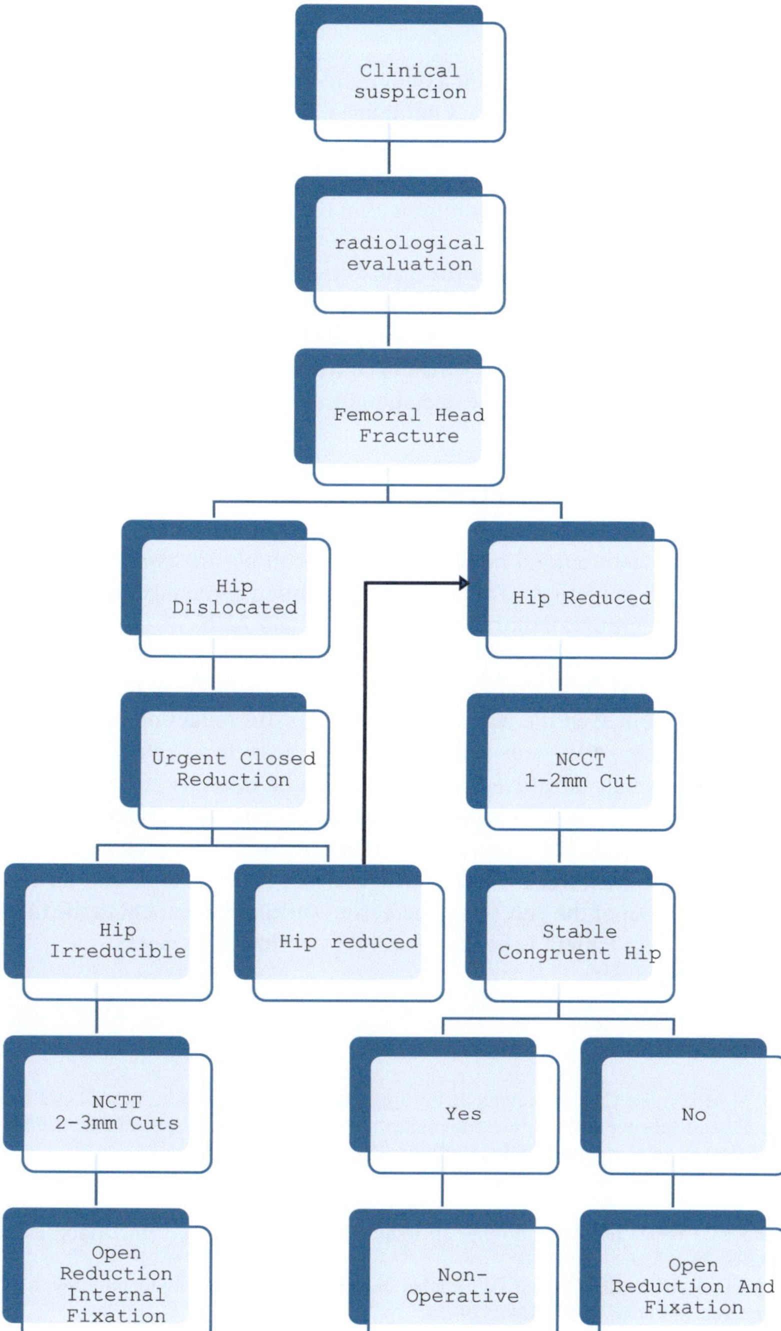

Fig. 3.8 Algorithm for emergency management of femoral head fractures

3.5 Summary

- The goal of treatment is to obtain a congruent and stable hip joint.
- Manage all cases as per the ATLS guidelines. Hip dislocations can be "distracting." Perform primary and secondary surveys to not miss out on other injuries.
- Plain radiographs of the pelvis with bilateral hips will help confirm the diagnosis. Attempt reduction of the hip joint within 6 h either in the emergency or operation theater.
- Reduction should be attempted for a maximum of two times in the ER under sedation.
- Always perform the standard pelvic X-rays and CT scan after reduction to check for fracture pattern and plan necessary treatment. Irreducible hips may require an urgent CT scan before being taken to the operation theater for open reduction and fixation.

3.6 Authors' Preferred Treatment

All cases of suspected femoral head fracture dislocations are assessed in the emergency as per ATLS guidelines. The aim of the emergency management is to reduce the hip joint to minimize femoral head ischemia and AVN. A plain X-ray of the pelvis with bilateral hip is done to confirm the dislocation. Closed reduction under sedation is attempted in the recovery via the Allis method. A maximum of two attempts are performed in the emergency. A successful reduction is followed by a repeat pelvic X-ray series and a thin-sliced CT scan to check for the fracture. Undisplaced and small infrafoveolar fractures can be treated conservatively, while displaced fractures in the weight-bearing region require open anatomic reduction and fixation. Indications for surgery include an irreducible hip, incongruent reduction, femoral neck fracture, incarcerated intraarticular fragment, and an unstable hip. A quick CT scan of the pelvis is done before shifting the patient to the OT to aid in surgical planning. Patient is kept non-weight-bearing for 6 weeks.

References

1. Kubo Y, Motomura G, Utsunomiya T, Fujii M, Ikemura S, Sonoda K, et al. Distribution of femoral head subchondral fracture site relates to contact pressures, age, and acetabular structure. AJR Am J Roentgenol. 2020;215(2):448–57.
2. Suraci AJ. Distribution and severity of injuries associated with hip dislocations secondary to motor vehicle accidents. J Trauma. 1986;26(5):458–60.
3. Tabuenca J, Truan JR. Knee injuries in traumatic hip dislocation. Clin Orthop Relat Res. 2000;377:78–83.
4. Clegg TE, Roberts CS, Greene JW, Prather BA. Hip dislocations--epidemiology, treatment, and outcomes. Injury. 2010;41(4):329–34.
5. Holt GE, McCarty EC. Anterior hip dislocation with an associated vascular injury requiring amputation. J Trauma Acute Care Surg. 2003;55(1):135.
6. Hougaard K, Thomsen PB. Coxarthrosis following traumatic posterior dislocation of the hip. JBJS. 1987;69(5):679.

7. ATLS Algorithms | Pocket ICU Management [Internet]. [cited 2024 Sept 27]. Available from: https://anesth.unboundmedicine.com/anesthesia/view/Pocket-ICU-Management/534159/all/ATLS_Algorithms?refer=true.
8. Foulk DM, Mullis BH. Hip dislocation: evaluation and management. J Am Acad Orthop Surg. 2010;18(4):199–209.
9. Alonso JE, Volgas DA, Giordano V, Stannard JP. A review of the treatment of hip dislocations associated with acetabular fractures. Clin Orthop Relat Res. 2000;377:32–43.
10. Nair AV, Nazar P, Sekhar R, Ramachandran P, Moorthy S. Morel-Lavallée lesion: a closed degloving injury that requires real attention. Indian J Radiol Imaging. 2014;24(3):288–90.
11. Chiron P, Reina N. Dislocation fracture of the femoral head in adult. EFORT Open Rev. 2022;7(6):375–83.
12. Graber M, Marino DV, Johnson DE. Anterior hip dislocation. In: StatPearls [Internet]. Treasure Island: StatPearls Publishing; 2024 [cited 2024 Sept 28]. Available from: http://www.ncbi.nlm.nih.gov/books/NBK507814/.
13. Tehranzadeh J, Vanarthos W, Pais MJ. Osteochondral impaction of the femoral head associated with hip dislocation: CT study in 35 patients. AJR Am J Roentgenol. 1990;155(5):1049–52.
14. Giordano V, Giordano M, Glória RC, de Souza FS, di Tullio P, Lages MM, et al. General principles for treatment of femoral head fractures. J Clin Orthop Trauma. 2019;10(1):155–60.
15. Yu JS. Easily missed fractures in the lower extremity. Radiol Clin North Am. 2015;53(4):737–55.
16. MR imaging of acetabular fractures: value in detecting femoral head injury, intraarticular fragments, and sciatic nerve injury. [Internet]. [cited 2024 Sept 28]. Available from: https://www.ajronline.org/doi/epdf/10.2214/ajr.163.4.8092028.
17. Menger MM, Braun BJ, Herath SC, Küper MA, Rollmann MF, Histing T. Fractures of the femoral head: a narrative review. EFORT Open Rev. 2021;6(11):1122–31.
18. McCarthy JC, Busconi B. The role of hip arthroscopy in the diagnosis and treatment of hip disease. Orthopedics. 1995;18(8):753–6.
19. Moed BR, Maxey JW. Evaluation of fractures of the femoral head using the CT-directed pelvic oblique radiograph. Clin Orthop Relat Res. 1993;296:161–7.
20. Droll KP, Broekhuyse H, O'Brien P. Fracture of the femoral head. J Am Acad Orthop Surg. 2007;15(12):716.
21. Tannast M, Pleus F, Bonel H, Galloway H, Siebenrock KA, Anderson SE. Magnetic resonance imaging in traumatic posterior hip dislocation. J Orthop Trauma. 2010;24(12):723–31.
22. Laorr A, Greenspan A, Anderson MW, Moehring HD, McKinley T. Traumatic hip dislocation: early MRI findings. Skeletal Radiol. 1995;24(4):239–45.
23. Epstein HC, Wiss DA, Cozen L. Posterior fracture dislocation of the hip with fractures of the femoral head. Clin Orthop Relat Res. 1985;201:9.
24. Kellam P, Ostrum RF. Systematic review and meta-analysis of avascular necrosis and posttraumatic arthritis after traumatic hip dislocation. J Orthop Trauma. 2016;30(1):10–6.
25. Spitler CA. Hip dislocations and femoral head fractures.
26. dela Cruz JE, Sullivan DN, Varboncouer E, Milbrandt JC, Duong M, Burdette S, et al. Comparison of procedural sedation for the reduction of dislocated total hip arthroplasty. West J Emerg Med. 2014;15(1):76–80.
27. Dursteler BB, Wightman JM. Etomidate-facilitated hip reduction in the emergency department. Acad Emerg Med. 2000;7(10):1165–6.
28. Bigelow HJ. Luxations of the hip-joint. Boston Med Surg J. 1870;82(4):65–7.
29. Allis OH. An inquiry into the difficulties encountered in the reduction of dislocations of the hip. Dornan; 1896. 200 p
30. Lefkowitz M. A new method for reduction of hip dislocations. Orthop Rev. 1993 Feb;22(2):253–6.
31. Waddell BS, Mohamed S, Glomset JT, Meyer MS. A detailed review of hip reduction maneuvers: a focus on physician safety and introduction of the Waddell technique. Orthop Rev [Internet] 2016 [cited 2024 Sept 27];8(1). Available from: https://www.ncbi.nlm.nih.gov/pmc/articles/PMC4821229/.

4 Anterior Surgical Approaches for Femoral Head Fractures

Ramesh Perumal, Agraharam Devendra, B. Roy Wilson Armstrong, Asif Imran, Jayaramaraju Dheenadhayalan, and Shanmuganathan Rajasekaran

4.1 Introduction

Femoral head fractures are uncommon and challenging injuries, often resulting from high-velocity trauma and frequently associated with posterior hip dislocation [1]. While various classification systems exist for these fractures, the Pipkin's classification, introduced in 1957, remains the most widely used [2, 3]. Pipkin's classification is based on the fracture's relation to the fovea and associated injuries to the femoral neck and acetabulum. Pipkin types I and II involve isolated head fractures, whereas types III and IV are associated with femoral neck and acetabular fractures, respectively. Though some studies suggest favorable outcomes with conservative treatment for congruent joints with type I and II fractures, most current literature advocates for open reduction in cases of displaced femoral head fractures. In cases of type I fractures where fixation is not feasible, excision of small infrafoveolar fragments may be considered as an alternative option [4]. Pipkin types III and IV typically require surgical intervention through safe surgical dislocation or other posterior approaches, discussed in other chapters of this book. A key debate, particularly for type I and II fractures, is whether to use an anterior or posterior approach. This chapter focuses on the anterior approach for treating femoral head fractures, providing a historical overview, surgical indications, detailed technique, and an analysis of its advantages and disadvantages.

R. Perumal (✉) · A. Devendra · B. R. W. Armstrong
A. Imran · J. Dheenadhayalan · S. Rajasekaran
Department of Orthopaedics and Trauma, Ganga Medical Centre and Hospitals Pvt. Ltd, Coimbatore, Tamil Nadu, India

R. K. Sen, S. K. Tripathy (eds.), *A Practical Guide to Management of Femoral Head Fracture-Dislocation*, https://doi.org/10.1007/978-981-96-9852-3_4

4.2 Significance of the Anterior Approach

The typical mechanism of injury for a femoral head fracture is traumatic posterior hip dislocation. In this scenario, a significant force is applied to the hip joint, causing the femoral head to dislocate posteriorly. As the head forcefully impacts and shears against the acetabular rim, it results in a fracture of the femoral head [5]. Choosing an anterior approach is sensible since the fracture is frequently anteroinferior, which makes it challenging to access and repair via the posterior approach. An ideal surgical approach should allow for clear and easy access to the target structures while minimizing damage to surrounding tissues. It should follow natural cleavage lines and fascial planes and, whenever feasible, pass between rather than through muscles. Additionally, it is essential to avoid harming key neurovascular structures. The anterior approach to the hip aligns well with these principles. It follows an internervous plane, with muscles on the medial side innervated by the femoral nerve and upper lumbar roots, while those on the lateral side are supplied by the superior gluteal nerve, making it an anatomically safe and efficient approach [6]. These benefits are further supported by findings from Singh et al., who demonstrated in a cadaveric study that while the SSD approach provides better visualization of the posterolateral quadrants, the anterior approach remains sufficient for most femoral head fractures [7].

4.3 Historical Evolution

The evolution of the anterior approach to the hip has a rich history, beginning in *1881* when German surgeon Carl Hueter introduced it as the first direct anterior approach. Initially, it was used primarily to treat conditions such as hip tuberculosis, developmental hip dysplasia, and femoroacetabular impingement [8]. In *1917*, Marius N. Smith-Petersen helped popularize the technique. Later, in *1949*, E.J. Gordon became the first to report the use of the anterior approach for fragment excision [9]. By *1981*, Hansen had successfully performed open reduction and internal fixation (ORIF) on anterior femoral head fragments [4]. However, in 1985, H.C. Epstein cautioned against using anterior approaches due to concerns about disrupting the anterior blood supply in cases where the posterior supply was already compromised [3]. In *1992*, M.F. Swiontkowski endorsed the anterior approach for Pipkin type I and II fractures, highlighting its ability to provide better visualization of fracture fragments, along with reduced blood loss, shorter operative times, and overall better outcomes [4]. More recently, in *2020*, Gavaskar and colleagues demonstrated that the modified Hueter approach offered significantly reduced surgical time, blood loss, and pain (as measured by 24-h VAS scores) when compared to surgical dislocation. This approach allows for direct access to fracture fragments without dislocating the hip joint and supports future total hip arthroplasty through the same incision, avoiding the complications associated with trochanteric osteotomy [10].

4.4 Surgical Anatomy

The mechanism of injury for femoral head fractures is associated with the position of the hip and the direction of force at the time of trauma. When the hip is flexed at 90 degrees with forced adduction, high-energy axial compression can lead to a pure dislocation. In a neutral adduction position, compression forces are perpendicular to the posterior wall, often causing a posterior wall fracture and potentially a suprafoveal fracture of the femoral head. Depending on the degree of adduction, the injury can result in various sizes of head fragments, with more adduction leading to smaller fragments. In some cases, the femoral neck may also fracture, either due to the trauma or during reduction attempts. When the leg is abducted during trauma, the posterior column of the acetabulum is more likely to fracture, or the acetabulum may protrude into the pelvic cavity, but the femoral head generally remains intact. The extent of adduction during injury determines the size and location of the femoral head fragments [11].

4.4.1 Lateral Femoral Cutaneous Nerve of the Thigh

Understanding the course of the lateral femoral cutaneous nerve (LFCN) is essential in performing the anterior approach to the hip. This knowledge helps in avoiding nerve injury, which could lead to complications such as meralgia paresthetica, a condition characterized by tingling, numbness, or burning pain on the outer thigh. **The anatomical variation and most common branching pattern will help surgeons in preserving the nerve and make them aware. LFCN can be found medial to the sartorius 86% of the time. The distance from the nerve to ASIS is also highly variable, creating a zone in which the LFCN might be found, ranging from 10 mm (most common) to 46 mm medially. The bifurcation pattern of the lateral femoral cutaneous nerve is also highly variable. The nerve may bifurcate in the thigh (most common), in the pelvis, and near the exit to the pelvis, or the LFCN may trifurcate or quadrifurcate.** The LFCN originates from the dorsal branches of the second and third lumbar nerve roots. It travels over the iliacus muscle, deep to its fascia, and crosses the iliac branch of the iliolumbar artery. After its course within the pelvis, the LFCN crosses the deep circumflex iliac artery and enters the anterior thigh, passing under, through, or above the inguinal ligament, typically about 1 cm medial to the anterior superior iliac spine (ASIS). Study by Grothaus [12] found that the nerve enters the thigh through an opening around 36 ± 20 mm (with a range of 6–73 mm) medial to the ASIS under the inguinal ligament. In approximately 30% of cases, the LFCN divides into branches before crossing the inguinal ligament. After entering the thigh, the nerve moves laterally and downward, forming an angle of about 63° (range: 20°–90°) with the inguinal ligament. It then splits into anterior and posterior branches around 5 cm below the ASIS on the surface of the sartorius muscle. The nerve crosses the lateral border of the sartorius muscle at a variable distance from the ASIS, usually between 2.2 cm and 11.3 cm distal to it. The nerve crosses the lateral border of the sartorius 12 ± 8 mm (range: 1–36 mm) medial to a vertical line drawn down from the ASIS. The anterior branch of the LFCN innervates the anterior thigh down to the knee, while the posterior branch supplies the lateral thigh up to the greater trochanter (Fig. 4.1).

4.5 Surgical Options for Femoral Head Fractures

The primary objectives of femoral head fracture treatment are to restore the anatomical integrity of the articular surface, preserve the blood supply, and achieve stable internal fixation. Selecting the appropriate surgical approach is crucial for optimal visualization and screw trajectory. Surgical approaches for femoral head

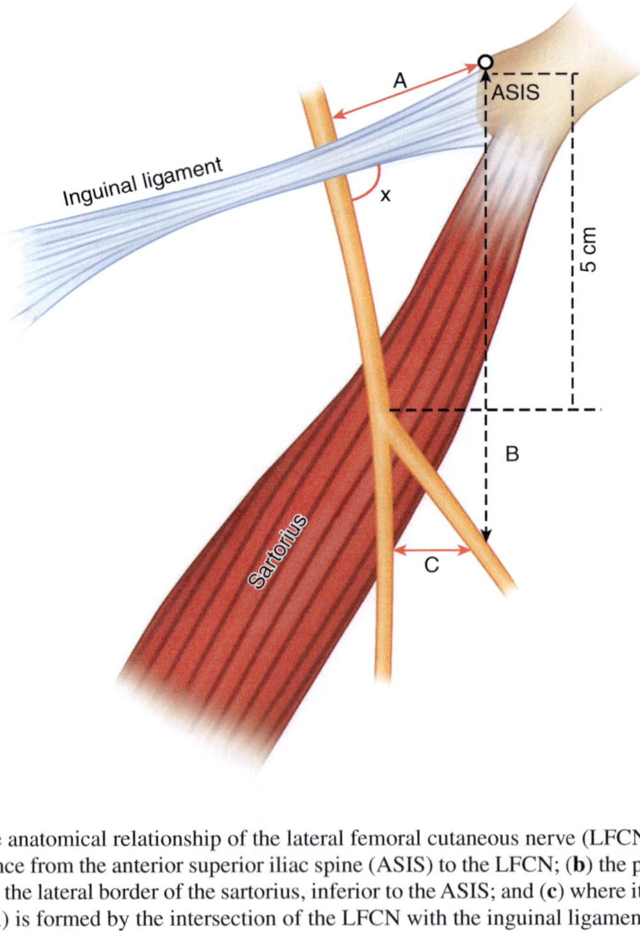

Fig. 4.1 The anatomical relationship of the lateral femoral cutaneous nerve (LFCN) of the thigh. (**a**) The distance from the anterior superior iliac spine (ASIS) to the LFCN; (**b**) the point where the nerve crosses the lateral border of the sartorius, inferior to the ASIS; and (**c**) where it crosses medially. Angle (x) is formed by the intersection of the LFCN with the inguinal ligament

fractures can be broadly categorized into anterior (Smith-Petersen/Hueter approach), anterolateral (Watson-Jones approach), medial (Wang anterior fenestration approach, Chiron medial hip approach), and posterior-based approaches. This chapter will delve into the anterior, anterolateral, and medial approaches (Figs. 4.2 and 4.3).

4.5.1 Modified Smith-Petersen Approach

The patient is positioned supine on a radiolucent table with a sandbag under the affected hip. The affected lower limb is also painted and draped to allow for movements of the hip like traction, flexion, and external rotation during the procedure (Table 4.1). The surgeon and the scrub nurse with the instruments stand on the affected side, while the assistant stands on the contralateral side to retract. Fluoroscopy is shown from the contralateral side. Anatomical landmarks such as the anterior superior iliac spine, the greater trochanter, and patella are marked. A 10–12 cm of skin incision begins 2 cm lateral and distal to ASIS pointing toward the

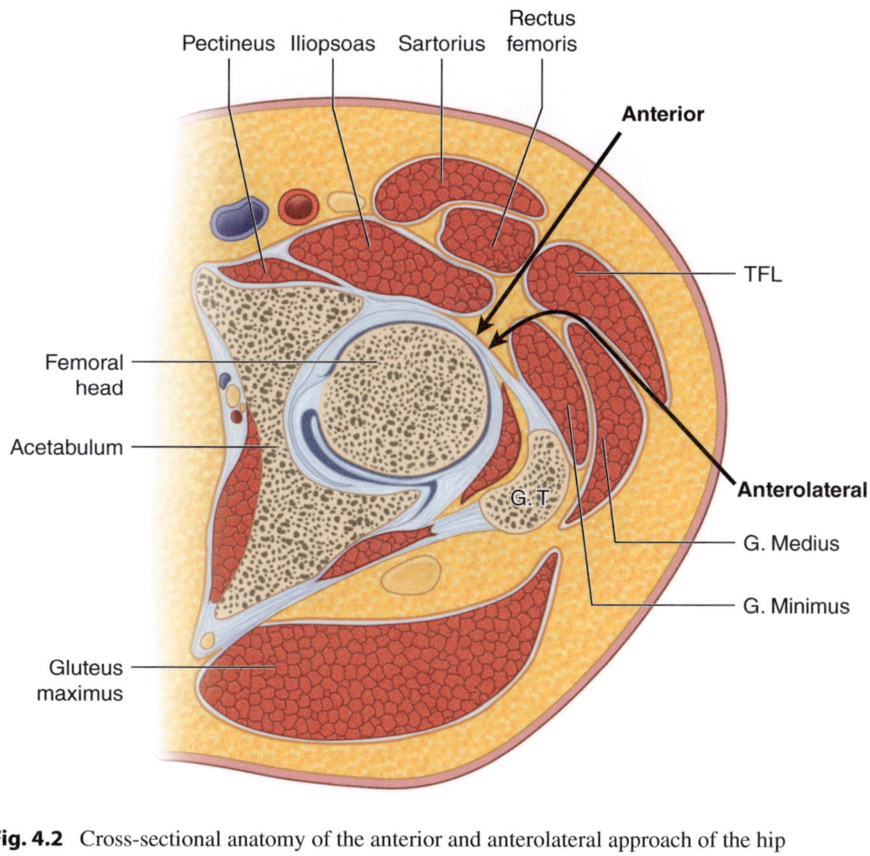

Fig. 4.2 Cross-sectional anatomy of the anterior and anterolateral approach of the hip

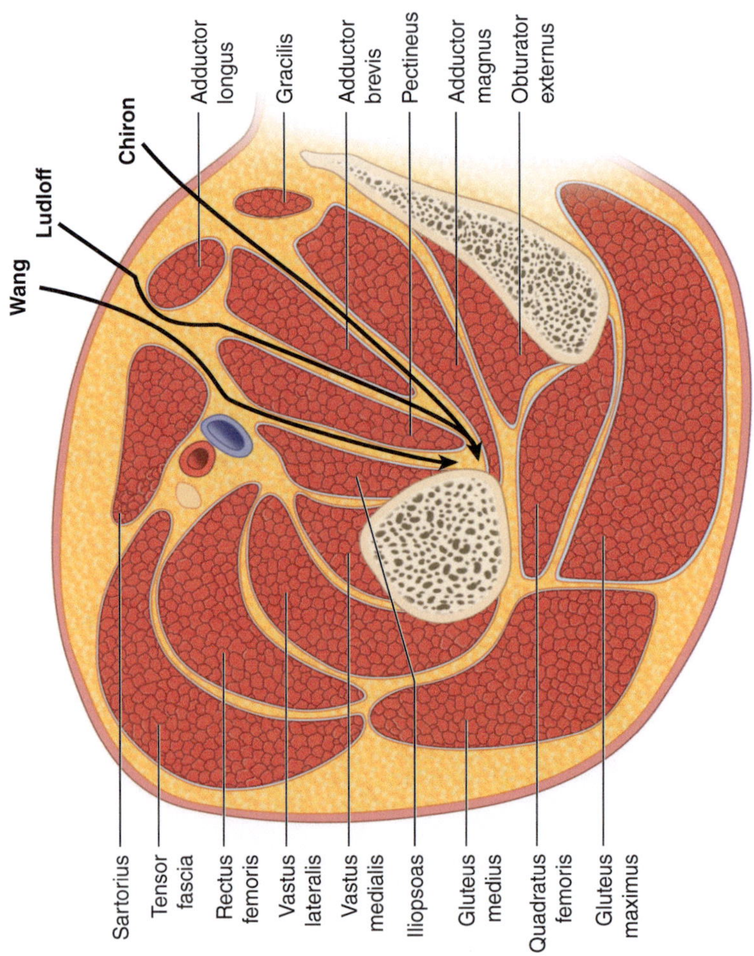

Fig. 4.3 Medial approaches to hip

Table 4.1 Preoperative planning

Imaging	Plain anteroposterior view of pelvis with both hip radiograph CT scan with 3D reconstruction
Anesthesia	Spinal anesthesia General anesthesia
Positioning	Supine position with radiolucent table

lateral border of patella over the muscle belly of tensor fascia lata. Following the skin incision, a translucent fascia is seen covering the muscle. The medial border of the tensor fascia lata muscle is identified, and fascia over there is divided. The lateral femoral cutaneous nerve of the thigh is identified and protected medially. Using blunt dissection within the fascial sheath, the interval between the tensor fascia lata and the sartorius muscles is developed. The self-retaining retractor is used to retract the sartorius medially and tensor fascia lata laterally; then the rectus femoris, which is incised and retracted, and the gluteus medius, which is retracted laterally. The ascending branche of lateral circumflex vessel is identified inferiorly and ligated. At this point, flexing the hip aids in muscle relaxation and enhances surgical exposure. The capsule is separated from the overlying rectus muscle using sharp dissection. The femoral neck is palpated, and Hohmann retractors are placed medially and laterally around it for better exposure. A T-shaped capsulotomy is performed, centered on the femoral neck, with care taken to avoid damaging the labrum. Placing Hohmann retractors deep to the capsule provides clear visualization of the femoral head. Flexion, abduction, and external rotation of the hip provides access to the fracture site. Small or comminuted fragments of the femoral head lodged in the acetabulum are removed, while larger fragments are anatomically reduced and temporarily stabilized with Kirschner wires. These are subsequently replaced by either headless or cannulated screws, with their heads countersunk beneath the cartilage. Soft tissue attachments to bone fragments are preserved to maintain blood supply to the femoral head. For closure, the arthrotomy, rectus femoris reattachment, superficial fascia, and skin are repaired in sequence (Fig. 4.4).

4.5.2 Rationale for Modifications and Their Benefits

This approach is simple, direct, and minimally invasive, providing adequate exposure for reduction and fixation without requiring muscle detachment. Neither the tensor fascia lata nor the abductors are released. Unlike the Smith-Petersen approach, which involves releasing the gluteus medius, minimus, tensor fascia lata, and performing osteotomies, this technique avoids such steps. The traditional Smith-Petersen approach involves an incision extending from the midpoint of the iliac crest to the anterior superior iliac spine (ASIS), then continuing 10–12 cm along the anterior edge of the tensor fascia lata toward the lateral border of the patella. To minimize the risk of lateral femoral cutaneous nerve (LFCN) injury, the modified Smith-Petersen approach lateralizes the incision, allowing the nerve to be easily spared. Additionally, the approach allows rapid access to the hip joint, enabling the surgeon to focus more on reduction and fixation (Table 4.2).

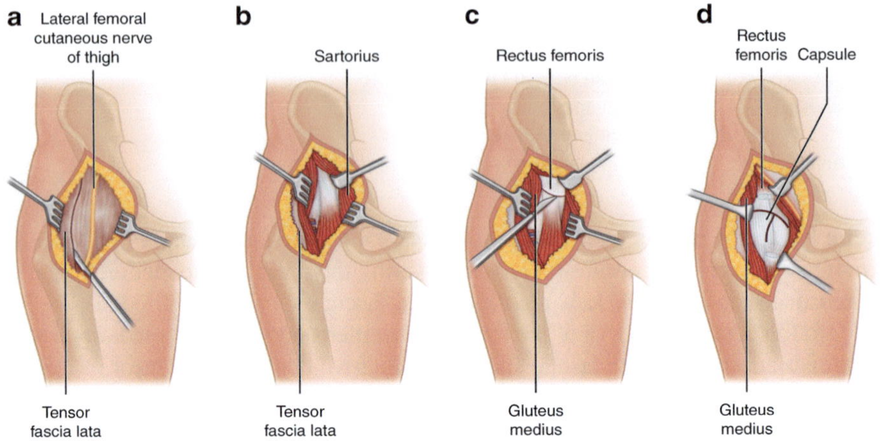

Fig. 4.4 Smith-Petersen approach: (**a**) Make an incision in the fascia overlying the tensor fasciae latae muscle. The lateral femoral cutaneous nerve is located medially along the fascia. (**b**) Bluntly dissect the interval between the sartorius and tensor fasciae latae, retracting the tensor fasciae latae laterally. (**c**) Incising the direct head of rectus femoris muscle enhances the visualization. (**d**) Making a T-shaped incision in the capsule

Table 4.2 Advantages and disadvantages of anterior approach

Advantages	Disadvantages
1. Safer for hip vascularity compared to posterior approaches	1. Increased risk of heterotopic ossification (HO) formation, reported up to 40%
2. Effective for Pipkin I and II fractures, where the fragment is typically anteroinferior, allowing fixation without full hip dislocation	2. Limited ability to inspect the acetabulum fully without extensive release of the tensor fascia lata (TFL) and gluteus medius
3. Utilizes true internervous and intermuscular planes, minimizing muscle damage	3. Up to 9% of patients may experience persistent anterolateral thigh numbness following the procedure
4. Avoids disruption and detachment of abductor muscles, reducing the incidence of postoperative limping	4. Does not allow for the management of concomitant posterior injuries, such as in Pipkin type IV fractures
5. Associated with reduced operative time, blood loss, and lower incidence of femoral head avascular necrosis (AVN)	5. Potential disruption of the remaining blood supply to the femoral head, especially if already compromised by a posterior dislocation

4.5.3 Medial Approach

This approach, primarily developed for developmental dysplasia of the hip, was first described by Ludloff in 1908 [13, 14]. Fergusson later modified it [14]. Additionally, two other medial approaches for femoral head fractures have been described: the direct medial approach by Chiron et al. [15] and the anterior fenestration approach by Wang et al. [16].

4.5.4 Wang Anterior Fenestration Approach

The approach requires a supine position with the limb positioned in flexion, abduction, and external rotation. A vertical incision begins below the inguinal crease on the medial side of the pulsating femoral artery, approximately 8–10 cm in length. After dissecting the subcutaneous tissue and deep fascia, the great saphenous vein is retracted. The femoral sheath and its contents are retracted laterally, and the adductor longus and pectineus are retracted medially, exposing the lesser trochanter. The iliopsoas muscle is then isolated and retracted upward, and the traversing branch of the medial circumflex femoral artery is identified and retracted downward. The hip joint capsule is incised, and the femoral head is exposed. With the limb maintained in flexion, abduction, and external rotation, the anterior inferior femoral head is exposed. Hip extension exposes the upper and inner quadrants of the femoral head, while flexion, abduction, and internal rotation expose the anterior outer quadrant. Extension in this position reveals the upper and outer quadrants of the femoral head. Fixation can be achieved with headless screws. Relevant images will confirm fracture reduction, and the capsule and wound are closed in layers with a drain (Fig. 4.3).

Hematoma formation may occur due to incomplete ligation of vascular channels, and the medial circumflex femoral artery may be injured during the procedure. There is a limited number of reported studies using this approach for fixing Pipkin type I and II fractures. This approach is not routinely used and requires a learning curve.

4.5.5 Chiron Medial Hip Approach

For this approach, limb should be kept in flexion abduction external rotation to make adductor longus and hip capsule to be taught. Incision starts from pubic tubercle along the adductor longus up to 8–10 cm and the plane developed between adductor longus and gracilis. Further, the deeper plane progresses between adductor brevis and magnus; then the lesser trochanter is reached where the tendon of iliopsoas is identified and retracted upward and outward [11, 15]. Hip capsule is reached and the traversing medial circumflex femoral artery is identified and retracted to expose the upper capsule and anterior wall of acetabulum. Hip capsule is opened by a vertical incision along the neck and extended up and down to expose the anteromedial femoral head, hip joint, and neck. Fixation can be performed with headless screws, and appropriate imaging can confirm the reduction and congruency of the hip joint. The author recommends that anteroinferior fragments of one-third to one-quarter size fragment can be reached through this approach for fixation or excision. Postoperative hematoma formation and injury to the medial circumflex femoral artery are potential risks during the procedure (Fig. 4.3).

4.5.6 Anterolateral Approach

Watson-Jones described the anterolateral approach for fractures of the femoral neck in 1936 [17]. In subsequent years, this approach has been adapted for femoral head fractures with hip dislocations. Several authors have reported its utility in Pipkin type II and III fractures, where the suprafoveal fragment and femoral neck can be addressed [18–20].

The patient is positioned supine, and the incision is centered over the trochanter, curving anteriorly for approximately 7–10 cm toward the gluteal tubercle of the iliac crest. Distally, it extends along the shaft of the femur. The tensor fascia lata is incised along its full length and retracted anteriorly. A deeper plane is developed between the gluteus medius and tensor fascia lata. Proximal extension should be limited to avoid injury to the superior gluteal neurovascular structures. Blunt dissection through this plane exposes the hip capsule, and releasing the vastus lateralis increases the exposure of the anterolateral part of the trochanter. Branches from the lateral circumflex iliac artery must be cauterized. Positioning the limb in external rotation further enhances exposure of the hip capsule. A T-shaped incision is placed over the capsule, with the horizontal limb positioned proximally for femoral head exposure and distally for femoral neck exposure. This approach allows for simultaneous exposure of the anterolateral femoral head and neck (Fig. 4.5).

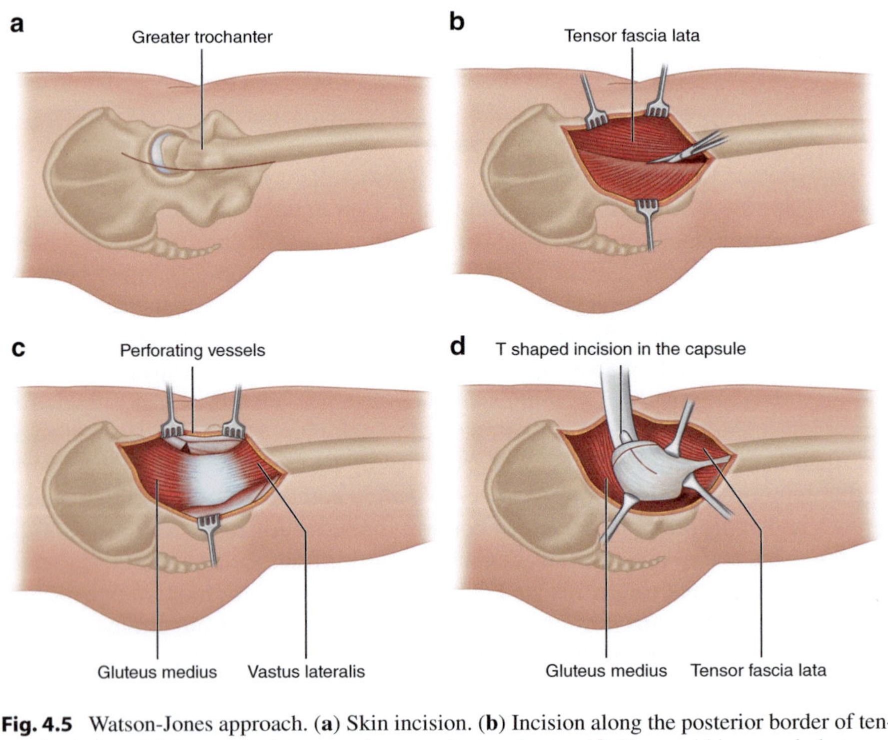

Fig. 4.5 Watson-Jones approach. (**a**) Skin incision. (**b**) Incision along the posterior border of tensor fascia lata. (**c**) Exposed gluteus medius, greater trochanter. (**d**) Exposed hip capsule between tensor fascia lata and gluteus medius

4.6 Indication

For Pipkin type I and II fractures, if the hip joint remains congruent after closed reduction and the fragment is located anteriorly or anteroinferior, anterior-based approaches are recommended for excision or fixation [21–23]. Additionally, unreduced anterior hip dislocation is also an indication for using the anterior approach [24]. Recently, Liu et al. found that combining the direct anterior and posterior approaches for treating Pipkin IV femoral head fractures led to better outcomes, including reduced postoperative pain, faster functional recovery, and shorter hospital stays, without increasing the risk of complications [25].

4.7 Author's Preferred Treatment

1. In cases of posterior dislocation with a posterior rim avulsion, after a successful closed reduction, it is essential to assess the stability of the hip joint using dynamic stress testing. If the hip is stable, Pipkin type I and II fractures can be treated with an anterior approach alone.
2. The author favors the anterior approach for managing Pipkin type I and II fractures, as well as unreduced anterior hip dislocations with or without femoral head fractures.
3. We prefer safe surgical dislocation when the fracture fragment is located posteriorly and/or accompanied by femoral head impaction.
4. For the skin incision, the author typically begins 2 cm lateral and distal to the ASIS, ensuring the identification of the lateral femoral cutaneous nerve (LCFN) to reduce the risk of nerve injury and subsequent meralgia paresthetica.
5. In all cases involving the anterior approach, we prefer to incise the rectus femoris and maintain knee flexion, which helps relax the muscles and enhances visualization. While various capsulotomy shapes—such as T, H, and I—are used, we prefer T-shaped capsulotomy, with the horizontal limb parallel to the acetabular labrum, taking care to avoid damaging the labrum, and the vertical limb centered along the neck.
6. For undisplaced large fracture fragments with a congruent joint, the author opts for fixation in situ without dislocation to minimize soft tissue and vascular damage. Whenever feasible, the soft tissue attachments to fracture fragments are preserved.
7. Although medial and anterolateral approaches have been described for femoral head fractures, the author consistently prefers the anterior approach for Pipkin type I and II fractures. Pipkin types III and IV are managed using the safe surgical dislocation method or the posterior approach, respectively.

4.8 Rehabilitation

Patients with type I infrafoveolar fractures are allowed to bear weight as tolerated from the first postoperative day. For type II fractures, non-weight-bearing is recommended for the first 6 weeks, followed by a gradual progression to partial weight-bearing after 6 weeks and full weight-bearing by 12 weeks. The authors do not routinely administer prophylaxis for heterotopic ossification.

4.9 Outcome and Complications

Martin Kloub conducted a comparison of functional outcomes based on the Thompson-Epstein criteria in 177 cases across 14 studies for ORIF of Pipkin type I and II fractures. The results showed that anterior approaches provided better overall outcomes. Among 138 fractures treated with anterior approaches, 41% had excellent outcomes, 34% had good outcomes, while 14% were fair and 11% poor. In contrast, posterior approaches in 39 fractures resulted in 31% excellent outcomes, 49% good, 13% fair, and 8% poor [26].

Heterotopic ossification (HO) and avascular necrosis (AVN) are complications associated with surgical approaches to the hip [27]. Previous studies have identified the anterior approach as a risk factor for heterotopic ossification (HO), while the posterior approach has been associated with a higher incidence of avascular necrosis (AVN) of the femoral head [26, 28, 29]. In Martin Kloub's analysis of 538 cases from 33 articles, the anterior approach (Hueter, Smith-Petersen) demonstrated a higher incidence of AVN, affecting 17.5% of cases, compared to 6.2% in the flip osteotomy and 15.6% in the Kocher-Langenbeck approach. Additionally, HO was more frequent in the anterior approach, occurring in 36.9% of cases, compared to 19.6% in the flip osteotomy and 19.5% in the Kocher–Langenbeck approach. Arthritis was reported in 23.3% of anterior approach cases, similar to 24% in the Kocher-Langenbeck approach but higher than the 8.1% seen with flip osteotomy. Fracture-related infections were rare, with no cases reported in the anterior group. These findings underscore the elevated risk of HO and AVN with the anterior approach, despite its effectiveness in treating femoral head fractures [26].

Variations in nerve anatomy and prolonged retraction can contribute to lateral femoral cutaneous nerve (LFCN) injury [30, 31]. Studies have reported an LFCN injury rate of approximately 23.3–31.9% during direct anterior approach to total hip arthroplasty [32]. However, Gavaskar et al. [10] observed a lower rate of 9%. A thorough understanding of the surgical anatomy and the use of a lateral-based incision can help minimize the risk of nerve injury.

4.10 Case Example

A 30-year-old man was involved in a road traffic accident in which his car was hit by another vehicle. He sustained a closed posterior dislocation of the left hip. There were no other systemic or limb injuries, and he presented 6 h after the accident. The dorsalis pedis pulse was palpable, and sciatic nerve function was intact. The dislocation was reduced under spinal anesthesia, and a post-reduction stress test was negative. Post-reduction computed tomography scans revealed a large Pipkin type I fracture located anteroinferiorly on the femoral head. The fracture was reduced and fixed with a headless screw through a Smith-Petersen approach. Postoperative radiographs demonstrated a reduced fracture and a congruent joint. The patient was initially placed on toe-touch weight-bearing for 6 weeks, followed by full weight-bearing along with active hip range-of-motion exercises. He resumed his original occupation within 4 months. At the 2-year follow-up, radiographs showed a united fracture with a congruent joint and no signs of avascular necrosis and heterotrophic ossification. The functional outcome was excellent (Figs. 4.6, 4.7 and 4.8).

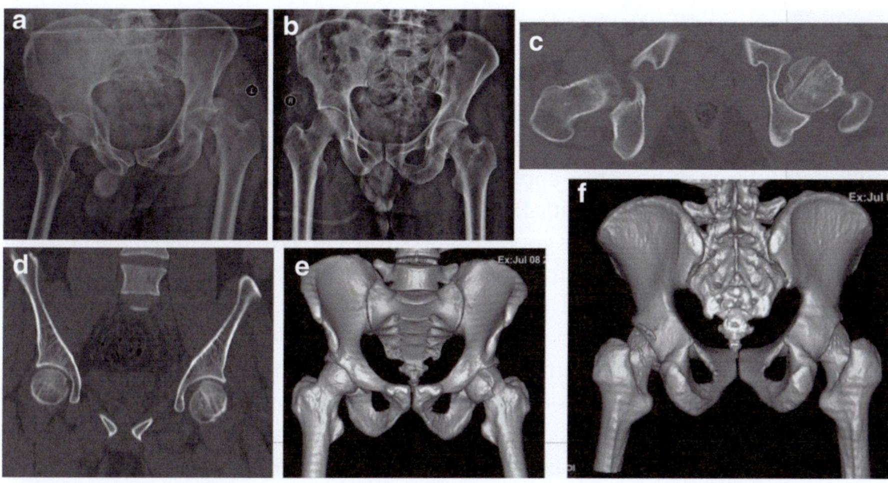

Fig. 4.6 A 30-year-old man was involved in a road traffic accident, where his car was hit by another vehicle, resulting in a left-sided posterior hip dislocation (**a**). The dislocation was successfully reduced (**b**) under spinal anesthesia. Post-reduction CT scans (**c–e**) reveal a large Pipkin type I fracture located anteroinferiorly on the femoral head. A 3D reconstruction image (**f**) shows a rim avulsion fracture of the posterior acetabular wall

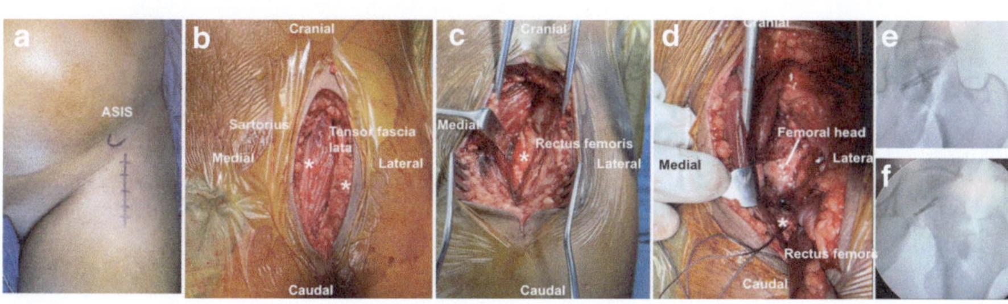

Fig. 4.7 (**a**) Identified anatomical landmark (ASIS) with the planned incision made 2 cm lateral and distal to the ASIS. (**b**) Plane created between the sartorius (asterisk) medially and tensor fascia lata (asterisk) laterally. (**c**) Deep plane visualized between the rectus femoris (medially) and gluteus medius (laterally), exposing the joint capsule. (**d**) Post-capsulotomy image showing the femoral head, with the tenotomized rectus femoris retracted. (**e and f**) Fluoroscopic images demonstrating the fixation of the femoral head with headless screws

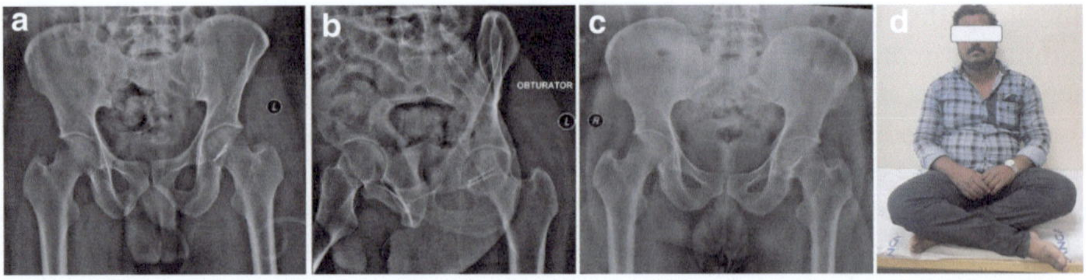

Fig. 4.8 Immediate postoperative radiographs (**a** and **b**) show fixation of the femoral head fracture with headless screws and a congruent hip joint. At the 2-year follow-up, radiographs (**c**) show a united fracture and a congruent joint, while clinical images (**d**) demonstrate a good functional outcome

4.11 Summary

The anterior approach for femoral head fractures, especially Pipkin types I and II, offers advantages in accessing anteroinferior fracture fragment sites that are difficult to reach through posterior approach. Historically developed by Carl Hueter in 1881 and later refined by Smith-Petersen, this approach has evolved to improve surgical outcomes. It allows for good visualization and fixation without the need for extensive muscle detachment, focusing on the preservation of important neurovascular structures like the lateral femoral cutaneous nerve. However, complications such as heterotopic ossification (36.9%) and avascular necrosis (17.5%) are more common with this approach compared to others, such as flip osteotomy or Kocher-Langenbeck. Despite these risks, the anterior approach remains a preferred option for Pipkin I and II fractures, providing effective outcomes while preserving soft tissue integrity. Overall, it is a reliable and efficient method when used appropriately.

4.12 Key Points

1. The anterior approach provides excellent access to anteroinferior femoral head fragments, minimizes muscle detachment, and follows a safer internervous plane, reducing risks to neurovascular structures.
2. The superficial plane is between the tensor fascia lata (TFL) and the sartorius muscles. The deep plane is between the rectus femoris and the gluteus medius muscles.
3. Studies indicate that the anterior approach yields better functional outcomes in treating Pipkin type I and II fractures, when compared to posterior approaches.
4. Despite its advantages, the anterior approach has a higher incidence of heterotopic ossification (HO) compared to posterior approaches, though posterior approaches have a higher risk of AVN.

Acknowledgement Nil.

Ethics Approval Approval was obtained from the institutional ethics committee. The procedures used in this study adhere to the tenets of the Declaration of Helsinki.

Consent to Participate and Publish Informed consent was obtained from all individual participants included in the study.

Author Contributions Perumal Ramesh: Validation, visualization, writing—review and editing

- Agraharam Devendra: Validation, visualization, writing—review and editing
- Asif Imran: Conceptualization, data curation, methodology, writing—original draft
- B Roy Wilson Armstrong: Supervision, validation
- Jayaramaraju Dheenadhayalan: Supervision, validation
- Shanmuganathan Rajasekaran: Resources, project administration

Conflicts of Interests The authors have no competing interests to declare that are relevant to the content of this article.

Declarations of Interest None.

Funding No funding was received for conducting this study.

References

1. Brumback RJ, Kenzora JE, Levitt LE, Burgess AR, Poka A. Fractures of the femoral head. Hip; 1987. p. 181–206.
2. Pipkin G. Treatment of grade IV fracture-dislocation of the hip. J Bone Joint Surg Am. 1957;39-A(5):1027–1042 passim.
3. Epstein HC, Wiss DA, Cozen L. Posterior fracture dislocation of the hip with fractures of the femoral head. Clin Orthop. 1985;201:9–17.
4. Swiontkowski MF, Thorpe M, Seiler JG, Hansen ST. Operative management of displaced femoral head fractures: case-matched comparison of anterior versus posterior approaches for Pipkin I and Pipkin II fractures. J Orthop Trauma. 1992;6(4):437–42.
5. Davis JB. Simultaneous femoral head fracture and traumatic hip dislocation. Am J Surg [Internet] 1950 ;80(7):893–895. Available from: https://www.sciencedirect.com/science/article/pii/0002961050904739. [cited 2024 Sept 10].
6. Lowell JD, Aufranc OE. The anterior approach to the hip joint. Clin Orthop Relat Res [Internet]. 1968 Dec [cited 2024 Sept 15];61:193. Available from: https://journals.lww.com/clinorthop/citation/1968/11000/the_anterior_approach_to_the_hip_joint.20.aspx.
7. Singh K, Weitlich JD, Zitsch BP, Schweser KM, Cook JL, Crist BD. Which surgical approach provides maximum visualization and access for open reduction and internal fixation (ORIF) of femoral neck fractures? Injury [Internet]. 2022 [cited 2024 Sept 15];53(3):1131–1136. Available from: https://www.sciencedirect.com/science/article/pii/S002013832100930X.
8. Rachbauer F, Kain MSH, Leunig M. The history of the anterior approach to the hip. Orthop Clin North Am. 2009;40(3):311–20.
9. Gordon EJ, Greiberg JA. Posterior dislocation of the hip with fracture of the head of the femur. J Bone Joint Surg Am. 1949;31A(4):869–72.

10. Gavaskar AS, Srinivasan P, Jeyakumar B, Raj RV, Sharath V, Narayan D. Surgical dislocation or the modified heuter anterior approach for Pipkin I and II femoral head fracture dislocations. J Orthop Trauma [Internet]. 2020 Dec [cited 2024 Sept 10];34(12):626. Available from: https://journals.lww.com/jorthotrauma/fulltext/2020/12000/surgical_dislocation_or_the_modified_heuter.2.aspx.
11. Chiron P, Lafontan V, Reina N. Fracture-dislocations of the femoral head. Orthop Traumatol Surg Res. 2013;99(1 Suppl):S53–66.
12. Grothaus MC, Holt M, Mekhail AO, Ebraheim NA, Yeasting RA. Lateral femoral cutaneous nerve: an anatomic study. Clin Orthop. 2005;437:164–8.
13. Koizumi W, Moriya H, Tsuchiya K, Takeuchi T, Kamegaya M, Akita T. Ludloff's medial approach for open reduction of congenital dislocation of the hip. A 20-year follow-up. J Bone Joint Surg Br. 1996;78(6):924–9.
14. Khalifa AA, Ahmed EM, Farouk OA. Surgical approaches for managing femoral head fractures (FHFs); what and how to choose from the different options? Orthop Res Rev. 2022;14:133–45.
15. Chiron P, Murgier J, Cavaignac E, Pailhé R, Reina N. Minimally invasive medial hip approach. Orthop Traumatol Surg Res [Internet]. 2014;100(6):687–9. [cited 2024 Sept 15]. Available from: https://www.sciencedirect.com/science/article/pii/S1877056814001601.
16. In Situ Reduction and Fixation of the Anterior Medial Fenestration Approach for Femoral Head Fracture – PubMed [Internet]. [cited 2024 Sept 15]. Available from: https://pubmed.ncbi.nlm.nih.gov/31762204/.
17. Watson-Jones R. Fractures of the neck of the femur. Br J Surg [Internet]. 2005 Dec 5 [cited 2024 Sept 15];23(92):787–808. Available from: https://academic.oup.com/bjs/article/23/92/787/6221606.
18. Harris WH. Traumatic arthritis of the hip after dislocation and acetabular fractures: treatment by mold arthroplasty. J Bone Jt Surg [Internet]. 1969 Jun [cited 2023 June 24];51(4):737–55. Available from: http://journals.lww.com/00004623-196951040-00012.
19. Müller M, Tohtz S, Dewey M, Springer I, Perka C. Evidence of reduced muscle trauma through a minimally invasive anterolateral approach by means of MRI. Clin Orthop [Internet]. 2010 Dec [cited 2024 Sept 15];468(12):3192–200. Available from: https://journals.lww.com/00003086-201012000-00008.
20. Sköldenberg O, Ekman A, Salemyr M, Bodén H. Reduced dislocation rate after hip arthroplasty for femoral neck fractures when changing from posterolateral to anterolateral approach: A prospective study of 372 hips. Acta Orthop [Internet]. 2010 Oct [cited 2024 Sept 15];81(5):583–587. Available from: https://actaorthop.org/actao/article/view/11106.
21. Kloub M, Holub K, Peml M, Urban J, Latal P. Closed reduction and minimally invasive screw osteosynthesis of Pipkin femoral head fractures. J Appl Biomed. 2023;21(1):1–6.
22. Shakya S, Chen J, Sun J, Xiang Z. Management and outcome of patients with femoral head fractures: the mid-term follow-up with injuries and associated prognostic factors. BMC Musculoskelet Disord. 2023;24(1):311.
23. Wang C guang, Li Y min, Zhang H feng, Li H, Li Z jun. Anterior approach versus posterior approach for Pipkin I and II femoral head fractures: A systemic review and meta-analysis. Int J Surg [Internet]. 2016 Mar [cited 2024 Sept 15];27:176–81. Available from: https://linkinghub.elsevier.com/retrieve/pii/S1743919116001102.
24. Tarchichi J, Daher M, Sakr I, Ghoul A, Zalaket J, Ghanem I, et al. Anterior hip dislocation: a current concepts review and proposal of management algorithm. Injury [Internet]. 2024 Feb 1 [cited 2024 Sept 15];55(2):111252. Available from: https://www.sciencedirect.com/science/article/pii/S0020138323009695.
25. Liu B, Zhao B, Zhang Q. Efficacy of direct anterior approach combined with direct posterior approach in Pipkin IV femoral head fractures. J Orthop Surg [Internet]. 2022 [cited 2024 Sept 15];17(1):160. Available from: https://josr-online.biomedcentral.com/articles/10.1186/s13018-022-03058-9.
26. Kloub M, Látal P, Giannoudis P. Techniques and results of reconstruction of femoral head fractures: An update. Injury [Internet]. 2024 Jun [cited 2024 Sept 15];55(6):111473. Available from: https://linkinghub.elsevier.com/retrieve/pii/S0020138324001608.

27. Henriques R, Ramalho D, Soares Do Brito J, Rocha P, Spranger A, Almeida P. Management of Pipkin Fractures Using a Safe Surgical Hip Dislocation. Case Rep Orthop [Internet]. 2019 Oct 23 [cited 2024 Sept 15];2019:1–6. Available from: https://www.hindawi.com/journals/crior/2019/3526018/.
28. Wang S, Li B, Li J, Zhang Z, Yang H, Liu L. Comparison of the modified Heuter approach and the Kocher-Langenbeck approach in the treatment of Pipkin type I and type II femoral head fractures. Int Orthop [Internet]. 2019 Nov [cited 2024 Sept 15];43(11):2613–20. Available from: http://link.springer.com/10.1007/s00264-019-04301-5.
29. Guo JJ, Tang N, Yang HL, Qin L, Leung KS. Impact of surgical approach on postoperative heterotopic ossification and avascular necrosis in femoral head fractures: a systematic review. Int Orthop. 2010;34(3):319–22.
30. Rudin D, Manestar M, Ullrich O, Erhardt J, Grob K. The Anatomical Course of the Lateral Femoral Cutaneous Nerve with Special Attention to the Anterior Approach to the Hip Joint. J Bone Jt Surg [Internet]. 2016 Apr 6 [cited 2024 Sept 15];98(7):561–7. Available from: https://journals.lww.com/00004623-201604060-00005.
31. Den Brave PS, Vas Nunes SE, Bronkhorst MWGA. Anatomical variations of the lateral femoral cutaneous nerve and iatrogenic injury after autologous bone grafting from the iliac crest. J Orthop Trauma [Internet]. 2015 Dec [cited 2024 Sept 15];29(12):549–553. Available from: https://journals.lww.com/00005131-201512000-00005.
32. Ukai T, Suyama K, Hayashi S, Omura H, Watanabe M. The anatomical features of the lateral femoral cutaneous nerve with total hip arthroplasty: a comparative study of direct anterior and anterolateral supine approaches. BMC Musculoskelet Disord [Internet]. 2022 Dec [cited 2024 Sept 15];23(1):267. Available from: https://bmcmusculoskeletdisord.biomedcentral.com/articles/10.1186/s12891-022-05224-w.

Surgical Hip Dislocation Using a Trochanteric Flip Osteotomy

5

Chand Muddali Bharath, C. A. Aswath, Prakash Ayyadurai, Parthasarathy Srinivasan, and Ashok S. Gavaskar

5.1 Introduction

Most popular surgical approaches tend to be muscle sparing, extensile, and use inter-nervous planes. With regard to access to the hip joint for hip-preserving procedures for traumatic and non-traumatic conditions, the approach should also take into account the complex vascular anatomy of the femoral head. On these lines, Crock in 1996 [1] suggested for the development of a safe, open approach with no disturbance to the blood supply of the femoral head. Surgical hip dislocation using a trochanteric osteotomy often termed safe surgical dislocation (SSD) is one such elegant approach to the hip joint providing circumferential exposure of the acetabular cavity, labrum, femoral head, and the retro-acetabular surface. The approach was the result of the intricate vascular studies performed by Prof. Reinhold Ganz based on the principle of preserving the major extra-osseous arterial supply to the femoral head. Though Prof. Ganz and his team have been performing safe surgical dislocation (SSD) from 1992, the procedure became well known only after publication of his seminal paper in 2001 [2].

SSD provides safe anterior and posterior hip exposure through a stable flip osteotomy of the greater trochanter with preservation of the hip abductor insertion. The impressive initial results from Prof. Ganz and colleagues, the description of the retinacular flap elevation technique [3], and several follow-up anatomical and vascular studies [4–6] supporting the use of the approach led to widespread use of SSD worldwide. Since 2001, the approach has become popular among orthopedic surgeons to expose the hip joint in pediatric and adult population to treat a wide variety of traumatic and non-traumatic conditions. Though considered safe, the technique of performing a SSD needs skill and familiarity with hip anatomy and involves a learning curve especially in pediatric patients. Smith et al. [7] emphasized that the

C. M. Bharath · C. A. Aswath · P. Ayyadurai · P. Srinivasan · A. S. Gavaskar (✉)
Institute of Orthopedics, Trauma & Spine Surgery, Rela Hospital, Chennai, India

R. K. Sen, S. K. Tripathy (eds.), *A Practical Guide to Management of Femoral Head Fracture-Dislocation*, https://doi.org/10.1007/978-981-96-9852-3_5

procedure should not be undertaken in the pediatric population by surgeons in the early part of the learning curve.

Among traumatic conditions, femoral head fracture fixation represents a great indication to perform SSD. The approach provides direct access to the site of the problem and enables direct reduction and fixation with appropriate implants without further damage to the femoral head vascularity. This chapter will focus on the rationale and use of SSD for different types of femoral head fractures with emphasis on technique, outcomes, and complications.

5.2 Relevant Vascular Anatomy of the Femoral Head

A sound knowledge of the vascular anatomy of the femoral head is crucial for performing SSD for all indications. The femoral head receives its major blood supply from the medial femoral circumflex artery (MFCA). The MFCA is often a branch from the profunda femoris or sometimes directly from the femoral artery. The MFCA then divides into five major branches, namely, superficial, deep, ascending, descending, and acetabular branches. Of the five branches, the deep branch of the MFCA is considered the most important vessel for supplying the femoral head. The deep branch can be seen inferior to the obturator externus between the pectineus and the psoas going toward the intertrochanteric crest. Posteriorly, the deep branch gives off its main division between the inferior gemellus and the quadratus muscles. The main division then travels posterior to the obturator externus and then upward anterior to the obturator internus and gemelli muscles. The artery perforates the hip capsule cranial to the superior gemellus and distal to the piriformis tendon. It then divides into three major retinacular branches, namely, superior, anterior, and inferior, which course intracapsular in the posterosuperior region of the femoral neck (Fig. 5.1). These retinacular branches pierce the femoral neck few millimeters proximal to the cartilaginous margin of the femoral head. Preservation of these capsular branches is considered important for maintaining vascularity of the femoral head [8].

5.2.1 SSD and Femoral Head Vascularity

Prof. Ganz and his team showed the anatomical distribution of the vascular foramina at the femoral head neck junction to be predominantly located superior and posterosuperior [4]. Only a few small vessels penetrated the anterior head accounting for a very minor supply to the femoral head. This makes the anterior capsulotomy and anterior dislocation much safer. In a randomized- controlled cadaveric study, Lorich et al. from the hospital for special surgery showed that the trochanteric flip osteotomy maintained almost full perfusion to the femoral head and head-neck junction in contrast to the conventional posterior approach, which almost completely compromised femoral head and head-neck perfusion [5]. Both the ascending branch of the MFCA and the inferior retinacular artery were found universally disrupted in all specimens. These findings were further strengthened in another study

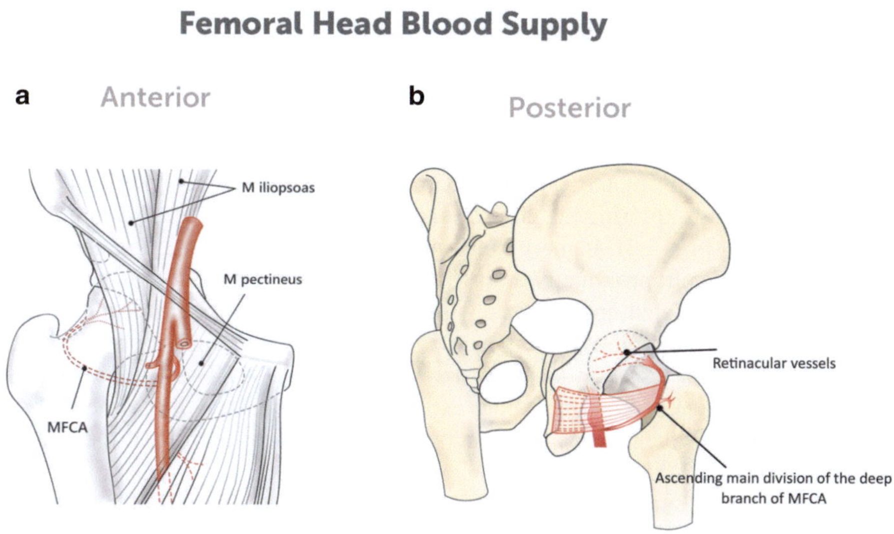

Fig. 5.1 (**a**) The anterior origin of the MFCA and its further course and branches. (**b**) The course of the deep branch of MFCA from posterior and its main ascending division before branching out as retinacular vessels

using laser Doppler flowmetry [6] by Ganz and his team where they showed there were transient reductions in blood flow after dislocation in specific hip positions, but the flow was completely restored within 30 minutes of hip reduction. Steffen and colleagues in their paper on hip resurfacing measured oxygenation of the femoral head through different surgical approaches [9]. They reported oxygenation to the head was better preserved with SSD than the posterior approach and also fluctuated less compared with the anterolateral approach.

5.3 Indications of SSD

SSD is used for a wide variety of pediatric and adult hip conditions [10]. With regard to femoral head fractures, the approach can be used for all four types classified according to the Pipkin system. For types I and II, SSD remains a commonly performed approach apart from the anterior-based surgical approaches and the posterior Kocher-Langenbeck (KL) approach. In these injuries, SSD provides additional opportunity to repair the hip labrum which is not possible with other anterior-based approaches. The hip labrum is found torn in more than 50% of type I and II fractures [11]. For type III, SSD offers several advantages if osteosynthesis is contemplated. Surgical approach for Pipkin type IV will depend on the acetabular fracture pattern. Though SSD is preferred for type IV injuries with associated posterior wall or column, the presence of other acetabular fracture patterns may dictate a different approach.

5.4 Surgical Approach

SSD is performed with the patient positioned lateral with the affected hip on top [12]. The surgical exposure is performed using a straight mid-lateral measuring 15–20 cm centered over the greater trochanter. The superficial exposure is performed either by splitting the gluteus maximus muscle between its anterior 1/3 and posterior 2/3 or by exploring the Gibson interval between the gluteus maximus and gluteus medius (Fig. 5.2). If the gluteus maximus muscle is split, care should be taken to limit the split proximally at the first crossing of the superior gluteal neuromuscular bundle located approximately 7–8 cm proximal to the tip of the greater trochanter. The distal limit of the exposure is indicated by the location of the gluteus maximus tendinous insertion to the proximal femoral shaft. The Gibson interval offers the advantage of more proximal exposure and avoids any inadvertent problems with injury to the neurovascular supply to the anterior portion of the gluteus maximus.

The deeper exposure can be divided into four parts: (i) retroacetabular exposure, (ii) trochanteric osteotomy, (iii) anterior exposure, and (iv) anterior capsulotomy.

5.4.1 Retroacetabular Exposure

The trochanteric bursa is teased gently, and the underlying muscular structures are visualized from the posterior border of the gluteus medius muscle proximally till the gluteus maximus tendon distally. The next step is to identify the sciatic nerve which is best done over the surface of the quadratus femoris muscle after teasing off the bursal layer. The nerve exits the greater sciatic notch and courses anteriorly to the piriformis muscle and posterior to the short external rotators and the quadratus femoris though variations are common. Positioning the hip in extension and knee in flexion facilitates retroacetabular exposure by relaxing the posterior musculature

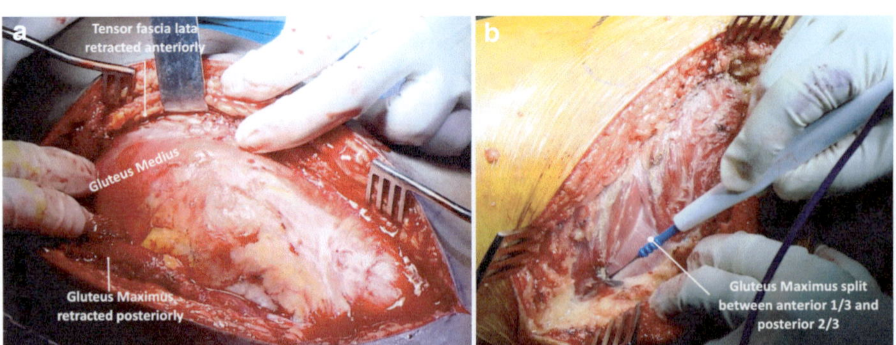

Fig. 5.2 (**a**) The Gibson interval between the gluteus maximus and the hip abductors. (**b**) The gluteus maximus split for the KL approach

and also eases tension on the sciatic nerve (Fig. 5.3). The nerve is not formally dissected further when dealing with isolated femoral head fractures (Pipkin I and II)..

5.4.2 Trochanteric Osteotomy

The osteotomy aims to flip the osteotomized fragment anteriorly retaining the muscle attachments of the hip abductors and vastus lateralis to facilitate an anterior hip dislocation without interrupting the femoral head blood supply. Preparation for the osteotomy begins with the identification and retraction of the posterior border of the gluteus medius anteriorly. This reveals the underlying piriformis tendon and the gluteus minimus insertion. The plane between the piriformis and gluteus minimus is developed, and the minimus is gently elevated from the posterosuperior hip capsule. This step is important to avoid the tethering of the gluteus minimus to the capsule hindering mobilization of the osteotomized fragment anteriorly. The osteotomy line is marked just anterior to the posterior most fibers of the gluteus medius aiming to exit just distal to the vastus lateralis origin (Fig. 5.4). The osteotomy can be performed in a straight line or as a step osteotomy [13]. A thin oscillating saw is used to perform the osteotomy. Pre-drilled K-wires to act as a saw guide and intraoperative fluoroscopy can be helpful for orientation. The hip is placed in around 20

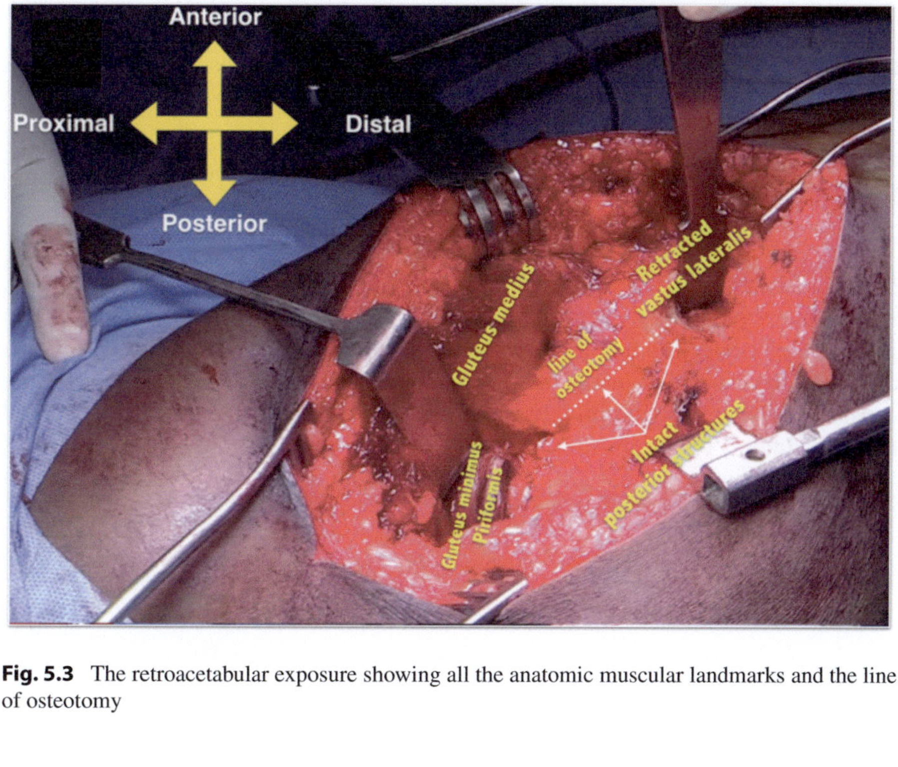

Fig. 5.3 The retroacetabular exposure showing all the anatomic muscular landmarks and the line of osteotomy

Trochanteric Osteotomy

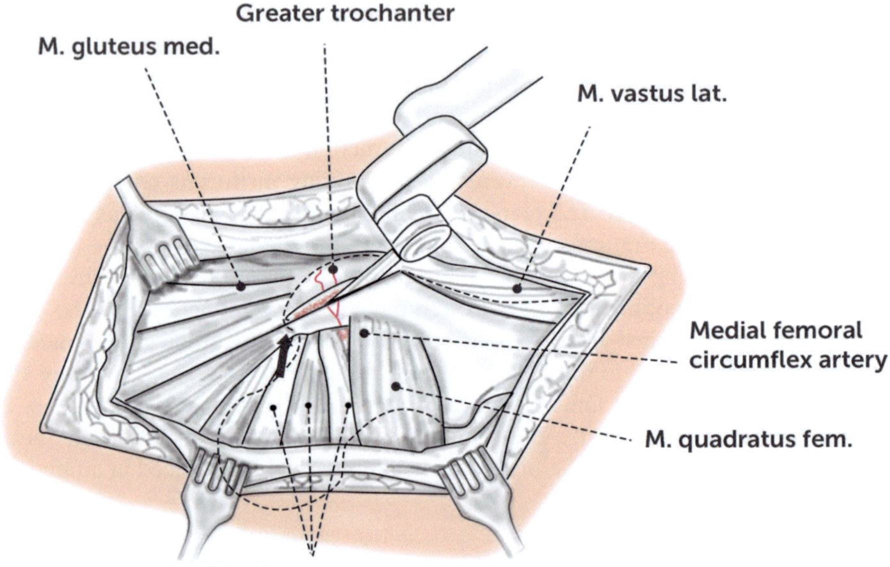

Fig. 5.4 The trochanteric osteotomy is performed just anterior to the posterior most fibers of the gluteus medius muscle (black arrow) aiming to exit distal to insertion of vastus lateralis

degrees of internal rotation to help orient the saw blade parallel to the floor. The osteotomy should ideally measure 1–1.5 cm in thickness..

5.4.3 Pitfalls

If the osteotomy is too thin, there is risk of breakage and also leaving behind most of the abductor insertion on the intact femur. This will need to be erased to reach the capsule, and repairing the muscles back could be difficult. The osteotomy should also exit lateral to the piriformis tendon, so that the piriformis tendon remains attached to the intact femur. This will ensure that the osteotomy is not too deep and does not interfere with the blood supply.

5.4.4 Anterior Exposure

The osteotomized fragment is gradually mobilized anteriorly which can be facilitated by a series of maneuvers. The remaining insertion of the vastus lateralis and some fibers of the vastus intermedius anteriorly in the distal aspect of the osteotomy and some residual fibers of the gluteus minimus proximally are erased, and the limb is gradually brought into a position of flexion, abduction, and external rotation. This position relaxes the hip abductors and places less tension on the vascular pedicle to the muscle posteriorly as the osteotomized fragment is gradually mobilized more anteriorly toward the anterior margin of the acetabulum. The anterior capsule is now visualized.

The reflected head of the rectus muscle is gradually teased off the anterior capsule, and spiked retractors can be positioned on the anterior column of the acetabulum and also superior and inferior to the femoral neck outside the hip capsule. This exposes the entire anterior capsule, and gentle hip rotation can help identify the exact location for the anterior capsulotomy.

5.4.5 Anterior Capsulotomy

The anterior capsule is split in a Z fashion as described by Ganz. The capsulotomy starts with an incision along the femoral neck axis from the intertrochanteric line distally till the acetabular rim proximally taking care not to injure the hip labrum. The distal limb of the Z begins from the distal limit of the first capsular incision coursing anteroinferiorly. It is important to remain anterior to the lesser trochanter in order to avoid any inadvertent injury to the MFCA. The proximal limb of the Z is performed last along the acetabular rim beginning at the proximal limit of the first capsular incision coursing posteriorly parallel to the hip labrum. This creates two capsular flaps, one superior and one inferior, which can be tagged, and the spiked retractors can now be positioned inside the hip capsule to expose the femoral head (Fig. 5.5). The head can now be dislocated gently by progressive external rotation with the hip flexed, facilitated by a bone hook if required..

5.5 Reduction and Fixation Techniques Through SSD

5.5.1 Pipkin I and II Injuries

Fractured head fragments, especially type I (infra-foveolar) fragments, are often attached to the ligamentum teres and are retained in the acetabular cavity after dislocation. The fragment may have to be detached from the ligamentum teres to facilitate reduction. Once the head is dislocated, spiked retractors are mounted on the anterior column and inferior to the transverse acetabular ligament along with a bone hook or another spiked retractor on the posteroinferior aspect of the acetabulum to retract the femoral head to inspect the acetabular cavity for the presence of major

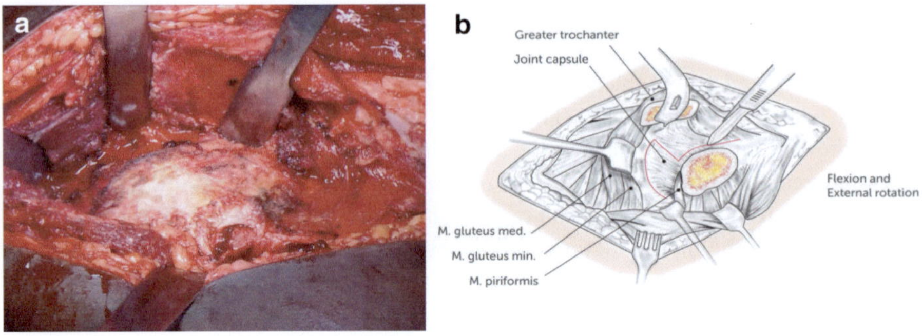

Fig. 5.5 (**a**) The exposed anterior capsule with the osteotomy fragment flipped anteriorly. (**b**) The schematic of the planned Z capsulotomy

posterior labral tears. If labral tear is present, it can be repaired before fracture fixation by using 3.5 mm suture anchors placed into the rim of the posterior wall. The number of anchors will depend on the size of the labral tear. Though SSD provides exposure for repair of the labral tear, there is no convincing evidence to support routine repair of the labrum in these injuries.

The fracture bed is cleaned of clots and debris and the fractured head fragment is reduced. The presence of comminution and impaction can complicate reduction. Small comminuted osteochondral fragments not amenable for fixation can be discarded. Excision of non-reconstructible fragments in the infra-foveolar region (type I) does not affect hip stability or increase peak stresses at the weight-bearing dome and is considered a safe procedure [14].

Larger fragments are reduced, are clamped using pointed clamps, and can be held in position by using 1.5 mm K-wires. For fixation, cannulated headless compression screws or mini-fragment countersunk screws (2 or 2.4 mm) can be used. During the process of drilling, the presence of active backbleeding from the head has been interpreted as a sign of viability of the femoral head [15]. Depending on the size of the fragment, two to four screws contained within the femoral head in all planes may be required for secure fixation (Fig. 5.6). Once fracture fixation is complete, the head can be reduced into the acetabulum, and fluoroscopic evaluation can be performed to validate reduction and fixation. The capsulotomy is then closed with interrupted absorbable sutures.

5.5.2 Chondral Defects due to Non-reconstructible Fragments

It could be often evident that after reduction and fixation of large head fragments, there are still reasonable sized gaps or defects due to sacrifice of delaminated non-reconstructible cartilage fragments. If they are in the non-weight-bearing region, they could be left as such without major long-term problems. If the defects are in supra-foveal weight-bearing region, several options are available for reconstruction. Options range from microfracture, reimplantation of delaminated chondral

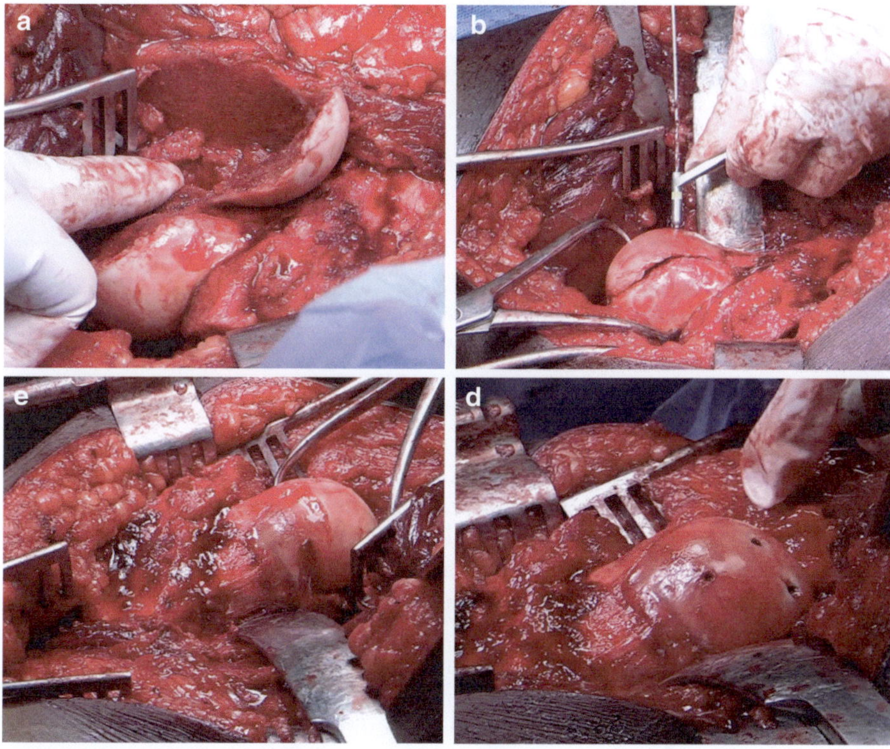

Fig. 5.6 The sequence of fracture stabilization with the SSD. (**a**) Identification and cleaning of the fracture bed. (**b**) Fracture reduction with a pointed clamp. (**c**) Active backbleeding from the femoral head is often interpreted as a sign of intact vascularity. (**d**) Fixation is performed with countersunk mini-fragment or headless screws

fragments along with microfracture, mosaicplasty, osteochondral autograft or allograft implantation procedures, and use of synthetic osteochondral scaffolds [16].

5.5.3 Osteotomy Repair

The osteotomy can be gently reduced using a small pointed clamp and secured in position by using a large pointed reduction clamp. Provisional fixation is performed using multiple 1.5 mm K-wires. Once reduction is confirmed satisfactory under fluoroscopy, fixation can be performed with multiple 2.7 or 3.5 mm fully threaded cortex screws (Fig. 5.7).

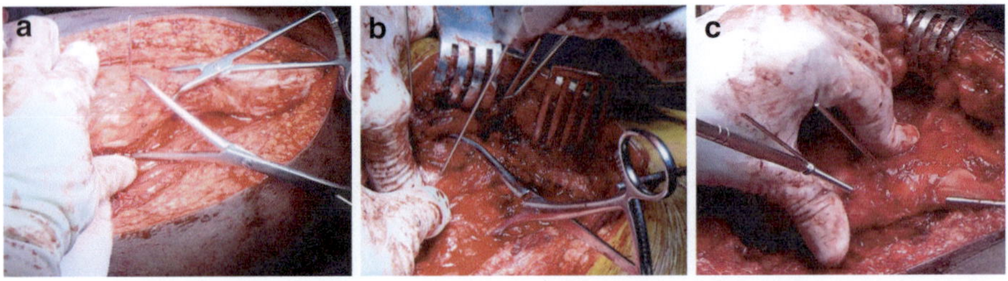

Fig. 5.7 (**a**) The osteotomy is reduced in multiple planes with the help of small and large pointed clamps. (**b**) K-wires can help temporarily hold the reduction before definitive fixation. (**c**) Fixation is performed with 2.7 or 3.5 mm fully threaded cortical screws

5.5.4 Pipkin III Injuries

SSD is one of the preferred approaches for Pipkin III injuries if osteosynthesis is chosen. It allows the head to be visualized circumferentially and also reduce the associated neck fracture under vision. In such injuries, the head fragments may have to be reconstructed outside the surgical field and re-implanted. Once reduced, further stabilization can be performed by using implants inserted from the lateral aspect of the proximal femur. Once stabilized, the hip has to be carefully reduced under vision in a very gentle manner to avoid loss of fixation at the femoral neck. Addition of an inferomedial plate along the calcar can also help improve stability of fixation, which can be performed easily in this setting since the head and entire neck is easily accessible with SSD.

5.5.5 Pipkin IV Injuries

In Pipkin IV injuries involving the posterior wall (commonest) or the posterior column, retro-acetabular exposure similar to the KL approach can be performed after fixation of the femoral head fragment as described previously. The capsulotomy and osteotomy can be left unrepaired till acetabular fixation so that in case if needed, the articular reduction after posterior wall/column fixation can be evaluated by re-dislocating the head anteriorly. In such cases, it is important to release the gluteus maximus tendon to ease tension on the sciatic nerve, and the nerve should be traced up to the greater sciatic notch and protected with the sleeve of triceps coxae muscles.

5.6 Published Results and Outcomes

Several authors have reported outcomes after internal fixation of femoral head fractures using SSD. Giannoudis et al. [17] in their recent systematic review reported SSD as the most preferred and practiced surgical approach for osteosynthesis of Pipkin types II and IV injuries. In the review with inclusion of 50 studies involving more than 1400 patients, SSD was the most common surgical approach used in type II injuries (59%) and also in type IV injuries (61%). Some of these data also include KL approach without an osteotomy. Though the authors did not indicate the exact numbers, they reported that majority of KL approaches included a flip osteotomy. SSD is also the second most popular among surgeons for treating Pipkin type I injuries after anterior-based Smith-Petersen or Hueter approaches [17]. Singh et al. reported in their cadaveric study that SSD provides the best possible visualization of the femoral head for fracture fixation [18]. The exposure was considered significantly better compared to Hueter and Smith-Petersen approaches.

Since these fractures are rare, most reports are retrospective case series with small number of patients and no control groups. The outcome measurement tools used in these reports are also widely variable. Henle et al. [19] reported good to excellent outcomes with SSD for femoral head fractures in 83% (10 of 12) patients using the Merle d'Aubigne scores. Gardner and colleagues described two cases elaborating the surgical technique where they had reported that fractures involving larger areas of the female head may be difficult to accurately visualize and reduce with other anterior surgical approaches [20]. Kloen et al. [21] in their comparative analysis reported significantly better outcome measures in higher number of patients with SSD compared to other anterior and posterior surgical approaches.

We reported our results with SSD for Pipkin I and II injuries in 28 patients [11]. Two patients underwent fragment excision and the remaining underwent internal fixation. The fracture and osteotomies healed in all patients. The mean modified Merle d'Aubigne scores were 16.5, and the mean Oxford hip scores were 42.6 at a mean follow-up of 3 years without any incidence of avascular necrosis. We reported a labral tear incidence of 54% and the tears were repaired. Our assessment found that the presence of a labral tear negatively influenced functional outcome, but repair did not increase complications.

The published evidence on Pipkin III injuries is scarce. Regardless of the surgical approach, the outcomes after osteosynthesis of Pipkin III injuries are universally poor [17]. SSD has been widely used for Pipkin IV injuries. While SSD offers the possibility of combining both femoral head and acetabular fixations through a single approach, the trochanteric flip also provides a more extensile visualization of the cranial and anterior portions of the retro-acetabular exposure compared to the KL approach [22] (Fig. 5.8). This makes it the approach of choice for addressing cranial posterior wall fractures with or without associated femoral head injuries. Solberg et al. [23] reported their results in a small group of Pipkin IV injuries treated with SSD. The authors reported good to excellent outcomes using the Epstein scores in 10 of 12 patients and a mean Merle d'Aubigne score of 15.6 at a mean follow-up of 24 months.

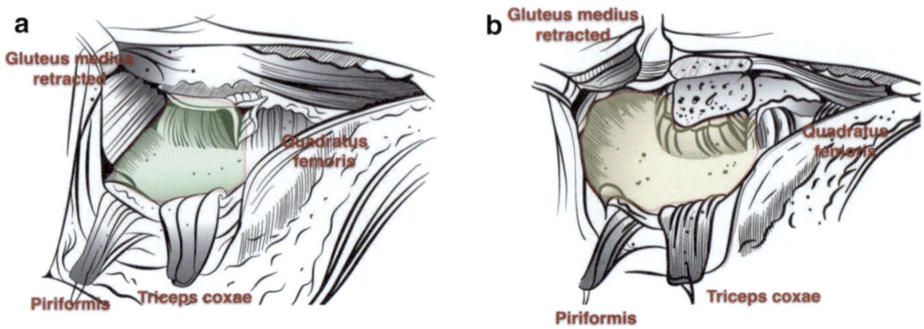

Fig. 5.8 (**a**) The amount of exposure (shaded in green) through a conventional KL approach. (**b**) The increase in exposure (shaded yellow) of the retroacetabular surface cranially and anteriorly when a trochanteric flip is performed

5.7 Author's Preference

We have used SSD extensively in our unit over the last 15 years. It is still our preferred surgical approach for Pipkin II injuries. We used to treat all Pipkin I and II injuries with SSD before but had gradually moved to the Hueter approach for reasons such as supine positioning, shorter surgical time, and blood loss. We reported on this few years ago and found no difference in outcome between the two surgical approaches for Pipkin I and II injuries [24]. We have again shifted back to SSD for type II injuries because SSD provides the best possible visualization of the head quadrants. In type II suprafoveal injuries, excellent exposure is important because we may need additional osteochondral filling procedures to address chondral defects apart from fixation of the main large fragments. These defects can be ignored in type I injuries. SSD also allows us to do a good labral repair which may improve outcome in type II injuries even though there is no convincing evidence to suggest that labral repair improves outcome in femoral head fractures. It is notable that type II injuries have larger posterosuperior labral tears compared to type I injuries where the tears are located posteroinferior majority of the times (Fig. 5.9)..

We prefer SSD for osteosynthesis of Pipkin III injuries. While these injuries could be really difficult technically to reduce and fix needing a really good exposure, it is also important not to jeopardize the blood supply further. We prefer to do a CT in these injuries prior to hip reduction. The CT can help to identify undisplaced neck fractures which can be stabilized during open reduction before hip reduction. This can make the procedure a lot easier and also help preserve blood supply. Displaced neck fractures can also be studied better before planning your surgical tactic through SSD.

SSD is our preferred approach for treating Pipkin IV injuries where the acetabular fracture needs primarily a posterior KL approach (Fig. 5.10). The exception would be small peripheral caudal posterior wall fractures which do not affect hip stability. In these injures, our preference is to fix the femoral head fracture from the Hueter approach and then do a stress examination for hip stability [25]. If the hip is

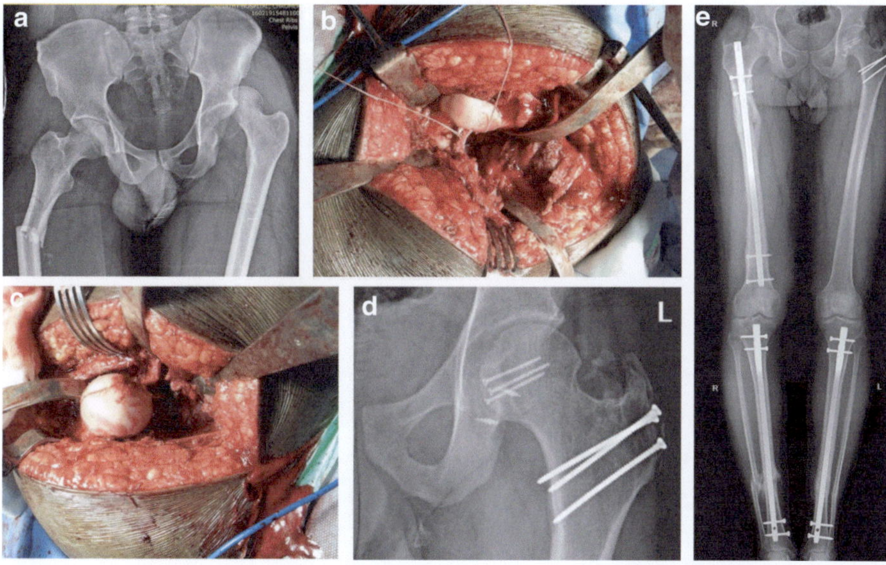

Fig. 5.9 Example of a multiply injured male with a type I Pipkin fracture. (a) His femoral head fracture was treated with SSD. (b) His labral tear was repaired. (c) His fracture was stabilized with countersunk screws. (d) At 2 years, the hip remains congruent, and head is vascular. (e) The overall limb alignment has been restored

unstable, the wall can be fixed through a KL approach though this is rarely needed. In some of these injuries involving large posterior wall fragments and capsular tears, it may be possible to fix some of the femoral head fractures through the KL exposure. If this is not possible, SSD is performed. In such cases, it is our preference to address the femoral head first before reduction and fixation of the posterior wall, column fractures, or other fractures. We also prefer to do a CT scan before hip reduction in Pipkin IV injuries to appreciate the amount of femoral head impaction, and some of these fractures may be really locked and perched on the posterior wall, and some injuries may have an associated undisplaced femoral neck fracture. Both these scenarios can complicate hip reduction if not appreciated prior.

5.8 Rehabilitation

Patients are mobilized out of bed early with support. Weight-bearing primarily depends on the injury pattern. Patients with Pipkin I injuries are allowed weight-bearing as tolerated regardless of excision or fixation of the fractured fragment. Patients with Pipkin II, III, and IV injuries are mobilized using a restricted weight-bearing protocol progressing from toe-touch weight-bearing to weight-bearing as tolerated over the period of 8–12 weeks with progression in fracture healing. Patients receive pharmacological thromboprophylaxis for a period of up to 3 weeks. We do not use any prophylaxis for heterotopic ossification.

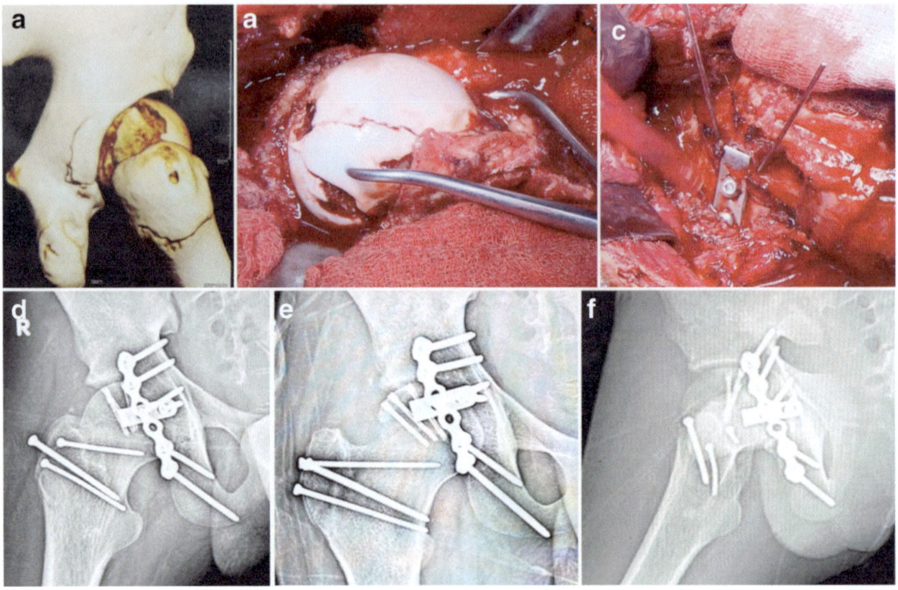

Fig. 5.10 Example of a Pipkin IV injury treated with SSD. (**a**) The suprafoveal head fracture and a posterior wall fracture. (**b**) Femoral head reduction. (**c**) Posterior wall fixation with spring plate and supplemental buttress plate. (**d–f**) Healed fractures in AP, obturator, and iliac oblique views, respectively

5.9 Complications

Prof. Ganz in his paper reported an overall complication rate of in 42% in a cohort of 213 patients [2]. The most common complication reported in his paper was heterotopic ossification (HO) accounting for 37% of patients (79 hips), but only 2 patients had Brooker grade III HO and had to undergo surgical treatment to improve hip mobility. Other complications reported include transient sciatic neuropraxia in two patients and sagging of the subcutaneous fat in seven patients with a KL type exposure. Sink et al. [26] in their multicenter study on complications after SSD reported an overall complication rate of 9% and 4.8% after excluding grade I and II HO. The failure of osteotomy fixation was reported to be around 1.5% in both papers with successful healing after revision fixation. Chronic lateral thigh pain not affecting function has been reported in up to 45% of patients. Both these studies did not report any incidence of AVN which is significant in that there was no iatrogenic occurrence of AVN due to the surgical approach in both these studies. The study by Sink et al. reiterates the safety of the approach at the hands of multiple surgeons.

While occurrence of AVN may be entirely due to insult occurring during the surgical approach in most non-traumatic conditions, femoral head fracture dislocations have an inherent risk of developing AVN due to injury itself. We reported an HO incidence of 18% and posttraumatic arthritis in 11% after using SSD for Pipkin I and II injuries [11]. No AVN was noted at 3 years follow-up. Scolaro et al. [25]

reported an AVN rate and degenerative arthritis incidence of 8.7% and conversion to hip arthroplasty in 10% patients in one of the largest series on femoral head fractures operated through multiple surgical approaches. Guo et al. [27] in their systematic review in 2010 reported that SSD is associated with less incidence of HO than other anterior approaches but more than the KL approach. The rates of AVN with SSD was comparable with other anterior approaches but lesser compared to the posterior approach. Kim et al. [28] in their more recent systematic review reported similar findings with regard to incidence of HO, but the incidence of AVN was similar between SSD and KL approaches.

5.10 Summary

SSD remains an important tool in the osteosynthesis of different types of femoral head fractures and fracture dislocations. SSD provides the best possible exposure of the femoral head fracture components without compromise in arterial supply to the femoral head. Associated injuries to the hip labrum and acetabulum can also be addressed through the same approach when needed. The published results with SSD have been consistently good with minimal complications. Most procedure-related complications are related to HO of mild-to-moderate grades not needing intervention. The procedure involves a learning curve and should be performed with sufficient training.

5.11 Key Points

- SSD through a trochanteric flip osteotomy is a safe and extensile approach to treat femoral head fracture dislocations.
- In the author's experience, SSD offers the best exposure with great safety window for osteosynthesis of Pipkin II, III, and most of the IV injuries.
- Clinical and cadaveric studies have repeatedly validated the non-interference of the approach with the dominant femoral head arterial supply.
- HO remains the most common complication after SSD in femoral head fracture fixation. Though rare, problems with osteotomy healing remains the only unique major procedure-related complication with the trochanteric flip osteotomy.
- AVN and degenerative arthritis are inherent to the injury, and their occurrence mainly depends on the injury and sometimes to surgeon (reduction quality) and patient factors (age, smoking, etc.).

References

1. Crock HV, Calne RY, Hughes S. An atlas of vascular anatomy of the skeleton and spinal cord. (No Title). 1996.

2. Ganz R, Gill TJ, Gautier E, Ganz K, Krügel N, Berlemann U. Surgical dislocation of the adult hip a technique with full access to the femoral head and acetabulum without the risk of avascular necrosis. J Bone Joint Surg Br. 2001;83(8):1119–24.
3. Ganz R, Huff TW, Leunig M. Extended retinacular soft tissue flap for intra-articular hip surgery: surgical technique, indications, and results of application. Instr Course Lect. 2009;58:241–55.
4. Lavingne M, Kalhor M, Beck M, Ganz R, Leaning M. Distribution of vascular foramina around the femoral head and neck junction: relevance for conservative intracapsular procedures of the hip. Orthop Clin North Am. 2005;36(2):171–6. viii
5. Lazzaro LE, Sculco PK, Pardee NC, Klinger CE, Dyke JP, Helfet DL, Su EP, Lorich DG. Assessment of femoral head and head-neck junction perfusion following surgical hip dislocation using gadolinium-enhanced magnetic resonance imaging: a cadaveric study. Randomised control trial. J Bone Joint Surg Am. 2013;95(23):e1821–8.
6. Notzli HP, Siebenrock KA, Hempfing A, Ramseier LE, Ganz R. Perfusion of the femoral head during surgical dislocation of the hip. Monitoring by laser Doppler flowmetry. J Bone Joint Surg Am. 2016;98(6):475–83. https://doi.org/10.2106/JBJS.15.00367.
7. Smith C, DiBartola AC, Fisher M, Klingele KE. Surgical hip dislocation in pediatric and adolescent patients. J Am Acad Orthop Surg. 2023;31(6):e287–97.
8. Gautier E, Ganz K, Krügel N, Gill T, Ganz R. Anatomy of the medial femoral circumflex artery and its surgical implications. J Bone Joint Surg Br. 2000;82(5):679–83.
9. Steffen RT, De Smet KA, Murray DW, Gill HS. A modified posterior approach preserves femoral head oxygenation during hip resurfacing. J Arthroplast. 2011;26(3):404–8.
10. Ross JR, Schoenecker PL, Clohisy JC. Surgical dislocation of the hip: evolving indications. HSS J. 2013;9(1):60–9.
11. Gavaskar AS, Tummala NC. Ganz surgical dislocation of the hip is a safe technique for operative treatment of Pipkin fractures. Results of a prospective trial. J Orthop Trauma. 2015;29(12):544–8.
12. Gavaskar A, et al. Trochanteric flip (Ganz) anterior hip dislocation for fixation of Pipkin fracture dislocations. JBJS Essent Surg Tech. 2020;10(3):e19.00040. https://doi.org/10.2106/JBJS.ST.19.00040.
13. Bastian JD, Wolf AT, Wyss TF, Nötzli HP. Stepped osteotomy of the trochanter for stable, anatomic refixation. Clin Orthop Relat Res. 2009;467(3):732–8. https://doi.org/10.1007/s11999-008-0649-x.
14. Chen Z-W, Lin B, Zhai W-L, Guo Z-M, Liang Z, Zheng J-P, Lian K-J, Ding Z-Q. Conservative versus surgical management of Pipkin type I fractures associated with posterior dislocation of the hip: a randomised controlled trial. Int Orthop. 2010;35(7):1077–81.
15. Sen RK, Tripathy SK, Goyal T, Aggarwal S, Kashyap S, Purudappa PP, Chandrappa MH. Complications and functional outcome of femoral head fracture-dislocation in delayed and neglected cases. Indian J Orthop. 2021;55(3):595–605.
16. Du D, Hsu P, Zhu Z, Zhang C. Current surgical options and innovation for repairing articular cartilage defects in the femoral head. J Orthop Translat. 2019;21:122–8.
17. Kloub M, Látal P, Giannoudis P. Techniques and results of reconstruction of femoral head fractures: an update. Injury. 2024;55(6):111473.
18. Singh K, Weitlich JD, Zitsch BP, Schweser KM, Cook JL, Crist BD. Which surgical approach provides maximum visualization and access for open reduction and internal fixation of femoral head fractures? J Orthop Trauma. 2022;36(Suppl 2):S12–6. https://doi.org/10.1097/BOT.0000000000002308.
19. Henle P, Kloen P, Siebenrock KA. Femoral head injuries: which treatment strategy can be recommended? Injury. 2007;38:478–88.
20. Gardner MJ, Suk M, Pearle A, Buly RL, Helfet DL, Lorich DG. Surgical dislocation of the hip for fractures of the femoral head. J Orthop Trauma. 2005;19:334–42.
21. Kloen P, Siebenrock KA, Raaymaers E, et al. Femoral head fractures revisited. Eur J Trauma. 2002;28:221–33. https://doi.org/10.1007/s00068-002-1173-4.

22. Phelps KD, Crickard CV, Li K, Harmer LS, McArthur EA, Robinson KS, Sims SH, Tsu JR. Why make the cut? Trochanteric slide osteotomy can improve exposure to the anterosuperior acetabulum. J Orthop Trauma. 2021;35:106–9.
23. Solberg BD, Moon CN, Franco DP. Use of a trochanteric flip osteotomy improves outcomes in Pipkin IV fractures. Clin Orthop Relat Res. 2009;467(4):929–33.
24. Gavaskar A, et al. Surgical dislocation or the modified Heuter anterior approach for Pipkin I and II femoral head fracture dislocations. J Orthop Trauma. 2020;34(12):626–31.
25. Scolaro JA, Marecek G, Firoozabadi R, Krieg JC, Routt MLC. Management and radiographic outcomes of femoral head fractures. J Orthop Traumatol. 2017;18(3):235–41.
26. Sink EL, Beaulé PE, Sucato D, Kim YJ, Millis MB, Dayton M, Trousdale RT, Sierra RJ, Zaltz I, Schoenecker P, Monreal A, Clohisy J. Multicenter study of complications following surgical dislocation of the hip. J Bone Joint Surg Am. 2011;93(12):1132–6.
27. Guo JJ, Tang N, Yang HL, Qin L, Leung KS. Impact of surgical approach on postoperative heterotopic ossification and avascular necrosis in femoral head fractures: a systematic review. Int Orthop. 2010;34(3):319–22.
28. Kim CH, Ma DS, Cho HC, Yoon YC. Comparison of postoperative complications between trochanter flip osteotomy and Kocher-Langenbeck approaches for the treatment of femoral head fractures: a systematic review and meta-analysis. Indian J Orthop. 2023;57(4):577–85.

Infra-foveal Femoral Head Fracture: Management Options and Outcome

6

Mehool Acharya

6.1 Etiology

The earliest recorded case of an articular femoral head fracture dates back to 1869 when John Birkett documented the injury during the autopsy of a 35-year-old woman who had sustained a fatal fall from a window. This case marked the initial understanding of these rare fractures [1].

Infra-foveal femoral head fractures, commonly referred to as Pipkin type I fractures, typically result from high-energy trauma, most frequently associated with motor vehicle accidents. These injuries occur when the hip is in a flexed and adducted position, a biomechanical state that increases joint laxity. The mechanism involves a posteriorly directed force transmitted through the femur, often in conjunction with a posterior hip dislocation.

6.2 Epidemiology

Pipkin type I fractures are a common subset of femoral head fractures. These injuries almost exclusively occur in the context of high-energy trauma, particularly associated with posterior hip dislocations, which frequently result from motor vehicle collisions [2]. Posterior dislocations account for approximately 90% of all traumatic hip dislocations, and associated femoral head fractures occur in an estimated 5–15% of such cases [3, 4].

Among the Pipkin classification types, type I fractures constitute about 15–27% of femoral head fractures, making them the second most common type only after Pipkin type II fractures [5, 6].

M. Acharya (✉)
Trauma and Orthopaedics, North Bristol NHS Trust, Bristol, UK

R. K. Sen, S. K. Tripathy (eds.), *A Practical Guide to Management of Femoral Head Fracture-Dislocation*, https://doi.org/10.1007/978-981-96-9852-3_6

Impression- or impaction-type fractures caused by anterior or central hip dislocations, or isolated fractures without dislocations, are less frequent, with CT scans revealing that impaction fractures are observed in about 63% of patients following posterior hip dislocations, compared to 12% of patients after anterior hip dislocations [7, 8].

Risk factors for these fractures are closely related to the mechanism of injury. Young males are disproportionately affected, and this may be related to their increased participation in high-velocity activities, such as extreme sports or vehicular trauma [9]. However, these fractures can also occur in older patients, often resulting from low-energy trauma due to age-related bone fragility, which can be missed without a high index of suspicion when examining radiographs [10, 11].

6.3 Diagnosis

Patients with femoral head fractures, often resulting from posterior hip dislocations, commonly present with a shortened limb positioned in flexion, adduction, and internal rotation. This classic presentation is highly indicative of a posterior dislocation (Fig. 6.1). However, the presence of associated fractures, such as those of the femoral neck or head, may obscure or alter this characteristic limb positioning [12].

Clinicians should approach these cases with a systematic evaluation. Following observation of the limb position, a rapid and thorough neurovascular examination is essential. This includes assessing pulses, capillary refill, and skin temperature. The neurological status of the limb should be evaluated meticulously, as sciatic nerve injury is a frequent complication of posterior hip dislocations. Signs and symptoms of motor or sensory deficits should be noted, as they can guide subsequent management [13].

Radiographic imaging is a cornerstone of diagnosis. An anterior-posterior (AP) pelvic radiograph is typically the initial investigation of choice and often provides

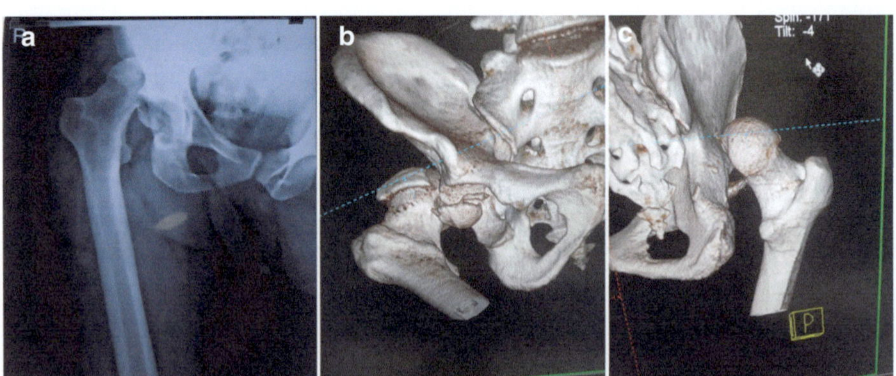

Fig. 6.1 Radiograph (**a**) and 3D CT (**b**, **c**) showing a posterior hip dislocation associated with infra-foveal femoral head fracture. (Picture curtsey: Dr. Sujit Kumar Tripathy)

evidence of fracture-dislocation. In cases of posterior hip dislocation, radiographs may show a superiorly displaced femoral head, a void in the acetabular socket, and disruption of Shenton's line. The affected femoral head may appear smaller than the contralateral side due to its posterior displacement, which reduces the magnification effect [14].

If the diagnosis is unclear, additional imaging is warranted. Computed tomography (CT) scans are especially valuable in polytrauma settings, offering detailed visualization of fracture patterns, fragment displacement, occult fractures, and associated injuries (Fig. 6.1). For isolated hip injuries, further radiographic views, including Judet oblique views and pelvic inlet and outlet views, can help clarify findings and ensure accurate assessment of the femoral head, acetabulum, and joint congruency once the dislocated hip has been reduced.

6.4 Special Investigations

Post-reduction computed tomography (CT) imaging is critical for comprehensive assessment following a femoral head fracture. CT scans provide detailed information on the location and morphology of fracture fragments, the degree of comminution, the presence of intra-articular loose bodies, and any associated acetabular or femoral neck fractures.

Routine CT evaluation is recommended after both closed and open reduction procedures. The data obtained from CT imaging guides further management decisions and helps ensure optimal treatment outcomes. CT scans should be conducted with a maximal slice thickness of 2 mm [15]. The size and location of the fracture fragment can be deducted from the CT scans by assessing it in the axial, sagittal, and coronal planes. Similarly, displacement of the fracture can be obtained from these views. Three-dimensional reconstructions can provide an idea about the size of the fragment in relation to the femoral head as well as the amount of displacement [16] (Fig. 6.2).

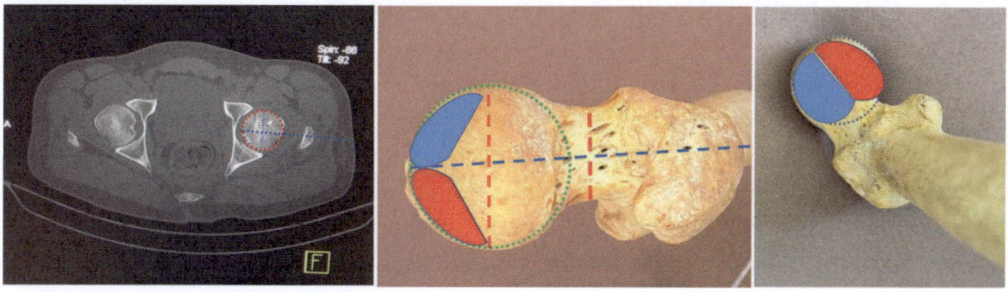

Fig. 6.2 An axial CT slice capturing the largest fracture fragment, along with accompanying dry bone photographs, illustrates the method for assessing fracture size and type. The classification of the fragment is determined by its position relative to the bisection line of the femoral head and neck. Specifically, if the main portion of the fragment is located in the blue area, it is classified as anterior-inferior (AI); if it falls in the red area, it is considered posterior-inferior. In this example, a large anterior-inferior (AI) fragment is clearly visible. (Figure curtsey: Dr. Sujit Kumar Tripathy)

Magnetic resonance imaging (MRI) is not usually indicated in the acute settings. However, it may be useful for detecting soft-tissue injuries, such as avulsions of the acetabular labrum, unexplained joint widening, or early signs of femoral head necrosis. These insights can be crucial for addressing complications and optimizing long-term prognosis.

6.5 Treatment

Management of Pipkin type I fractures involves a spectrum of approaches ranging from conservative treatment to different surgical techniques. A paradigm shift in recent years has favored surgical interventions due to improved outcomes and advancements in technology [17].

6.6 Immediate Reduction

Hip dislocations with associated femoral head fractures are surgical emergencies. Immediate reduction is crucial to restore blood flow to the femoral head and minimize the risk of avascular necrosis (AVN). Closed reduction under sedation or anesthesia should be attempted promptly. Whether the closed reduction is performed in the emergency room or in the operating theater will depend on local policies, guidelines, and resources. Following successful reduction, radiographs and CT scans are mandatory to evaluate residual displacement, joint congruency, and fracture morphology.

If closed reduction is contraindicated (e.g., in cases of concomitant femoral neck fracture) or fails due to soft-tissue interposition or large fracture fragments, open reduction is indicated. Delay in reduction must be avoided as it significantly increases the risk of femoral head necrosis.

6.6.1 Examination Under Anesthesia (EUA)

If hip instability is suspected, then EUA should be performed following closed reduction. Traditionally, the patient is placed in a supine position on a radiolucent table. The hip is brought into gradual flexion upto 70 to 90 degree then slight adduction with internal rotation. A force can be applied in the direction of dislocation, and fluoroscopic images can be obtained to detect any subluxation or incongruence; this would be more evident in the obturator oblique view [18].

6.7 Conservative Treatment

Historically, conservative treatment was the preferred approach for Pipkin type I fractures. Patients were often managed with prolonged bed rest with or without axial traction after closed reduction.

Currently, conservative management can be considered in cases where a closed reduction achieves a congruent joint with minimal residual displacement and no intra-articular fragments or in patients with lower demand and those that are deemed not fit for an anesthesia. Post-reduction protocols include touch weight-bearing or partial weight-bearing with crutches for up to 6 weeks, avoiding adduction and internal rotation beyond neutral for up to 2 months. Regular radiographic follow-up is essential to monitor the maintenance of reduction and hip congruency. Follow-up and progression to full weight-bearing and full unrestricted activities will be dependent on patient factors, fracture configuration, and local protocols. However, the aim should be to try and get the patient fully weight-bearing by 3–4 months and progress to unrestricted activities under the supervision of the physiotherapist.

6.8 Surgical Treatment

6.8.1 Irreducible Dislocations

When a hip dislocation cannot be reduced by closed reduction—due to factors such as a concomitant femoral neck fracture, rotation of a fracture fragment around the still attached ligamentum teres, femoral head button holed through soft tissues, or an interposed osteochondral fragment—urgent open reduction in the operating room becomes necessary [19].

While a preoperative CT scan is recommended to better define the pathology and guide surgical planning, it is crucial to avoid significant delays, as prolonged dislocation dramatically increases the risk of femoral head osteonecrosis. If an open reduction is required, it is ideal to do this through an approach which will allow reduction and definitive treatment of the fracture at the same time.

6.8.2 Open Reduction and Internal Fixation (ORIF)

ORIF can be considered the gold standard for managing Pipkin type I fractures with incongruent reduction or instability [17, 20]. The surgical approach is tailored to the injury pattern.

Despite the lack of clear guidelines on what fragment size is amenable to fixation, the authors believe that fragments larger than 2 cm can be fixed using internal fixation techniques such as headless compression screws or Herbert screws to achieve stable reduction without damaging the articular cartilage. Bioabsorbable pins are an alternative, allowing fixation without interfering with MRI imaging or causing metal artifacts. Smaller fragments located outside the weight-bearing zone may be excised if fixation is not feasible. Free articular fragments must be removed from the joint to avoid cartilage grinding and third body wear.

6.8.2.1 Approaches

Surgical approaches for Pipkin type I fractures are broadly categorized into anterior and posterior approaches, each offering specific advantages depending on the fracture pattern and dislocation direction. The choice of approach is guided by the location of the fracture fragments, associated injuries, and surgeon expertise.

Anterior Approaches

- *Direct Anterior Hueter/Smith-Petersen Approach*

The direct anterior Hueter/Smith-Petersen approach is commonly favored for Pipkin type I fractures, as they usually have anteriorly or medially located fragments. By utilizing the intermuscular and internervous plane between sartorius and tensor fascia latae (TFL) muscles, this approach provides excellent access for internal fixation. Its minimally invasive nature allows precise visualization of the femoral head, especially for anterior fractures, and facilitates accurate reduction of fracture fragments (Fig. 6.3).

This approach was first described by Carl Hueter, a German surgeon, in 1881 [21] and later popularized by Marius N. Smith-Petersen, earning its alternate name, the Smith-Petersen approach [22].

Advantages

1. Preservation of Hip Vascularity: This approach minimizes the risk to the hip's blood supply compared to posterior approaches [5].
2. Targeted Access: Ideal for isolated femoral head fractures (Pipkin types I and II), particularly when the main fragment is located anteromedially. Full hip dislocation is often unnecessary [23].
3. True Internervous and Intermuscular Planes: The dissection avoids muscle detachment, reducing postoperative complications.

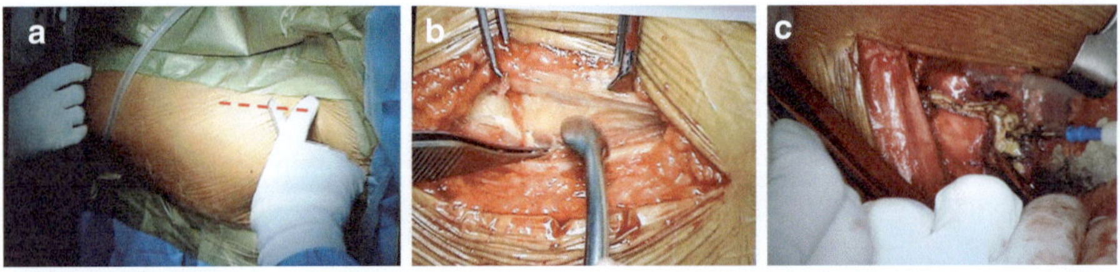

Fig. 6.3 Intraoperative picture of the direct anterior approach for Pipkin I fractures. (**a**) A longitudinal incision is made in a caudal direction, positioned approximately 2 cm lateral to the distal anterior superior iliac spine, following the line of the tensor fascia lata. (**b**) The tensor fascia lata is then retracted laterally, while the underlying fascia along with the sartorius and rectus femoris muscles are mobilized medially. (**c**) Z-shaped anterior capsulotomy is performed to fully expose the femoral neck

4. Lower Risk of Limping: The abductor muscles remain intact, resulting in less postoperative limping.
5. Efficiency: Studies have demonstrated reduced operative time, blood loss, and a lower incidence of femoral head avascular necrosis (AVN) with this approach compared to the posterior approach [24, 25].

Disadvantages
1. Heterotopic Ossification (HO): Increased risk of HO formation, reported in up to 40% of cases [26].
2. Potential for Vascular Compromise: The ascending branch of the lateral femoral circumflex artery (LFCA), which supplies the femoral head to a lesser degree compared to the medial circumflex femoral artery, may be at risk, especially following posterior dislocations.
3. Limited Visualization: This approach provides restricted access to the entire labrum unless extensive release of the TFL and gluteus medius is performed.
4. Thigh Numbness: The lateral femoral cutaneous nerve is directly in the surgical field and if it is stretched or damaged can result in persistent anterolateral thigh numbness in up to 9% of cases [27].
5. Inaccessibility to Posterior Injuries: Concomitant posterior injuries, such as those seen in Pipkin type IV fractures, cannot be addressed with this approach.

Anterolateral (Watson-Jones)

Advantages
1. Inter-muscular plane: Between the tensor fascia latae medially and gluteus medius and minimus laterally
2. Ideal for Pipkin type I and II with anterior fragments
3. Avoids need for trochanteric osteotomy and risk of subsequent non-union [28]

Disadvantages
1. Less familiar approach to most surgeons
2. Higher incidence of HO compared to anterior approaches
3. Limited access: Inability to access posterior fragments or assess posterior acetabular labrum

Posterior Approaches

- Posterior approaches such as the Kocher-Langenbeck are ideal for fractures associated with posteriorly located fragments, associated acetabular fractures involving the posterior wall or column, posteriorly based capsular-labral injuries requiring repair, or when excision is planned. However, when further visualization of anterior structures is needed simultaneously in order to reduce or fix more anteriorly based fractures, a digastric **trochanteric osteotomy** and a safe surgical hip dislocation can be employed as an extension of the posterior approach. This technique involves taking the greater trochanter forward and performing an anterior dislocation of the femoral head in order to provide 360° access to the femoral head and acetabulum.

A. **Incision Placement**

   A linear incision is made starting from the midpoint along a line drawn between the posterior edge of the tip of the greater trochanter and the posterior superior iliac spine, extending to the posterior border of the greater trochanter. This precise incision placement facilitates optimal access to the surgical site.
B. **Muscle Dissection**

   The gluteus maximus is carefully split along its natural fiber orientation. Once divided, the muscle is retracted laterally on both sides, which significantly enhances the exposure of the deeper anatomical structures.
C. **Exposure of the Surgical Field**

   With the lateral retraction complete, the superior segment of the greater sciatic foramen is revealed. During this process, the superior gluteal vessels and nerves are meticulously preserved and dissected free along the periosteum. This careful handling ensures their protection while allowing full visualization of the bone fragment from the posterior wall of the acetabulum.

Mostafa et al. have shown that the trochanteric osteotomy improves visualization. Importantly, this approach preserves the integrity of the gluteus medius and minimus, maintaining hip stability and function postoperatively. While outcomes with this technique are comparable to standard approaches, the improved access facilitates precise screw fixation and ensures optimal reduction.

Advantages

1. **Extension with Trochanteric Osteotomy:** A digastric trochanteric osteotomy enables dislocation of the femoral head, providing 360° access for reduction and fixation [29].
2. **Lower Risk of HO Compared to Anterior Approaches:** Some studies suggest that the posterior approach has a lower incidence of HO compared to anterior approaches [26, 30].

Disadvantages

Highest Risk of AVN Among all surgical approaches, the posterior approach carries the highest incidence of AVN, attributed to the risk of damaging the medial femoral circumflex artery during dissection, even higher than the use of a trochanteric osteotomy to improve access while attempting to preserve blood supply. Reported AVN incidence is 16.9% for the standard posterior approach and 12.5% for the trochanteric flip osteotomy [30].

Medial Approach

The medial approach was first introduced by Ludloff in 1908 for the surgical treatment of developmental hip dysplasia. [31] In 1973, Ferguson modified and popularized the technique, offering more precise anatomical guidelines [32]. Ludloff's original description broadly described an interval between the adductor longus and sartorius muscles superficially and between the iliopsoas and pectineus muscles in the deeper layers. Ferguson's modification shifted the approach posteriorly, utilizing a superficial plane between the gracilis and adductor longus and a deeper interval between the adductor brevis and adductor magnus muscles.

In a novel adaptation, Chiron et al. described a "modified medial hip approach" tailored for anterior-inferior femoral head fractures. This method employs a more anterior interval, dissecting between the muscle bellies of the adductor longus, brevis, and pectineus posteriorly, and their aponeuroses anteriorly, offering direct access to specific fracture types [33]. Furthermore, a study utilizing this modified Ludloff approach reported good outcomes with fewer complications compared to other procedures, suggesting it may be a promising technique for managing Pipkin IV femoral head fractures [34].

Advantages

1. Minimal dissection and blood loss
2. Direct access to the fracture site, particularly in Pipkin type I fractures, with additional exposure to key anatomical structures such as the femoral neck base, lesser trochanter, and anterior aspects of the acetabulum and labrum [34, 35]·
3. A much less incidence of heterotopic ossification compared to the anterior and posterior approach [34]·

Disadvantages

1. Technically challenging for surgeons unfamiliar with the approach

6.8.3 Fixation Techniques

Regardless of the chosen approach, reduction involves direct reduction under vision and to temporarily maintain the reduction with multiple Kirschner wires. Definitive fixation typically involves the use of countersunk screws or headless compression screws (Fig. 6.4). Headless screws allow subchondral placement, avoiding additional damage to the articular cartilage. Bioabsorbable screws have also been employed, reducing imaging artifacts and allowing for earlier detection of complications such as AVN [36]

6.8.4 Arthroscopic Techniques

Advances in hip arthroscopy have introduced minimally invasive options for Pipkin type I fractures. Arthroscopy allows precise reduction, fixation, and debridement of loose fragments while minimizing soft-tissue damage and morbidity. The technique is particularly beneficial for young patients, offering early rehabilitation and reduced risk of heterotopic ossification. Furthermore, it allows debridement and washout of small fragments, which were previously neglected. Arthroscopy-assisted treatment

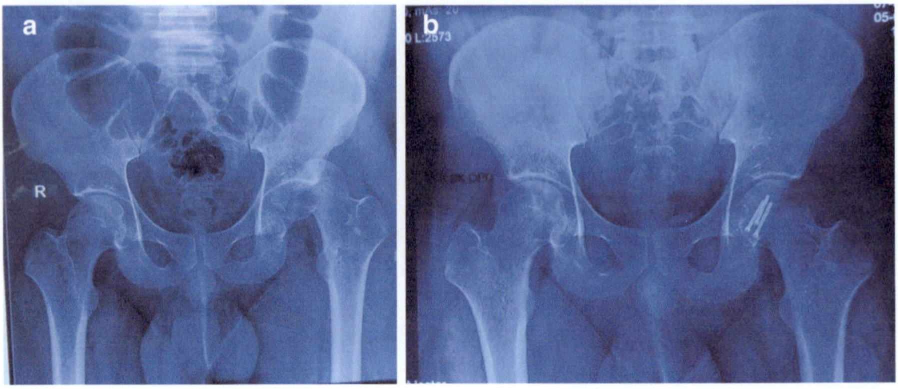

Fig. 6.4 Pipkin type I fracture (**a**) fixed with headless compression screws through Hueter approach (**b**)

of femoral head fractures allows detection and repair of any labral and osteochondral injuries. Furthermore, since hip arthroscopy is less invasive and muscle-sparing, heterotopic ossification is less likely to develop [37]. However, it is important to note that percutaneous techniques, including those used in arthroscopic-assisted fixation, carry an inherent risk of neurovascular injury [38].

Arthroscopic mosaicplasty and osteochondral autologous transfer have shown promising results in preserving joint function after significant trauma. However, the evidence is limited to case reports and small studies, indicating the need for multicentric trials to validate these approaches.

6.8.4.1 Advantages

1. **Minimally Invasive Approach:** Arthroscopic fixation avoids the extensive soft tissue dissection in open surgery. This reduced surgical morbidity may lead to less postoperative pain and a shorter recovery period [39].
2. **Preservation of Femoral Head Blood Supply:** By avoiding the need for surgical hip dislocation, the arthroscopic technique helps preserve the vascular supply to the femoral head, thereby potentially reducing the risk of avascular necrosis [40].
3. **Effective Joint Debridement:** Direct arthroscopic access permits thorough debridement of the joint—removing hematoma, loose fragments, and other debris—which may improve overall joint function.
4. **Capability for Labral and Capsular Repair:** This approach not only addresses the bony fracture but also enables simultaneous repair of associated posterior capsule–labral injuries that may not have been viewed by the anterior approach [39].

6.8.4.2 Disadvantages

1. **Technical Complexity and Steep Learning Curve:** This procedure is technically demanding and requires proficiency in both hip arthroscopy and trauma surgery.

2. **Risk of Neurovascular Injury:** There remains an inherent risk of neurovascular injury if the guidewire or fixation devices are not accurately positioned, as evidenced by reports of iatrogenic injuries [38].

6.8.5 Excision of Fragments

In cases where fragments are too small or comminuted to be fixed, excision may be considered. Earlier literature recommended fragment removal when it constituted less than one-third of the femoral head. Current evidence suggests that fragments smaller than 1 cm and that are not amenable to fixation can be excised without compromising outcomes; however, in all other circumstances, fixation yields better results than excision [17].

A 2016 meta-analysis indicated that ORIF yields better functional outcomes compared to fragment excision. Precise reduction of the chondral articular plane is critical for restoring anatomy and achieving optimal results [26].

6.8.6 Total Hip Arthroplasty

Secondary or delayed arthroplasty has been reported in Pipkin type I fractures due to posttraumatic arthritis or AVN [5, 6]. Primary arthroplasty—although not well documented—can be a viable option in the elderly with significant femoral head impaction.

6.9 Outcomes

Complications such as posttraumatic osteoarthritis and heterotopic ossification were reported in a subset of postoperative cases [9]. These findings highlight the critical importance of selecting the appropriate surgical approach and timing of intervention to minimize complications and optimize outcomes. Early intervention, precise imaging, and careful surgical planning are essential to preserving vascular integrity and achieving anatomical reduction in cases requiring surgical management [9].

6.10 Future Prospects

A shift toward operative treatment for Pipkin type I fracture has been definitely observed in the literature over the past few years [17]. However, more studies are needed to address the parameters that would favor conservative treatment over fixation or over fragment excision. Till now, the decision depends on the surgeon's assessment and expertise and an overall assessment of the fracture size and displacement, rather than precise parameters, such as those of other hip fractures and fractures of the acetabulum.

Furthermore, the introduction of hip arthroscopy in management of Pipkin type I fracture can allow the surgeon to fix the fracture under direct visualization, together with addressing the labral injury. Further studies are yet to determine the clinical significance of this compared to the traditional approaches [41]).

Impaction injuries to the femoral head have been difficult to diagnose, and the exact nature of how these should be treated and followed up is not well documented. As our experience with the diagnosis, documentation, and follow-up of these injuries increases, our understanding of their importance and the specific effect of them on the outcome will also become clear.

References

1. Birkett J. Description of a dislocation of the head of the femur, complicated with its fracture; with remarks. 1869. Clin Orthop Relat Res. 2007;458:10–1. Epub 2007/05/03.
2. Thompson VP, Epstein HC. Traumatic dislocation of the hip; a survey of two hundred and four cases covering a period of twenty-one years. J Bone Joint Surg Am. 1951;33-a(3):746–78; passim. Epub 1951/07/01.
3. Epstein HC, Wiss DA, Cozen L. Posterior fracture dislocation of the hip with fractures of the femoral head. Clin Orthop Relat Res. 1985;201:9–17. Epub 1985/12/01.
4. Hougaard K, Thomsen PB. Traumatic posterior fracture-dislocation of the hip with fracture of the femoral head or neck, or both. J Bone Joint Surg Am. 1988;70(2):233–9. Epub 1988/02/01.
5. Scolaro JA, Marecek G, Firoozabadi R, Krieg JC, Routt MLC. Management and radiographic outcomes of femoral head fractures. J Orthop Traumatol. 2017;18(3):235–41. Epub 2017/02/12.
6. Enocson A, Wolf O. Pipkin fractures: epidemiology and outcome. Eur J Trauma Emerg Surg. 2022;48(5):4113–8. Epub 2022/03/26.
7. Menger MM, Braun BJ, Herath SC, Kuper MA, Rollmann MF, Histing T. Fractures of the femoral head: a narrative review. EFORT Open Rev. 2021;6(11):1122–31. Epub 2021/12/16.
8. McCarthy JC, Busconi B. The role of hip arthroscopy in the diagnosis and treatment of hip disease. Orthopedics. 1995;18(8):753–6. Epub 1995/08/01.
9. Shakya S, Chen J, Sun J, Xiang Z. Management and outcome of patients with femoral head fractures: the mid-term follow-up with injuries and associated prognostic factors. BMC Musculoskelet Disord. 2023;24(1):311. Epub 2023/04/21.
10. Shaikh A, Desai M, Kantanavar R, Shah K. Femoral head fracture without associated hip dislocation. Arthroplast Today. 2021;8:145–9. Epub 2021/03/23.
11. Mody BS, Wainwright AM. Fracture of the femoral head without associated hip dislocation following low-energy trauma. Arch Orthop Trauma Surg. 1996;115(5):300–2. 1996/07/01.
12. Dawson-Amoah K, Raszewski J, Duplantier N, Waddell BS. Dislocation of the hip: a review of types, causes, and treatment. Ochsner J. 2018;18(3):242–52. Epub 2018/10/03.
13. Hillyard RF, Fox J. Sciatic nerve injuries associated with traumatic posterior hip dislocations. Am J Emerg Med. 2003;21(7):545–8. Epub 2003/12/05.
14. Whitehouse GH. Radiological aspects of posterior dislocation of the hip. Clin Radiol. 1978;29(4):431–41. Epub 1978/07/01.
15. Meesters AML, Kraeima J, Banierink H, Slump CH, de Vries J, Ten Duis K, et al. Introduction of a three-dimensional computed tomography measurement method for acetabular fractures. PLoS One. 2019;14(6):e0218612. Epub 2019/06/20.
16. Richardson P, Young JW, Porter D. CT detection of cortical fracture of the femoral head associated with posterior hip dislocation. Am J Roentgenol. 1990;155(1):93–4.

17. Bettinelli G, Placella G, Moharamzadeh D, Belluati A, Salini V. Articular femoral head fracture management: a meta-analysis of literature. Indian J Orthop. 2021;55(Suppl 2):304–13. Epub 2021/07/27.
18. Firoozabadi R, Spitler C, Schlepp C, Hamilton B, Agel J, Routt MC, et al. Determining stability in posterior wall acetabular fractures. J Orthop Trauma. 2015;29(10):465–9. Epub 2015/05/06.
19. Pipkin G. Treatment of grade IV fracture-dislocation of the hip. J Bone Joint Surg Am. 1957;39-A(5):1027–42 passim. Epub 1957/10/01.
20. Chen ZW, Lin B, Zhai WL, Guo ZM, Liang Z, Zheng JP, et al. Conservative versus surgical management of Pipkin type I fractures associated with posterior dislocation of the hip: a randomised controlled trial. Int Orthop. 2011;35(7):1077–81. Epub 2010/08/04.
21. Hueter C. Fünfte abtheilung: die verletzung und krankheiten des hüftgelenkes, neunundzwanzigstes capitel. Grundriss der chirurgie. 1883;2(129):e200.
22. Smith-Petersen MN. Approach to and exposure of the hip joint for mold arthroplasty. J Bone Joint Surg Am. 1949;31a(1):40–6. Epub 1949/01/01.
23. Massie WK. Fractures of the hip. JBJS. 1964;46(3):658–90.
24. Swiontkowski MF, Thorpe M, Seiler JG, Hansen ST. Operative management of displaced femoral head fractures: case-matched comparison of anterior versus posterior approaches for Pipkin I and Pipkin II fractures. J Orthop Trauma. 1992;6(4):437–42. Epub 1992/01/01.
25. Stannard JP, Harris HW, Volgas DA, Alonso JE. Functional outcome of patients with femoral head fractures associated with hip dislocations. Clin Orthop Relat Res. 2000;377:44–56. Epub 2000/08/16.
26. Wang CG, Li YM, Zhang HF, Li H, Li ZJ. Anterior approach versus posterior approach for Pipkin I and II femoral head fractures: a systemic review and meta-analysis. Int J Surg. 2016;27:176–81. Epub 2016/02/09.
27. Del Core MA, Gross B, Ahn J, Wallace SB, Starr A. Clinical and radiographic outcomes of femoral head fractures associated with traumatic hip dislocations. Strategies Trauma Limb Reconstr. 2019;14(1):6–10. Epub 2019/01/01.
28. Sifi N, Bouguenna R. Relevance of the Watson-Jones anterolateral approach in the management of Pipkin type II fracture-dislocation: a case report and literature review. J Trauma Inj. 2024;37(2):161–5. Epub 2024/10/09.
29. Henriques R, Ramalho D, Soares do Brito J, Rocha P, Spranger A, Almeida P. Management of Pipkin fractures using a safe surgical hip dislocation case. Rep Orthop. 2019;2019:3526018. Epub 2019/11/28.
30. Guo JJ, Tang N, Yang HL, Qin L, Leung KS. Impact of surgical approach on postoperative heterotopic ossification and avascular necrosis in femoral head fractures: a systematic review. Int Orthop. 2010;34(3):319–22. Epub 2009/08/15.
31. Ludloff K. The open reduction of the congenital hip dislocation by an anterior incision. JBJS. 1913;2(3):438–54.
32. Ferguson AB Jr. Primary open reduction of congenital dislocation of the hip using a median adductor approach. J Bone Joint Surg Am. 1973;55(4):671–89. Epub 1973/06/01.
33. Chiron P, Lafontan V, Reina N. Fracture-dislocations of the femoral head. Orthop Traumatol Surg Res. 2013;99(1 Suppl):S53–66. Epub 2013/01/30.
34. Abdelazeem A, Fahmy M, Abdelazeem H. Modified Ludloff's medial approach for management of Pipkin's type I femoral head fracture. Int Orthop. 2021;45(6):1591–8. Epub 2020/06/20.
35. Chiron P, Murgier J, Cavaignac E, Pailhé R, Reina N. Minimally invasive medial hip approach. Orthop Traumatol Surg Res. 2014;100(6):687–9. Epub 2014/08/29.
36. Yin XY, Liu Y, Liu WG, Yin QF. Arthroscopic fixation with absorbable suture anchors for Pipkin type I femoral head fractures—letter V technique. Arthroscopy Techniques. 2024;13:103090.
37. Ong C, Hall M, Youm T. Surgical technique: arthroscopic treatment of heterotopic ossification of the hip after prior hip arthroscopy. Clin Orthop Relat Res. 2013;471(4):1277–82. Epub 2012/10/12.
38. Nakano N, Khanduja V. Complications in hip arthroscopy. Muscles Ligaments Tendons J. 2016;6(3):402–9. Epub 2017/01/10.

39. Aprato A, Buzzone M, Di Benedetto P, Massè A. Surgical hip dislocation vs arthroscopy for fixation of subfoveal femoral head fractures. Acta Biomedica. 2021;92:e2021016.
40. Hsu SL, Chen CY, Ko JY, Hsu CH, Liu HC, Lu YD. Hip arthroscopy-assisted reduction and fixation for femoral head fracture dislocations: clinical and radiographic short-term results of seven cases. J Orthop Surg (Hong Kong). 2019;27(3):2309499019881865. Epub 2019/10/24.
41. Soylemez MS, Kemah B, Poyanli O. Arthroscopy-assisted reduction and fixation of femoral head and acetabulum fractures: a systematic review of the literature. Orthop Surg. 2022;14(4):652–62. Epub 2022/03/17.

Suprafoveal Fractures

7

Axel Gänsslen, Tilman Graulich, Richard A. Lindtner, Dietmar Krappinger, and Jan Lindahl

7.1 Introduction and Historical Knowledge

Pipkin fractures are most commonly traumatic fracture-dislocations of the hip joint involving intraarticular fractures of the femoral head. These fractures may occur in isolation or in association with femoral neck or acetabular fractures. In rare instances, femoral head fractures may be associated with intertrochanteric fractures [31].

The first known description of this injury was provided by Birkett in 1869 [5]. He reported the case of a 35-year-old woman with multiple injuries after falling from a height of 25 ft. The patient died shortly after admission due to severe head trauma. Examination of her left hip revealed a slightly shortened, internally rotated leg and crepitus during rotation. The injury was later identified as a Pipkin type II fracture, with the femoral head fragment still attached to the ligament of the head of the femur (ligamentum teres).

A. Gänsslen (✉)
Department of Trauma Surgery, Hannover Medical School, Hannover, Germany

University Hospital, Johannes Wesling Hospital, Minden, Germany

T. Graulich
Department of Trauma Surgery, Hannover Medical School, Hannover, Germany
e-mail: graulich.tilman@mh-hannover.de

R. A. Lindtner · D. Krappinger
Department of Orthopaedic and Trauma Surgery, Medical University Innsbruck, Innsbruck, Austria
e-mail: richard.lindtner@i-med.ac.at; dietmar.krappinger@tirol-kliniken.at

J. Lindahl
Department of Orthopaedics and Traumatology, Helsinki University Hospital, University of Helsinki, Helsinki, Finland
e-mail: jan.lindahl@hus.fi

R. K. Sen, S. K. Tripathy (eds.), *A Practical Guide to Management of Femoral Head Fracture-Dislocation*, https://doi.org/10.1007/978-981-96-9852-3_7

Jan Bartoníček has made significant contributions to the understanding of the historical evolution of femoral head fractures [3]. Over the decades that followed, a series of case reports further documented these injuries, with suprafoveal fracture patterns being most frequently described.

In 1872, Moxon reported a posterior-superior hip dislocation associated with what would now be classified as a Pipkin type II fracture [47].

In 1885, Bernhard Moritz Carl Ludwig Riedel described a similar posterior-superior dislocation with a Pipkin type II fracture [54].

Braun, in 1891, detailed an ischial dislocation accompanied by a combined Pipkin type I and II injury, which notably involved a split of the ligamentum teres [7].

The first radiographic documentation of femoral head fractures was provided by Durant in 1904, who identified such injuries in three separate cases [12].

In 1912, Morávek reported a case with a delayed diagnosis, where a femoral head fracture was only recognized 7 years after the injury [45].

Hinsdale, in 1923, presented a case involving an iliac dislocation and a Pipkin type II fracture, treated by fragment excision, which led to excellent hip function postoperatively [24].

Riedel was the first to describe surgical treatment for a femoral head fracture [54]. After failed closed reduction in a 15-year-old boy, he used a lateral approach with greater trochanter osteotomy. Two large femoral head fragments were reduced into the acetabulum, but the patient eventually developed hip ankylosis.

In 1939, Moore reviewed the etiology, types, clinical features, diagnosis, treatment, and prognosis of femoral head fractures; however, he did not specifically describe classical suprafoveal fractures [44]. Similarly, the classifications proposed by Thompson/Epstein and Stewart/Milford did not differentiate between femoral head fracture subtypes [63, 68].

It was not until 1957 that Garrett Pipkin introduced a classification system for femoral head fractures, which remains widely used in current clinical practice [51].

7.2 Mechanism of Injury

In a detailed biomechanical investigation, Chiron et al. [9] identified that femoral head fractures most commonly result from high-energy trauma, such as the so-called dashboard injury mechanism. This scenario typically involves a hip positioned in 90° flexion, as seen in frontal motor vehicle collisions. The degree of limb adduction or abduction at the time of impact plays a critical role in determining the location and morphology of the resulting femoral head fragment.

The authors described three distinct injury mechanisms based on hip positioning that can lead to suprafoveal fracture patterns:

- Hip in 90° flexion with neutral adduction: This positioning directs axial compressive forces perpendicularly to the posterior acetabular wall, resulting in a posterior dislocation with an associated wall fracture. Simultaneously, medially directed shear forces act on the femoral head, causing a suprafoveal fracture consistent with Pipkin type II, often with the fragment retained within the joint due to an intact ligamentum teres.

- Hip in 90° flexion with moderate adduction: Compared to neutral adduction, this configuration shifts shear forces toward the anterior-inferior quadrant of the femoral head, typically at or just above the fovea capitis, leading to variant Pipkin fracture patterns.
- Hip in flexion with abduction: Under these conditions, the impact is more likely to produce posterior column or central acetabular fractures, typically without involvement of the femoral head.

Though relatively uncommon, sciatic nerve injuries can occur in conjunction with these trauma patterns. Even in isolated dislocations or femoral head fractures (incidence $\approx 1\%$), experimental modeling has demonstrated that the sciatic nerve undergoes mechanical stretching in all tested positions involving 90° of hip flexion [9].

7.3 Classification of Femoral Head Fractures

Multiple classification systems exist for femoral head fractures, particularly focusing on suprafoveal variants. Among these, the **Pipkin classification** is the most widely used. A *suprafoveal fracture* is defined as a femoral head fracture located superior to the fovea capitis, typically occurring in the setting of a dislocation, with or without associated femoral neck or acetabular rim fractures. Pipkin's system, proposed in 1957, was developed based on standard radiographs, without the use of computed tomography (CT) or magnetic resonance imaging (MRI) [51].

To enhance the clinical utility of the Pipkin system, **Brumback et al.** [6] introduced a more detailed classification that includes anterior and central dislocation types, the degree of posterior acetabular involvement, and hip joint stability (Table 7.1). Suprafoveal fracture types within this system include:

More recently, **Chiron et al.** introduced a CT-based classification system to better assess fracture morphology, taking into account fragment size, location, and

Table 7.1 Brumback classification (focused on suprafoveal types)

Type	Description
2A	Posterior hip dislocation with suprafoveal femoral head fracture with minimal or no acetabular fracture and a stable hip joint after reduction
2B	Posterior hip dislocation with suprafoveal femoral head fracture and significant acetabular fracture with hip instability
3A	Hip dislocation (any direction) with femoral neck fracture, without head fracture
3B	Hip dislocation (any direction) with both femoral neck and femoral head fractures
4	Anterior dislocation with femoral head fracture
5	Central fracture-dislocation with femoral head fracture

associated injuries such as acetabular or femoral neck fractures [9] (Table 7.2).

Table 7.2 Chiron CT-based classification

Type	Description
1	Osteochondral fragments
2	¼ femoral head fragment
3	1/3 femoral head fragment
4	½ femoral head fragment
5	Superior femoral head collapse (impaction)

Each Chiron type is further subclassified as:

- **A**: Isolated femoral head fracture
- **B**: With associated acetabular fracture
- **C**: With associated femoral neck fracture

In a recent fracture mapping study, **Wu et al.** [74] proposed a new classification based on the direction of hip dislocation and associated impaction zones. Their analysis identified three main patterns:

- **Superior-lateral impaction fractures** (similar to Chiron type V), often linked to central dislocations
- **Anterior-inferior involvement**, corresponding to Pipkin type I and some type II fractures
- **Central femoral head fractures**, seen with central dislocations or certain anterolateral Pipkin variants

Interestingly, posterior dislocations rarely showed superior impaction injuries, in contrast to anterior or central dislocation patterns.

7.4 Diagnostic Evaluation

Initial assessment of patients with suspected femoral head fractures should follow established polytrauma protocols, such as the Advanced Trauma Life Support (ATLS) guidelines, as these injuries are commonly caused by high-energy trauma.

Posterior hip dislocation is the most frequent presentation. Clinically, patients typically exhibit a shortened, flexed limb held in adduction and internal rotation. A thorough **neurovascular examination** is essential, with particular attention to the sciatic nerve, which is at risk of injury [55].

A **standard anteroposterior (AP) pelvis X-ray** or **trauma-focused CT scan** should be obtained promptly to confirm the diagnosis before any reduction attempt. After **emergency closed reduction under general anesthesia**, a **post-reduction CT scan** is strongly recommended to evaluate joint congruity, detect associated fractures, and guide further management [39, 43].

Timely reduction is critical. Delayed reduction increases the risk of avascular necrosis (osteonecrosis) of the femoral head [1, 27, 41].

In cases of **irreducible dislocation**, urgent **open reduction** is required [28, 42, 70]. Causes of irreducibility include interposition of an avulsed ligamentum teres, osteochondral fragments, labrum, or other soft tissues.

There is a **risk of iatrogenic femoral neck fracture** during forceful closed reduction attempts [15, 50, 51, 55, 66, 67]. Unlike classical posterior dislocations (flexed, adducted, and internally rotated hip), **irreducible dislocations** often present with a fixed flexion posture, neutral or internal rotation, and marked shortening [37, 42, 50].

Magnetic resonance imaging (MRI) can be valuable in detecting subtle intra-articular injuries, including **labral tears**, **joint subluxation**, and **joint space widening**, the latter suggesting soft-tissue interposition [11].

7.5 Epidemiological Data

Pipkin fractures are relatively rare injuries, and as a result, epidemiological data remain limited. The incidence is low, and most institutions and individual surgeons encounter only a small number of cases. However, several studies with sample sizes greater than 40 patients provide valuable insights into the distribution, treatment, and outcomes of these fractures [14, 34, 38, 57–59, 69].

In a multicenter investigation by Lederer et al. [38], a total of 46 patients with Pipkin fractures were evaluated, comprising 13 type I, 14 type II, 2 type III, and 17 type IV injuries. Similarly, a retrospective study by Kloen et al. [50], which included 59 patients with a minimum follow-up of 5 years (mean: 9.4 years, range: 5–21 years), identified 43 type II and 16 type IV fractures. Notably, 83% of these patients (n = 49) presented with a hip dislocation. Within the subgroup of type II fractures, nine patients underwent open reduction and internal fixation (ORIF) and seven received primary total hip replacement (THR). The ORIF group showed good to excellent outcomes in 67% of cases, as assessed both clinically and radiographically using the Epstein criteria.

A larger cohort study by Scolaro et al. [58] reviewed 147 cases, including 40 type I, 62 type II, 7 type III, and 23 type IV fractures. An additional 15 cases exhibited femoral head impaction injuries.

Enocson et al. [14] analyzed 47 Pipkin fractures, reporting 7 type I, 13 type II, 1 type III, and 26 type IV fractures. Although different treatment strategies were employed, the study did not provide detailed data stratified by fracture type.

In a more recent retrospective series, Shakya et al. [59] included 50 patients, identifying 18 type I, 10 type II, 8 type III, and 14 type IV fractures. Among those with type II injuries, 80% were treated with ORIF, 10% received conservative management, and 10% underwent primary THR. Notably, type III fractures demonstrated the highest rate of conversion to THR, occurring in 25% of cases.

Table 7.3 Demographic distribution of Pipkin fractures in large clinical series

Author	Year	Study period	Total cases	Cases/year	Type I	Type II	Type III	Type IV	Unknown
Kloen [50]	2002	1970–1990	33	1.57	10	8	1	14	–
Sahin [34]	2003	1980–1994	57	3.8	19	26	9	3	–
Lederer [38]	2007	1982–2005	46	1.92	13	14	2	17	–
Tonetti [69]	2010	1972–2008	110	3.06	37	16	4	45	8
Scolaro [58]	2017	2000–2013	147	10.5	40	62	7	23	15
Enocson [14]	2022	2013–2022	47	4.7	7	13	1	26	–
Shakya [59]	2023	2011–2018	50	6.25	18	10	8	14	–
Total	–	–	**490**	–	**144**	**149**	**32**	**142**	**23**

Several clinical studies comprising more than 30 patients have contributed to our understanding of the epidemiology and treatment outcomes of Pipkin fractures. These injuries remain uncommon, and most institutions encounter them infrequently. The compiled data suggest that **Pipkin types I, II, and IV occur at similar frequencies**, whereas **type III fractures are consistently rare** across all cohorts (Table 7.3) [14, 34, 38, 57–59, 69].

This analysis confirms the **notable underrepresentation of type III fractures**, which remain the least commonly observed subtype in large series.

Further insights were provided by a **meta-analysis by Giannoudis et al. (2009)** [57], involving **450 patients**, which emphasized **open reduction and internal fixation (ORIF)** as the preferred treatment for **Pipkin type II fractures**. Interestingly, this analysis did **not reveal statistically significant differences in clinical outcomes among Pipkin types** when evaluated using the **Thompson and Epstein scoring system**. These findings support the importance of considering **individual injury patterns and patient-specific factors** when choosing the most appropriate treatment strategy.

7.6 Treatment

The optimal management of **Pipkin type II fractures** remains a subject of ongoing debate. **Giannoudis et al.** [21] reported that smaller femoral head fragments are associated with worse clinical outcomes. More recently, evidence has favored **surgical intervention over conservative treatment**, and **open reduction and internal fixation (ORIF)** has shown superior results compared to fragment excision in displaced Pipkin type I and II fractures [4].

Fragment excision, particularly in type II fractures, may alter joint biomechanics by increasing central and superior pressure forces across the hip joint [25]. A **finite element analysis** demonstrated that **Herbert screw fixation** provides superior stability compared to standard cortical screws for these injuries [16], a finding supported by a clinical study involving 68 patients [65].

Since 2000, data from **125 Pipkin type II fractures** have been reported in the literature with sufficient clinical detail [2, 8, 10, 17, 23, 26, 33–36, 46, 48, 49, 52, 53, 56, 60–62, 71, 73, 75].

Patient Demographics

- **Mean age**: 38.3 years (Range: 14–71 years)
- **Sex**: 75.6% male
- **Injury mechanism**: High-energy trauma in all documented cases ($n = 65$)
- **Hip dislocation**: Posterior dislocation in all patients with recorded data ($n = 92$).

Treatment Modalities

1. **Conservative Management**
    - Performed in 19 patients after closed reduction
    - Mean **Thompson-Epstein (T/E) score**: 2.68 (fair result)
    - Functional outcomes:
        - Excellent: 3
        - Good: 4
        - Fair: 8
        - Poor: 4
    - Only **36.8%** achieved good or excellent results
    - All poor outcomes were associated with **avascular necrosis (AVN)**; one required **secondary THR**
2. **Fragment Excision**
    - Performed in 17 patients
    - Mean T/E score: 2.31
    - Functional outcomes:
        - Excellent: 4
        - Good: 8
        - Fair: 2
        - Poor: 3
    - **68.7%** had good or excellent results
3. **Open Reduction and Internal Fixation (ORIF)** (Fig. 7.1)
    - Most common treatment ($n = 83$)

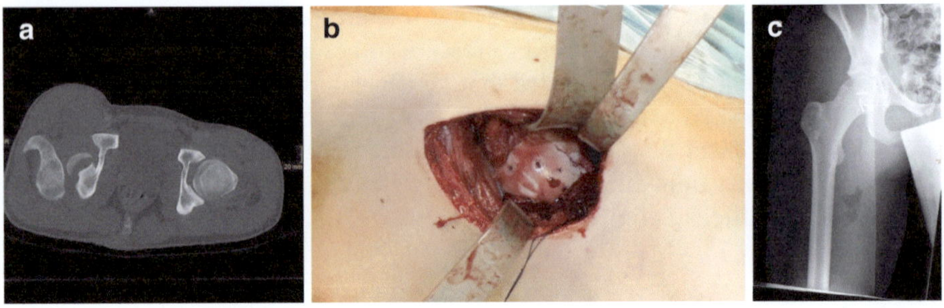

Fig. 7.1 CT scan demonstrating a posterior hip dislocation with an associated suprafoveal femoral head fracture (**a**). Intraoperative image (**b**) shows fragment fixation via the direct anterior approach. Postoperative anteroposterior (AP) radiograph (**c**) confirms stable fixation following screw osteosynthesis

- Mean T/E score: **1.78**
- Functional outcomes:
  - Excellent: 34
  - Good: 37
  - Fair: 8
  - Poor: 4
- **85.5%** achieved good or excellent outcomes
- Only **one case** required secondary THR; **no primary THRs** were performed

Surgical Approaches Used in ORIF (n = 64 Cases with Approach Documented)

- Anterior/Smith-Petersen: 18
- Watson-Jones: 3
- Kocher-Langenbeck: 3
- Kocher-Langenbeck + Ganz (surgical hip dislocation): 27
- Percutaneous: 10
- Lateral ± trochanteric osteotomy: 3

Influence of Surgical Approach on Outcomes
The eight approaches were grouped into four categories:

- **Anterior (or anterolateral)**
- **Posterior**
- **Posterior with surgical hip dislocation (Ganz approach)**
- **Lateral**

Mean T/E scores (lower = better function) by approach:

- **Anterior**: 1.71
- **Ganz approach**: 1.77
- **Posterior**: 1.6
- **Lateral**: 2.67

While anterior and Ganz approaches provided the most favorable functional outcomes, isolated lateral approaches were associated with poorer results. Over the past two decades, there has been a clear shift toward **posterior approaches combined with surgical hip dislocation (Ganz technique)**, reflecting the trend toward enhanced exposure and preservation of the femoral head's vascular supply.

Our analysis demonstrated that conservative treatment for Pipkin type II fractures is associated with inferior outcomes and is therefore not considered an appropriate management strategy. The optimal results were achieved with open reduction and internal fixation (ORIF), with more than 85% of cases resulting in good to excellent functional outcomes (Fig. 7.1). In select cases—such as elderly patients, those presenting late, or individuals with severely comminuted and non-reconstructible Pipkin II fractures—primary total hip arthroplasty (THA) may offer a more effective management strategy (Fig. 7.2).

7.7 Clinical Implications

For **Pipkin type II fractures**, internal fixation using **screw osteosynthesis** remains the treatment of choice, with the most favorable outcomes observed when either an **anterior-based approach** or a **Ganz surgical hip dislocation technique** is employed (Fig. 7.1). While some Pipkin type II injuries may also involve the femoral neck (thus reclassifying them as **Pipkin type III**), the **extent of displacement of the femoral neck component** is the primary determinant of prognosis [19].

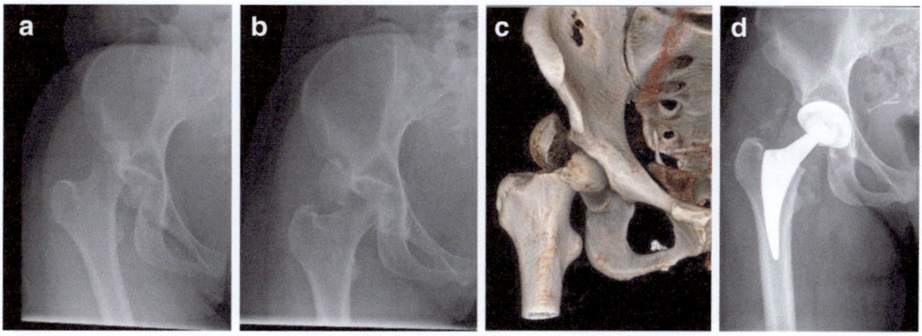

Fig. 7.2 A 34-year-old female involved in a motor vehicle accident (MVA) presented with a posterior-superior fracture-dislocation of the right hip (**a**), initially appearing as an infrafoveal femoral head fracture. Following closed reduction, imaging with standard X-ray and 3D CT (**b**, **c**) revealed a suprafoveal fracture. Given the poor prognosis associated with the fracture configuration, a primary total hip replacement (THR) was performed (**d**)

In the context of **Pipkin type IV fractures**, clinical outcomes appear to correlate with the type of femoral head involvement. Specifically, patients whose femoral head injury resembles a **type I fracture** tend to experience better results than those with **type II-like patterns** [18]. Similar to type III fractures, **Pipkin type IV injuries** are associated with increased rates of long-term complications, including **avascular necrosis (AVN)**, **heterotopic ossification (HO)**, **posttraumatic osteoarthritis**, and **nerve dysfunction** [21]. Supporting this, **Engel et al.** [13] documented that over **50%** of patients with Pipkin type IV fractures required **secondary total hip arthroplasty (THR).**

While no consensus has been established regarding the superiority of the **anterior** versus the **Ganz (posterior surgical dislocation)** approach for femoral head reconstruction, both techniques are consistently associated with **better functional results** when compared to alternative surgical options.

7.8 Surgical Approach Considerations

The choice of surgical approach in femoral head fracture management continues to be debated and should be **individualized based on patient- and injury-specific parameters**. These include the **fracture morphology**, **presence of concomitant injuries**, **surgeon expertise**, and **institutional resources**. The **Ganz approach**, which involves controlled surgical dislocation of the hip, has gained traction due to its ability to provide **comprehensive visualization of the femoral head and acetabulum** while preserving critical **vascular structures** [29].

A variety of surgical approaches have been utilized, each with distinct indications and anatomical advantages [29]:

- **Anterior approaches**: Direct anterior (Hueter) and Smith-Petersen
- **Lateral approaches**: Anterolateral (e.g., Watson-Jones) and direct lateral (e.g., McFarland/Osborne, Hardinge)
- **Posterior approaches**: Kocher-Langenbeck and Ganz surgical hip dislocation (via Kocher-Langenbeck or Gibson)
- **Medial approaches**: Less commonly used, but may be suitable for specific indications
- **Minimally invasive technique**: Hip arthroscopy, typically reserved for limited fragment removal or diagnostic purposes

Several variables influence the choice of approach:

- **Size and orientation** of any associated acetabular wall or rim fracture
- Degree of **hip joint instability**
- **Surgeon experience** and familiarity with specific techniques
- **Concurrent injuries**, including femoral neck or acetabular involvement
- **Availability of specialized tools**, such as arthroscopy equipment [21, 22, 30]

A key consideration is the **risk of AVN**, which can result either from the **initial trauma** or from **iatrogenic injury** to the blood supply during surgery. Reported rates of AVN after Pipkin fractures range from **7% to 24%**, regardless of the surgical approach used [30, 64].

Some concern exists regarding **anterior approaches**, especially in the setting of posterior dislocations, where further compromise to the **medial femoral circumflex artery (MFCA)** may occur during anterior arthrotomy [73]. However, it should be noted that **posterior approaches** are not without risk, as the **deep branch of the MFCA** may also be injured during these procedures [20].

Ultimately, the selected approach should provide **adequate exposure for accurate reduction and fixation** while minimizing risks of **vascular injury** and **postoperative complications** [29]. For example, a **systematic review and meta-analysis** comparing anterior and posterior approaches found that **posterior approaches were associated with a lower incidence of heterotopic ossification** in Pipkin type I and II fractures [72]. Additionally, a more recent meta-analysis reported **no significant difference in clinical outcomes between the traditional Kocher-Langenbeck and Ganz surgical dislocation techniques** [32].

In conclusion, for **Pipkin type II fractures**, the **location of the primary fracture fragment** should guide the **surgical approach**, aiming to balance **optimal visualization**, **vascular preservation**, and **favorable long-term joint function**.

7.9 Author's Preferred Treatment

Based on current scientific evidence and clinical experience, the authors advocate **open reduction and internal fixation (ORIF)** as the treatment of choice for **suprafoveal femoral head fractures**.

The **Kocher-Langenbeck approach combined with surgical hip dislocation (Ganz)** is preferred. This approach not only facilitates anatomic reduction of the femoral head fracture but also allows for the direct management of associated intra-articular pathologies such as **labral tears**, **osteochondral defects**, and **loose bodies** (Fig. 7.3).

7.10 Complications

Despite advances in surgical technique, complications following femoral head fractures, particularly **suprafoveal (Pipkin type II)** fractures, remain significant. Although specific complication rates for suprafoveal injuries are limited in the literature, overall complication data from broader femoral head fracture series include

- **Avascular necrosis (AVN)** of the femoral head: Reported in up to **26.7%** of cases [40]

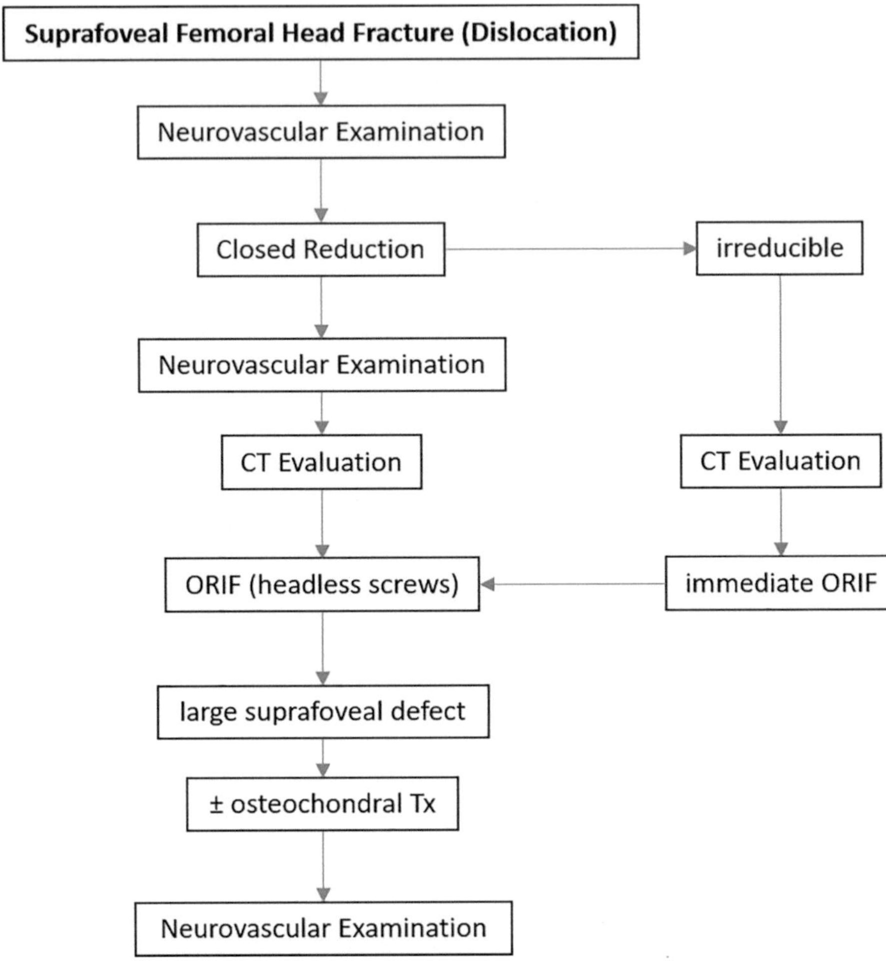

Fig. 7.3 Favored treatment algorithm with open reduction and internal fixation (ORIF) of suprafoveal femoral head fractures

- **Posttraumatic osteoarthritis**: May result from direct cartilage damage at the time of injury or from residual joint incongruity; observed in up to **43.6%** of patients [40]
- **Heterotopic ossification (HO)**: Especially common with the **anterior approach**, with reported rates up to **56.7%** [40, 72]
- **Nerve injuries**, particularly involving the **sciatic nerve**, may occur, though less frequently reported

7.11 Conclusions

Pipkin fractures are rare, high-energy injuries, most frequently seen in **young to middle-aged males under the age of 40**. Due to their infrequent occurrence, individual surgeon experience is often limited.

The **Pipkin classification** remains the standard for describing femoral head fracture patterns, while other classification systems serve primarily academic or research purposes.

- The **majority of Pipkin fractures**, particularly type II, are best managed with **ORIF**, which provides superior outcomes compared to fragment excision or nonoperative treatment.
- **Conservative management** in Pipkin type II fractures has demonstrated **poorest functional outcomes**.
- **ORIF** for type II fractures has shown **over 85% good to excellent results** across multiple series.
- **Both anterior and posterior surgical approaches** yield comparable functional outcomes and complication rates.
- Over the last decade, there has been a **clear shift toward the Ganz surgical dislocation technique**, reflecting its advantages in visualizing and preserving the femoral head while addressing associated injuries.

In summary, **anatomic reduction and stable fixation using a well-planned surgical approach**, tailored to fracture morphology and associated injuries, remains the cornerstone of successful treatment for Pipkin type II femoral head fractures.

References

1. Ahmed G, Shiraz S, Riaz M, Ibrahim T. Late versus early reduction in traumatic hip dislocations: a meta-analysis. Eur J Orthop Surg Traumatol. 2017;27:1109–16.
2. Alexa O, Puha B, Popescu D, Malancea RI, Veliceasa B. Treatment options in Pipkin fracture-dislocations of the femoral head: cases review. J Surg. 2016;12:23–7.
3. Bartoníček J, Rammelt S. History of femoral head fracture and coronal fracture of the femoral condyles. Int Orthop. 2015;39:1245–50.
4. Bettinelli G, Placella G, Moharamzadeh D, Belluati A, Salini V. Articular femoral head fracture management: a meta-analysis of literature. Indian J Orthop. 2021;55(Suppl 2):S304–13.
5. Birkett J. Description of a dislocation of the head of the femur, complicated with its fracture; with remarks. Med Chir Trans. 1869;52:133–8.
6. Brumback RJ, Kenzora JE, Levitt LE, Burgess AR, Poka A. Fractures of the femoral head. Hip. 1987:181–206. PMID: 3546215.
7. Busch F. Mehrere Fälle seltener Knochenverletzungen. Arch Klin Chir. 1891;10:703–19.
8. Chen Z, Lin B, Zhai W, Guo Z, Liang Z, Zheng J, Lian K, Ding Z. Conservative versus surgical management of Pipkin type I fractures associated with posterior hip dislocation of the hip: a randomised controlled study. Int Orthop. 2011;35:1077–81.
9. Chiron P, Lafontan V, Reina N. Fracture-dislocations of the femoral head. Orthop Traumatol Surg Res. 2013;99S:S53–66.

10. De Mauro D, Rovere G, Smakaj A, Marino S, Ciolli G, Perna A, Battiato C, El Ezzo O, Liuzza F. Gibson approach and surgical hip dislocation according to Ganz in the treatment of femoral head fractures. BMC Musculoskelet Disord. 2021;22:961.
11. Droll K, Broekhuyse H, O'Brien P. Fracture of the femoral head. J Am Acad Orthop Surg. 2007;15:716–27.
12. Durand D. Les fractures de la tête fémorale. Bul Soc Chir Lyon. 1903;6:376–82.
13. Engel J, Johnsen P, Patel N, Satpathy J, Mounasamy V. Pipkin type IV femoral head fractures: a case series and review of literature. Eur J Orthop Surg Traumatol. 2021;31:791–5.
14. Enocson A, Wolf O. Pipkin fractures: epidemiology and outcome. Eur J Trauma Emerg Surg. 2022;48:4113–8.
15. Epstein H. Posterior fracture-dislocations of the hip; long-term follow-up. J Bone Joint Surg. 1974;56A:1103–27.
16. Freitas A, Demeneghi N, Barin F, Battaglion L, Pires R, Giordano V. Pipkin type-II femoral head fracture – a biomechanical evaluation by the finite-element method. Rev Bras Ortop (Sao Paulo). 2023;58:507–13.
17. Galois L, Pfeffer F, Kermarrec I, Traversari R, Mainhard D, Delagoutte J. Posterior dislocation of the hip with concomitant ipsilateral fractures of both the femoral head and shaft: a case report. Eur J Orthop Surg Traumatol. 2001;11:129–31.
18. Gänsslen A, Grechenig S. Chapter 24: Femoral head fractures: Pipkin IV. In: Gänsslen A, Lindahl J, et al., editors. Acetabular fractures. Stuttgart: Thieme-Verlag; 2018. p. 320–5.
19. Gänsslen A, Lindtner R, Krappinger D, Franke J. Pipkin fractures: fracture type-specific management. Arch Orthop Trauma Surg. 2024;144:4601. https://doi.org/10.1007/s00402-024-05576-z.
20. Gautier E, Ganz K, Krugel N, Gill T, Ganz R. Anatomy of the medial femoral circumflex artery and its surgical implications. J Bone Joint Surg Br. 2000;82:679–83.
21. Giannoudis P, Kontakis G, Christoforakis Z, Akula M, Tosounidis T, Koutras C. Management complications and clinical results of femoral head fractures. Injury. 2009;40:1245–51.
22. Giordano V, Giordano M, Gloria R. General principles for treatment of femoral head fractures. J Clin Orthop Trauma. 2019;10:155–60.
23. Henle P, Kloen P, Siebenrock K. Femoral head injuries: which treatment strategy can be recommended? Injury. 2007;38:478–88.
24. Hinsdale G. Fracture of head of femur, with dislocation on dorsum of ilium. JAMA J Am Med Assoc. 1923;80:469.
25. Holmes W, Solberg B, Bay B, Laubach J, Olson S. Biomechanical consequences of excision of displaced Pipkin femoral head fractures. Poster #62, OTA October 24 1999.
26. Hosny H, Mousa S, Salama W. Management of femoral head fracture by Ganz surgical dislocation of the hip. J Orthop Traumatol. 2022;23:24. https://doi.org/10.1186/s10195-022-00643-w.
27. Hougaard K, Thomson P. Traumatic posterior fracture-dislocation of the hip with fractures of the femoral head or neck, or both. J Bone Joint Surg. 1988;70A:233–9.
28. Johnson E. Irreducible fracture-dislocation of the hip: a severe injury with a poor prognosis. J Orthop Trauma. 1999;13:228–9.
29. Khalifa A, Ahmed E, Farouk O. Surgical approaches for managing femoral head fractures (FHFs); what and how to choose from the different options? Orthop Res Rev. 2022;14:133–45.
30. Khalifa A, Refai O, Farouk O, Abdelnasser M. Management of femoral head fractures through surgical hip dislocation (SHD): a demanding but safe technique. Arch Orthop Trauma Surg. 2021;141:1701–10.
31. Khan M, Wright V, Prayson M. Ipsilateral intertrochanteric and Pipkin fractures: an unusual case. Am J Orthop. 2007;36:E53–5.
32. Kim C, Ma D, Cho H, Yoon Y. Comparison of postoperative complications between trochanter flip osteotomy and Kocher–Langenbeck approaches for the treatment of femoral head fractures: a systematic review and meta-analysis. Indian J Orthop. 2023;57:577–85.
33. Kim J, Chang J, Bae J, Kim J. Outcomes of treatment for femoral head fractures with hip dislocation. J Korean Hip Soc. 2010;22:298–304.

34. Kloen P, Siebenrock K, Raaymakers E, Marti R, Ganz R. Femoral head fractures revisited. Eur J Trauma. 2002;28:221–33.
35. Kloub M, Holub K, Peml M, Urban J, Latal P. Closed reduction and minimally invasive screw osteosynthesis of Pipkin femoral head fractures. J Appl Biomed. 2023;21:1–6.
36. Kokubo Y, Uchida K, Takeno K, Yayame T, Miyazaki T, Negoro K, Nakajima H, Sugita D, Takeura N, Yoshida A, Baba H. Dislocated intra-articular femoral head fracture associated with fracture-dislocation of the hip and acetabulum: report of 12 cases and technical notes on surgical intervention. Eur J Orthop Surg Traumatol. 2013;23:557–64.
37. Lawrence D, Smitaman E, Baumgartner M, Haims A. A rare but radiographically recognizable cause of an irreducible hip fracture-dislocation. Clin Imaging. 2013;37:595–7.
38. Lederer S, Tauber M, Karpik S, Bogner R, Auffahrt A, Resch H. Hüftkopffrakturen – eine Mulicenterstudie. Unfallchirurg. 2007;110:513–20.
39. Lehmann W, Spering C. Pipkin-Frakturen. Unfallchirurg. 2022;125:313–23.
40. Marshall S, Leary E, Crist B. Femoral head fractures systematic review and meta-analysis. Ann Surg Case Rep. 2024;7(1):1085.
41. McKee M, Garay M, Schemitsch E, Kreder H, Stephen D. Irreducible fracture-dislocation of the hip: a severe injury with a poor prognosis. J Orthop Trauma. 1998;12:223–9.
42. Mehta S, Routt M. Irreducible fracture–dislocations of the femoral head without posterior wall acetabular fractures. J Orthop Trauma. 2008;22:686–92.
43. Menger M, Braun B, Herath S, Küper M, Rollmann M, Histing T. Fractures of the femoral head: a narrative review. EOR. 2021;6. https://doi.org/10.1302/2058-5241.6.210034.
44. Moore J. Fractures of the upper end of the femur including fracture dislocations at the hip joint. Am J Surg. 1939;44:117–34.
45. Morávek A. Odštěpná zlomenina hlavice kosti stehenní [Split fracture of the femoral head]. Cas Lek Cesk. 1912;51:106–8.
46. Mostafa M. Femoral head fractures. Int Orthop. 2001;25:51–4.
47. Moxon A. Compound dislocation of hip-joint, the bone thrust through skin. Med Times Gaz. 1872;44(1):92.
48. Oransky M, Martinell N, Sanzarello I, Papapietro N. Fractures of the femoral head: a long term follow-up study. Muskuloskeletal Surg. 2012;96:95–6.
49. Özcan M, Copuroglu C, Saridogan K. Fractures of the femoral head: what are the reasons for poor outcome? Ulus Travma Acil Cerrahi Derg. 2011;17:51–6.
50. Park K, Lee K, Na B, Yoon T. Clinical and ardiographic outcomes of femoral head fractures: excision vs. fixation in Pipkin type I: what is the optimal choice for femoral head fracture? J Orthop Res. 2015;20:702–7.
51. Pipkin G. Treatment of grade IV fracture dislocation of the hip. J Bone Joint Surg. 1957;39A:1027–42.
52. Prokop A, Helling H, Hahn U, Udomkaewkanjana C, Rehm K. Biodegradable implants for Pipkin fractures. Clin Orthop Relat Res. 2005;432:226–33.
53. Rajagopal T, Kanse P. Percutaneous fixation for Pipkin type II femoral head fracture associated with posterior dislocation of the hip. SICOT Online Reports E045. 2003.
54. Riedel B. Längsfraktur von Schenkelkopf und – Hals. Bericht über die Verh Dtsch Ges Chir XIV. Congr Beilage Zbl Chir. 1885;12(24):92–3.
55. Roeder L, DeLee J. Femoral head fractures associated with posterior hip dislocations. Clin Orthop. 1980;147:121.
56. Rojas-Sayol R, De Caso J, Valera M. Arthroscopic-assisted percutaneous fixation of a femoral head fracture (Pipkin II): a case report. JBJS Case Connect. 2022;12. https://doi.org/10.2106/JBJS.CC.22.00194.
57. Sahin V, Karakas E, Aksu S, Atlihan D, Turk C, Halici M. Traumatic dislocation and fracture-dislocation of the hip: a long-term follow-up study. J Trauma. 2003;54:520–9.
58. Scolaro J, Marecek G, Firoozabadi R, Krieg J, Routt M. Management and radiographic outcome of femoral head fractures. J Orthop Traumatol. 2017;18:235. https://doi.org/10.1007/s10195-017-0445-z.

59. Shakya S, Chen J, Sun J, Xiang Z. Management and outcome of patients with femoral head fractures: the mid-term follow-up with injuries and associated prognostic factors. BMC Musculoskelet Disord. 2023;24:311.
60. Sifi N, Bouguenna R. Relevance of the Watson-Jones anterolateral approach in the management of Pipkin type II fracture-dislocation: a case report and literature review. J Trauma Inj. 2024;37:161–5.
61. Song H, Cho J, Lee Y, Park D, Han K. New surgical algorithm for femoral head split fractures. J Orthop Sci. 2012;17:710–6.
62. Stannard J, Harris J, Volgas D, Alonso J. Functional outcome of patients with femoral head fractures associated with hip dislocations. Clin Orthop. 2000;377:44–56.
63. Stewart M, Milford L. Fracture-dislocation of the hip. An end-result study. J Bone Joint Surg. 1954;36-A:315–42.
64. Stirma G, Uliana C, Valenza W, Abagge M. Surgical treatment of femoral head fractures through previously controlled hip luxation: four case series and literature review. Rev Bras Ortop. 2018;53:337–41.
65. Sun Z, Jiang L, Chen R, Zhao L, Li X. Clinical effects of direct anterior internal fixation with Herbert screws on hip joint function and quality of life in patients with Pipkin II femoral head fractures. Arch Orthop Trauma Surg. 2023;143:63–70.
66. Sy M, Kinkpe C, Dakoure P, Dieme C, Sane A, Ndiaye A, Dansokho A, Seye S. Femoral neck fracture complicating orthopedic reposition of a dislocated hip: four cases. Rev Chir Orthop Reparatrice Appar Mot. 2005;91:173–9.
67. Tannast M, Mack P, Klaeser B, Siebenrock K. Hip dislocation and femoral neck fracture: decision-making for head preservation. Injury. 2009;40:1118–24.
68. Thompson V, Epstein H. Traumatic dislocation of the hip. J Bone Joint Surg. 1951;33A:746–78.
69. Tonetti J, Ruatti S, Lafontan V, Loubignac F, Chiron P, Sari-Ali H, Bonnevialle P. Is femoral head fracture-dislocation management improvable: a retrospective study in 110 cases. Orthop Traumatol Surg Res. 2010;96:623–31.
70. Uzel A, Laflamme G, Rouvillain J. Irreducible Pipkin II femoral head fractures: is transgluteal approach the best strategy? Orthop Traumatol Surg Res. 2010;96:695–701.
71. Uzel A, Mazzola C, Lebreton G, Wilson G, Rouvillain J. Hip subluxation associated with Pipkin II fracture: an injury to look for before reduction. Musculoskelet Surg. 2009;93:33–5.
72. Wang C, Li Y, Zhang H, Li H, Li Z. Anterior approach versus posterior approach for Pipkin I and II femoral head fractures: a systemic review and meta-analysis. Int J Surg. 2016;27:176–81.
73. Wang J, Cai L, Xie L, Chen H, Guo X, Yu K. 3D printing-based Ganz approach for treatment of femoral head fractures: a prospective analysis. J Orthop Surg Res. 2019;14:338.
74. Wu S, Li R, Wang W, Zhang Y, Mei J. Fracture line distribution in femoral head fractures: a complement to Pipkin, Brumback, and AO/OTA classifications. Radiol Med. 2022;127:1235–44.
75. Yoon T, Rowe S, Chung J, Song E, Jung S, Anwar I. Clinical and radiographic outcome of femoral head fractures: 30 patients followed for 3–10 years. Acta Orthop Scand. 2001;72:348–53.

Femoral Head and Neck Fracture

8

Manish Sharma and Ramesh Kumar Sen

8.1 Introduction

Femoral head fractures are uncommon injuries that almost always occur in association with hip dislocations [1–3]. According to studies, including those by Epstein et al., nearly 90% of hip dislocations are posterior. Among these, femoral head fractures have an incidence of approximately 5–15% [2, 4]. A review by Alonso et al. revealed that about two-thirds of these injuries occur in young adults [5, 6]. Separate studies by Giannoudis et al. and Andres Enocson et al. identified motor vehicle accidents as the primary cause of femoral head fractures in younger individuals, while falls from height are the leading cause in elderly individuals with osteoporotic bones [6, 7]. This trend is expected to rise due to an increase in vehicle accidents and an aging population with reduced bone quality [4, 7]. Gullberg et al. predicted in 1997 that the global incidence of hip fractures would double by 2025 compared to 1990, with a further doubling anticipated by 2050 [9].

The discovery of femoral head fractures dates back to 1869, when Birkett first identified them during a postmortem examination, sparking enduring interest among orthopedic surgeons [8]. In 1957, Garrett Pipkin classified femoral head fractures into 4 types after studying 25 cases. Among these, type III Pipkin fractures involve an ipsilateral head and neck of the femur (IHNF) fracture. Literature on type III Pipkin fractures is limited, reflecting their rarity and the challenges in understanding their incidence, mechanism, and management [10].

IHNF fractures, the rarest subtype of femoral head fractures, have an incidence of approximately 8.6% and are almost exclusively associated with high-energy trauma [6]. Kyeon-Hyeon Park et al. reported instances where neck of the femur

M. Sharma
Indira Gandhi Medical College, Shimla, India

R. K. Sen (✉)
Institute of Orthopedic Surgery, Max Super Speciality Hospital, Mohali, Punjab, India

R. K. Sen, S. K. Tripathy (eds.), *A Practical Guide to Management of Femoral Head Fracture-Dislocation*, https://doi.org/10.1007/978-981-96-9852-3_8

fractures occurred iatrogenically during attempts to reduce irreducible hip dislocations [13, 15]. Although these fractures are the least common among the Pipkin types, they are associated with the highest complication rates. Managing these intracapsular fractures is particularly challenging due to their complexity and the high risk of complications. They are often accompanied by additional injuries to the hip joint, femur, or knee, necessitating a high degree of clinical suspicion for early diagnosis and timely intervention [5, 6].

8.2 Mechanism of Injury

Ipsilateral head and neck of the femur (IHNF) fractures typically result from high-energy trauma, most commonly motor vehicle accidents, followed by falls from significant heights. In vehicular collisions, the "dashboard injury" mechanism is the predominant cause, where the limb is subjected to both axial compression and shear forces. Axial compression results in posterior hip dislocation and femoral head fracture, while shear forces drive the femoral head against the iliac wing, causing a femoral neck fracture [6, 7, 10, 33]. When the limb is abducted beyond the neutral position and flexed less than 60 degrees, these forces become concentrated at the opposing bony surfaces of the hip joint, leading to Pipkin type III fractures [19].

In elderly individuals with osteoporotic bones, low-energy trauma, such as simple falls, may suffice to cause these injuries, as noted by Andres Enocson et al. and Thompson and Epstein [7, 16]. Additionally, Kyeon-Hyeon Park et al. reported iatrogenic cases of Pipkin type III fractures during attempts to reduce irreducible hip dislocations. In their study, five out of nine cases developed fresh femoral neck fractures due to excessive force during reduction, where the femoral head was impinged against the sharp acetabular rim [13, 15].

Recently, Pipkin type III fractures have also been reported as sports injuries in activities such as skiing, football, and paragliding [17, 18]. Upadhyay et al. highlighted that anatomical variations, such as decreased femoral anteversion, predispose individuals to posterior hip dislocations and femoral head fractures [14].

Thus, factors such as limb position, bone quality, and the magnitude of force at the time of impact are critical determinants of injury severity and pattern.

8.3 Classification

In 1951, Thompson and Epstein classified hip dislocations into five types, with type V being associated with fractures of the femoral head [16]. In 1954, Stewart and Milford introduced a four-grade system for posterior hip dislocations, where grade IV included cases with associated fractures of the ipsilateral femoral head or neck [20]. Garrett Pipkin refined this further in 1957, dividing Stewart and Milford's grade IV into four subtypes based on the fracture line's relationship to the fovea capitis and additional fractures of the femoral neck or acetabulum. Pipkin's classification is as follows (Table 8.1):

Table 8.1 Pipkin classification

Type	Description
Type I	Fracture line below fovea/ligamentum teres
Type II	Fracture line above fovea/ligamentum teres
Type III	Type I/II with ipsilateral femoral neck fracture
Type IV	Type I/II with acetabular fracture

Table 8.2 Brumback classification

Type	Description
Type 1A	Posterior dislocation with fracture of infero-medial femoral head; minimal or no acetabular rim fracture (stable hip)
Type 1B	Type 1A with significant acetabular rim fracture (unstable hip)
Type 2A	Posterior dislocation with fracture of supero-medial femoral head; minimal or no acetabular rim fracture (stable hip)
Type 2B	Type 2A with significant acetabular rim fracture (unstable hip)
Type 3A	Hip dislocation with femoral neck fracture
Type 3B	Type 3A with associated femoral head fracture
Type 4A	Anterior dislocation with indentation-type femoral head fracture
Type 4B	Anterior dislocation with trans-chondral shear fracture of femoral head
Type 5	Central fracture-dislocation with femoral head fracture

Table 8.3 Chiron classification

Type	Description
Type I	Osteochondral fragment
Type II	1/4th head fragment
Type III	1/3rd head fragment
Type IV	1/2 head fragment
Type V	Superior collapse
Group A	Isolated
Group B	With acetabular fracture
Group C	With femoral neck fracture

Type III fractures are the rarest among Pipkin types, with an incidence of approximately 8.6% [6].

In 1987, Brumback et al. proposed a more detailed classification, considering factors like joint instability, direction of dislocation, and severity of associated acetabular fractures. They categorized ipsilateral femoral head and neck fractures as type 3B [21] (Table 8.2).

In 2013, Chiron introduced a CT-based classification, focusing on the size of the femoral head fragment and grouping fractures based on associated acetabular or neck fractures. Ipsilateral head and neck fractures fall into group C [22] (Table 8.3).

Table 8.4 AO/OTA classification of the femoral head

Type	Description
31C1	Split fracture
31C1.1	Ligamentum teres avulsion
31C1.2	Infra-foveal split fracture
31C1.3	Supra-foveal fracture
31C2	Depression fracture
31C2.1	Chondral lesion
31C2.2	Impaction fracture
31C2.3	Split depression fracture

The AO/OTA classification describes femoral head fractures as either split or depression fractures but does not specifically address the combination of ipsilateral head and neck fractures [23] (Table 8.4).

While Pipkin's classification remains the most widely used, it lacks detail on fragment size, joint instability, and acetabular involvement. Brumback's classification addresses these gaps, providing better prognostic value [6, 24].

8.4 Blood Supply

The femoral head primarily receives its blood supply through retrograde circulation, predominantly from the medial circumflex femoral artery (MCFA), with additional contributions from the lateral circumflex femoral artery (LCFA). Both arteries originate from the profunda femoris branch of the femoral artery. The antegrade blood supply is provided by the foveal artery (or artery of ligamentum teres), which is a branch of the obturator artery.

The larger, deep branch of the MCFA and the smaller, ascending branch of the LCFA anastomose at the base of the femoral neck to form the extracapsular arterial ring [25]. From this ring, four ascending cervical or retinacular vessels—anterior, posterior, medial, and lateral—travel along the surface of the femoral neck. Among these, the lateral retinacular vessels are the most clinically significant. These retinacular vessels contribute to the formation of a subsynovial intracapsular arterial plexus as they approach the articular surface of the femoral head.

From this arterial plexus, medial and lateral epiphyseal vessels arise, penetrating the femoral head. The lateral epiphyseal vessels, in particular, anastomose with the medial epiphyseal vessels and metaphyseal vessels to supply the majority of the femoral head, accounting for approximately two-thirds of its blood supply, with a minor contribution from the artery of ligamentum teres [26, 27].

The anatomical proximity of the lateral retinacular vessels to the femoral neck renders them susceptible to injury during trauma, forceful reduction maneuvers, or surgical interventions. Disruption of these vessels is a significant risk factor for avascular necrosis (AVN) of the femoral head, especially in cases of Pipkin type III fractures, which are associated with a high likelihood of compromised blood supply [11, 12].

8.5 Clinical Presentation

8.5.1 History

The evaluation of a patient with any fracture-dislocation involving the hip joint begins with a thorough history and documentation of the injury mechanism [6]. Patients typically report pain in the hip joint accompanied by restricted movement. It is crucial to ascertain whether the patient was able to stand, bear weight, or ambulate following the injury. Additionally, document whether any manipulation was performed at the injury site before reaching the healthcare facility.

Understanding the magnitude of trauma can provide insights into the possibility of associated polytrauma, which may require prioritization over musculoskeletal injuries during resuscitation. Pre-injury ambulatory status, existing comorbidities, current medications (including anticoagulants), and relevant medical history such as cancer or pulmonary embolism should be meticulously recorded. This comprehensive history lays the groundwork for effective examination and management.

8.6 Examination

8.6.1 Inspection

In cases of Pipkin type III fracture-dislocation, the limb's attitude often deviates from that typically seen in a posterior hip dislocation. While the dislocated femoral head may rest posteriorly against the acetabular edge, the fracture of the femoral neck disrupts continuity. As a result, the usual presentation of internal rotation, adduction, and limb shortening seen in posterior dislocations may not be evident. Instead, with a completely displaced femoral neck fracture, the limb may appear shortened and externally rotated.

In cases where the femoral neck fracture is undisplaced, the clinical picture may mimic that of an isolated hip dislocation, with the femoral head positioned at the acetabular rim [13]. The extent and pattern of injury marks, abrasions, bruises, and swelling should be correlated with the severity of trauma. Pay attention to tell-tale signs such as knee injuries indicative of dashboard impact or heel injuries suggestive of falls from height or motor vehicle accidents [6, 7, 28].

8.6.2 Palpation

Gentle palpation of the hip region often reveals tenderness. The dislocated femoral head may be palpable as a globular mass in the buttock. However, assessing limb movement or range should be avoided to prevent exacerbating the injury. The heel-palm test may indicate a femoral neck fracture. Care should be taken to avoid displacing an undisplaced femoral neck fracture during reduction maneuvers [13].

8.6.3 Neurological and Vascular Assessment

Thoroughly document the status of distal neurovascular structures. Special attention should be given to the sciatic nerve, as it is commonly affected in Pipkin type III fracture-dislocations [3, 11, 18]. Any signs of neurological impairment or vascular compromise must be promptly identified and addressed.

This structured approach ensures a comprehensive evaluation, aiding in accurate diagnosis and optimal management of these complex injuries.

Patients with fracture-dislocations of the hip should always be evaluated for associated injuries, particularly pelvic and acetabular fractures, knee joint injuries, and trauma to the head, chest, and pelvis, which are frequently encountered in motor vehicle accidents. In such cases, resuscitation should follow the ATLS protocol when indicated. For patients presenting after a significant fall from height, assessment should focus on potential injuries to the heels, ankle joints, lumbosacral spine, and cervical spine [6, 7, 28].

8.6.4 Diagnostic Workup

Ipsilateral femoral head and neck fracture-dislocations are rare and present diagnostic challenges. Initial imaging should include plain radiographs of the pelvis in AP view and frog-leg lateral projections of the proximal femur. If the diagnosis remains uncertain, additional views such as Judet oblique, inlet, and outlet projections are recommended.

A high-resolution CT scan is the gold standard for diagnosis and treatment planning. It provides critical information about fracture morphology, displacement, comminution, head impaction against the acetabular rim, intra-articular fragments, and reduction congruency. CT scans are ideally performed both post-injury and post-osteosynthesis. In certain cases, MRI is useful to detect non-congruent reduction and joint instability caused by interposed labral or chondral fragments [4, 23].

For a comprehensive medical evaluation, laboratory tests such as complete blood count, renal and liver function tests, metabolic panels, coagulation profiles, chest X-ray (CXR), and ECG are required for pre-anesthetic preparation. In elderly patients, additional cardiology and pulmonology assessments may be necessary to ensure optimal preoperative status.

8.6.5 Prognosis

Pipkin type III fracture-dislocations have the poorest prognosis among the Pipkin classifications due to their complex fracture morphology [29]. These injuries result from high-energy trauma and often involve significant damage to surrounding soft tissues. The anatomical location of the blood vessels along the femoral neck makes them highly susceptible to injury, frequently resulting in osteonecrosis of the femoral head [6, 11, 32].

Vascular damage can be exacerbated by iatrogenic factors during reduction or surgical fixation [15]. Additionally, the complexity of these fractures makes achieving anatomical reduction and stable fixation challenging, with high rates of fixation failure [13, 37]. This underscores the need for meticulous surgical planning and technique to optimize outcomes.

8.7 Management

Being a rare injury, the management protocol of type III Pipkins fracture dislocation is still controversial. Initial treatment is aimed at early attempt to reduce the joint as soon as possible to alleviate pain and lower the chances of avascular necrosis of the head of the femur [1, 6]. Reduction is done under anesthesia with adequate analgesia. In difficult irreducible dislocations, the dislocated head is often stuck at the sharp edge of acetabular wall as observed by Park et al. in their study. They experienced that further forceful attempts to reduce the joint led to occurrence of fresh fracture of the neck of the femur in five out nine patients who initially had fracture of the femur head with posterior dislocation. Therefore, in irreducible dislocations, low threshold toward open reduction of the joint is recommended in such cases [13, 15].

The choice of definitive treatment in the form of osteosynthesis or primary total hip replacement depends on the fracture morphology, associated injuries, quality of bone, age of the patient, and the surgeon's preference. Droll et al. stated that the decision of osteosynthesis depends on the size and location of the femoral head fracture fragment along with degree of comminution. Observation by Henle et al. suggested that fracture fragments of the femoral head of size less than 1 cm or fragments in the non-weight-bearing zone of the head can be safely excised, otherwise, anatomic reduction and osteosynthesis is preferred [33]. While considering open reduction and internal fixation as the initial treatment, the time taken from injury to the reduction of joint becomes important [38]. A meta-analysis report by Ahmed et al. and work by Giannoudis observed that prolonged dislocations cause vasospasm and increase in intracapsular pressure which results in damage to the blood vessels supplying the head of the femur and progression to osteonecrosis of the femur head [34]. Hip joint reduction done within 6 h of dislocation reduces the chances of developing osteonecrosis from 15.6% to 5.1% as shown by Wang et al. [35]. For open reduction and fracture fixation of Pipkin type III fracture dislocation, either anterior or posterior approach may be used. With the anterior approach, there is lesser damage to the blood vessels supplying the femoral head but is associated with higher incidence of developing heterotopic ossification [13, 36]. Zhao et al. observed that the anterior approach is more suitable for Pipkin type I and II fracture dislocations than the more complex type III. Similarly, Park et al. stated that it is difficult to approach an irreducible hip dislocation by the anterior approach, where the head of the femur is stuck against the acetabular wall. Standard posterior Kocher-Langenbeck approach gives good exposure but is associated with damage to vascularity and higher incidence of osteonecrosis of the femur head [24, 33]. Ganz et al. described a novel posterior-based approach of safe surgical dislocation with flip osteotomy of the greater trochanter using either Gibson or Kocher-Langenbeck approach. It gives 360° access to the femoral head and acetabulum during surgery. Ganz et al. found no radiological evidence of osteonecrosis of the femur head in 213 cases operated by this approach during postoperative follow-up ranging from a period of 2–7 years [38]. Although this approach carries a risk of heterotopic ossification and non-union of the trochanteric osteotomy, with excellent exposure of the joint, it is the preferred approach for osteosynthesis in Pipkin type III injuries [30, 38]. Nevertheless, due to the complex nature of fracture, reconstruction is often difficult, and further damage to the vascularity is imperative. The results of ORIF are unpredictable, and the incidence of osteonecrosis is high even after the best possible effort. Mukhopadhaya et al. observed a good functional outcome at 5 years follow-up in a 25-year-old patient with Pipkin type III injury, managed by open reduction and internal fixation. On the contrary, Scolaro et al. reported the development of osteonecrosis of the head of the femur in six out of the seven cases of Pipkin type III, operated with open reduction and internal fixation [29]. Tonetti et al. performed THA in three out of the four cases due to development of osteonecrosis following initial open reduction and internal fixation [37]. Park et al. reported iatrogenic Pipkin type III fractures in five of the nine cases. They did primary THA in three and treated two with open reduction and internal fixation. Both these patients in the osteosynthesis group were converted to delayed THA later due to non-union and osteonecrosis of the head [13]. Failure rate of 58% was experienced in the open reduction and internal fixation group by Shanxi et al. in 12 patients with Pipkin type III who underwent THA later due to failed fixation and osteonecrosis [31]. Therefore, several authors have advocated that primary treatment with total hip arthroplasty becomes a preferred choice of treatment in Pipkin type III fracture dislocation [1, 32, 39]. Studies by Healy et al. and Wani et al. have stressed on the suboptimal functional outcomes in THA done after previous osteosynthesis for displaced neck fractures when compared to primary THA [40, 41]. Even then, these fracture dislocations are mostly seen in the younger age group with average age of patient being around 38.9 years; initial treatment should be aimed at joint preservation [5, 6, 19]. Multiple studies carried out by Swaroop et al. have reported a 20 years survivorship of prosthesis to be around 41–66% after THA in patients less than 35 years [42–44]. Therefore, literature is still vague, with no clear guidelines regarding the standard treatment options in the young adults where this injury is most commonly seen [31, 32]. Therefore, in younger patients with Pipkin type III, open reduction and internal fixation may be recommended as the first line of treatment, with proper counselling regarding chances of developing complications and possible conversion to THA later. In contrast, primary THA is a more suitable treatment option in the elderly patients with good functional outcomes [6, 10, 11, 13, 31, 33].

8.7.1 Author's Preference

A quick general assessment and resuscitation as per the trauma protocol is carried in the emergency department upon receiving any patient with hip dislocation. Relevant investigations are done both for diagnosis and treatment planning. These injuries are invariably associated with posterior dislocation of the hip joint for which open reduction is done. In young patients, hip preservation surgery is advised with thorough counselling regarding all the possible complications, whereas in patients above 50 years, primary total hip arthroplasty is preferred.

8.7.1.1 Open Reduction and Internal Fixation

With the patient in lateral decubitus position, posterior-based Kocher-Langenbeck approach to hip joint is used. The surgery is aimed at reduction of the hip joint followed by reduction and fixation of the fracture head and neck of the femur. The fragments of the femoral head are identified, and anatomical reduction is done using screws. In case there is difficulty in reducing the fracture fragments in situ, the reconstruction of the head may be carried outside on the table. Once the reconstruction of the femur head is complete, it is aligned, and anatomical reduction with the neck of the femur is achieved. Fixation of the fracture neck of the femur is done using cancellous screws. To aid anatomical fixation, sometimes, retrograde drilling of the neck of the femur may be done followed by antegrade insertion of the screws. Femoral head fracture fragments not involving the weight-bearing area and less than 1 cm in size may be excised (Fig. 8.1).

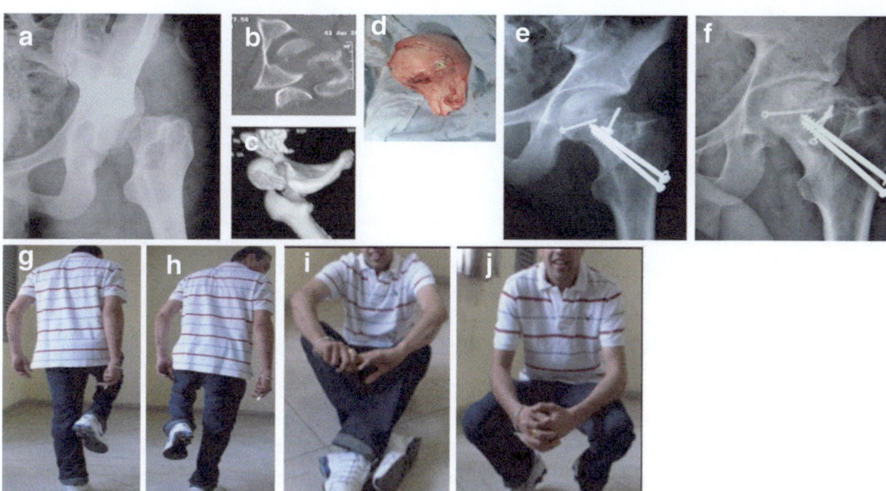

Fig. 8.1 (**a**) Left-sided fracture of the femur head and neck with hip dislocation in a 26-year-old male. (**b**) Axial CT section shows dislocated femoral head and fracture neck of the femur. (**c**) 3D-CT scan image of the fracture. (**d**) Reconstruction of the femur head on the OT table. (**e**) Reconstruction of the femur head and neck. (**f**) Five-year follow-up radiograph shows avascular necrosis and joint collapse; however, the patient is able to manage most of his daily activities (**g**, standing; **h**, weight-bearing; **i**, cross-leg sitting: **j**, squatting)

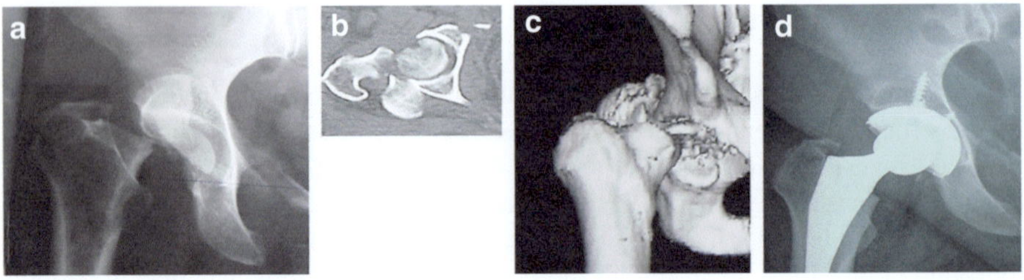

Fig. 8.2 (**a**) Fracture femur head and neck with hip dislocation in a 58-year-old man. (**b**) Axial CT section of the hip. (**c**) 3D-CT scan image of the fracture. (**d**) Primary total hip arthroplasty was performed

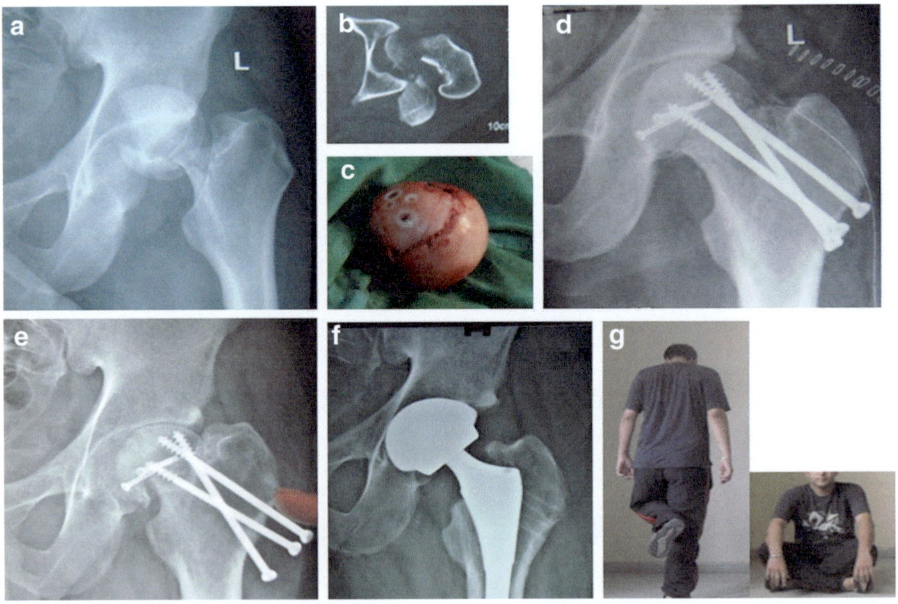

Fig. 8.3 (**a**) Fracture femur head and neck with hip dislocation in a19-year-old adult. (**b**) Axial CT section. (**c**) Reconstruction of the femur head was done on the OT table. (**d**) Reduction and fixation of the fracture head and neck of the femur. (**e**) Two years later, osteonecrosis of the femoral head with collapse occurred. (**f**) Delayed total hip arthroplasty. (**g**) Functional outcome

8.7.1.2 Total Hip Arthroplasty

In badly comminuted fractures of the head of the femur those are not amenable to reconstruction and in patients above 50 years of age, primary total hip arthroplasty is the preferred treatment with desirable functional outcome (Fig. 8.2). Delayed hip arthroplasty is done for failed reduction, non-union, osteonecrosis of femoral head, or secondary osteoarthrosis of the hip joint after open reduction and internal fixation (Fig. 8.3).

8.8 Summary

Motor vehicle accidents and fall from height are the most common mechanisms causing these fracture dislocations. A detailed and careful clinical assessment, supplemented with relevant investigations in the form of X-rays, CT scans, and 3D reconstruction images, is important for classifying these injuries. A high degree of suspicion is recommended while diagnosing such rare injury types. The management in the form of open reduction and internal fixation or primary total hip arthroplasty is based mainly upon the fracture morphology, any associated injuries, bone quality, age of the patient, and surgeons' preference. A poor outcome of open reduction and internal fixation has shifted the focus toward primary total hip arthroplasty especially in the elderly [31]. In contrast, in the younger population, considering the longevity of total hip arthroplasty prosthesis, fracture osteosynthesis may be recommended. With high complication rates involved in open reduction and internal fixation surgery, the importance of counselling the patient regarding the future need for total hip arthroplasty is crucial [19, 31].

References

1. Hougaard K, Thomsen PB. Traumatic posterior fracture-dislocation of the hip with fracture of the femoral head or neck, or both. J Bone Joint Surg Am. 1988;70-A:233–9.
2. Epstein HC, Wiss DA, Cozen L. Posterior fracture dislocation of the hip with fractures of the femoral head. Clin Orthop Relat Res. 1985;201:9–17.
3. Roeder LF Jr, DeLee JC. Femoral head fractures associated with posterior hip dislocation. Clin Orthop Relat Res. 1980;147:121–30.
4. Droll KP, Broekhuyse H, O'Brien P. Fracture of the femoral head. J Am Acad Orthop Surg. 2007;15(12):716–27. https://doi.org/10.5435/00124635-200712000-00005.
5. Alonso JE, Volgas DA, Giordano V, Stannard JP. A review of the treatment of hip dislocations associated with acetabular fractures. Clin Orthop Relat Res. 2000;377:32–43.
6. Giannoudis PV, Kontakis G, Christoforakis Z, Akula M, Tosounidis T, Koutras C. Management, complications and clinical results of femoral head fractures. Injury. 2009;40(12):1245–51.
7. Enocson A, Wolf O. Pipkin fractures: epidemiology and outcome. Eur J Trauma Emerg Surg. 2022;48(5):4113–8.
8. Birkett J. Description of a dislocation of the head of the femur, complicated with its fracture; with remarks. 1869. Clin Orthop Relat Res. 2007;458:10–1.
9. Gullberg B, Johnell O, Kanis JA. World-wide projections for hip fracture. Osteoporos Int. 1997;7:407–13. https://doi.org/10.1007/PL00004148.
10. Pipkin G. Treatment of grade IV fracture-dislocation of the hip. J Bone Joint Surg Am. 1957;39-A:1027–42.
11. Marchetti ME, Steinberg GG, Coumas JM. Intermediate-term experience of Pipkin fracture-dislocations of the hip. J Orthop Trauma. 1996;10(7):455–61. https://doi.org/10.1097/00005131-199610000-00002.
12. Romeo NM, Firoozabadi R. Classifications in brief: the Pipkin classification of femoral head fractures. Clin Orthop Relat Res. 2018;476:1114–9.
13. Park K, Kim J, Oh C, Kim J, Oh J, Kyung H. A treatment strategy to avoid iatrogenic Pipkin type III femoral head fracture-dislocations. Arch Orthop Trauma Surg. 2016;136(8):1107–13. https://doi.org/10.1007/s00402-016-2481-1.

14. Upadhyay SS, Moulton A, Burwell RG. Biological factors predisposing to traumatic posterior dislocation of the hip: a selection process in the mechanism of injury. J Bone Joint Surg (Br). 1985;67-B:232–6.
15. Keong MW, Razak H, Koon WM, Ping CC. Case report of a rare Pipkin type III femoral head fracture. J Orthop Case Rep. 2019;9:11–5.
16. Thompson VP, Epstein HC. Traumatic dislocation of the hip: a survey of two hundred and four cases covering a period of twenty-one years. J Bone Joint Surg Am. 1951;33-A:746–78.
17. Alice W, et al. Pipkin IV fracture dislocation of the hip in a football athlete—a case report. Trauma Case Rep. 2024;52:101072.
18. Nolte P-C, et al. Reconstruction of a fracture of the posterior acetabular wall with Pipkin fracture and lesion of the sciatic nerve after dorsal hip dislocation. Unfallchirurg. 2020;123(5):413–8.
19. Mukhopadhaya J, et al. Functional outcome of Pipkin type III fracture managed by osteosynthesis through trochanteric flip osteotomy in a young patient after 5 years follow-up—a case report and literature review. J Orthop Case Rep. 2021;11(8):101–6.
20. Stewart MJ, Milford LW. Fracture-dislocation of the hip: an end-result study. J Bone Joint Surg Am. 1954;36-A:315–42.
21. Brumback RJ, Kenzora JE, Levitt LE, Burgess AR, Poka A. Fractures of the femoral head. Hip. 1987:181–206.
22. Chiron P, Lafontan V, Reina N. Fracture-dislocations of the femoral head. Orthop Traumatol Surg Res. 2013;99:S53.
23. Muller ME, Nazarian S. Classification of fractures of the femur and its use in the AO. Rev Chir Orthop Reparatrice Appar Mot. 1981;67:297–309.
24. Stannard JP, Harris HW, Volgas DA, Alonso JE. Functional outcome of patients with femoral head fractures associated with hip dislocations. Clin Orthop Relat Res. 2000;377:44–56.
25. Gray H. Anatomy of the human body. 20th ed. Philadelphia: Lea and Febiger; 1918.
26. Chung S. The arterial supply of the developing proximal end of the human femur. J Bone Joint Surg Am. 1976;58-A:961–70.
27. Elizabeth OJ, et al. Vascular anatomy and microcirculation of skeletal zones vulnerable to osteonecrosis: vascularization of the femoral head. Orthop Clin N Am. 2004;35:285–91.
28. Bettinelli G, Placella G, Moharamzadeh D, Belluati A, Salini V. Articular femoral head fracture management: a meta-analysis of literature. Indian J Orthop. 2021;55(Suppl 2):304–13.
29. Scolaro JA, Marecek G, Firoozabadi R, Krieg JC, Routt MLC. Management and radiographic outcomes of femoral head fractures. J Orthop Traumatol. 2017;18(3):235–41. https://doi.org/10.1007/s10195-017-0445-z.
30. De Mauro D, Rovere G, Smakaj A, et al. Gibson approach and surgical hip dislocation according to Ganz in the treatment of femoral head fractures. BMC Musculoskelet Disord. 2021;22(S2):961.
31. Wang S, Xiaojun Y, Li B. Pipkin type III femoral head fracture: which treatment strategy can be recommended? J Orthop Traumatol. 2023;24:28.
32. Lederer S, Tauber M, Karpik S, Bogner R, Uffarth AA, Resch H. Fractures of the femoral head. A multicenter study. Unfallchirurg. 2007;110(6):513–20. https://doi.org/10.1007/s00113-007-1246-2.
33. Henle P, Kloen P, Siebenrock KA. Femoral head injuries: which treatment strategy can be recommended? Injury. 2007;38-A(4):478–88.
34. Ahmed G, Shiraz S, Riaz M, Ibrahim T. Late versus early reduction in traumatic hip dislocations: a meta-analysis. Eur J Orthop Surg Traumatol. 2017;27(8):1109–16.
35. Wang SX, Li BH, Zhang ZD, Yu XJ, Liu L. Early versus delayed hip reduction in treating femoral head fracture combined with posterior hip dislocation: a comparative study. BMC Musculoskelet Disord. 2021;22(1):1057.
36. Zhao B, Li H, Yan J, Han LR, Yang XF. Pipkin type III femoral head fracture-dislocation combined with complicated acetabular fracture: a rare case report and literature review. Medicine. 2017;96(50):e9214.

37. Tonetti J, Ruatti S, Lafontan V, Loubignac F, Chiron P, Sari-Ali H, et al. Is femoral head fracture-dislocation management improvable: a retrospective study in 110 cases. Orthop Traumatol Surg Res. 2010;96:623–31.
38. Ganz R, Gill TJ, Gautier E, Ganz K, Krugel N, Berlemann U. Surgical dislocation of the adult hip a technique with full access to the femoral head and acetabulum without the risk of avascular necrosis. J Bone Joint Surg Br. 2001;83(8):1119–24.
39. Tosounidis T, Aderinto J, Giannoudis PV. Pipkin type-III fractures of the femoral head: fix it or replace it? Injury. 2017;48(11):2375–8.
40. Healy WL, Iorio R. Total hip arthroplasty: optimal treatment for displaced femoral neck fractures in elderly patients. Clin Orthop Relat Res. 2004;429(429):43–8.
41. Wani IH, Sharma S, Latoo I, Salaria AQ, Jan M. Primary total hip arthroplasty versus internal fixation in displaced fracture of femoral neck in sexa- and septuagenarians. J Orthop Traumatol. 2014;15(3):209–14.
42. Swarup I, Shields M, Mayer EN, Hendow CJ, Burket JC, Figgie MP. Outcomes after total hip arthroplasty in young patients with osteonecrosis of the hip. Hip Int. 2017;27(3):286–92.
43. Swarup I, Lee YY, Christoph EI, Mandl LA, Goodman SM, Figgie MP. Implant survival and patient-reported outcomes after total hip arthroplasty in young patients with juvenile idiopathic arthritis. J Arthroplast. 2015;30(3):398–402.
44. Swarup I, Sutherland R, Burket JC, Figgie MP. Total hip arthroplasty in young patients with post-traumatic arthritis of the hip. Hip Int. 2017;27(6):546–50.

Femoral Head and Acetabular Fractures (Pipkin Type IV Injuries)

9

Arvind Kumar and Vivek Trikha

9.1 Introduction

Simultaneous femur-head fractures and hip dislocation acetabular fractures are rare and complicated injuries. These difficult injuries occur due to high-energy trauma of both the acetabulum and the femur-head [1]. Their management demands a comprehensive understanding of hip anatomy, meticulous diagnostic evaluation, and a strategic approach to surgical intervention. Despite advances in orthopedic trauma care, these fractures remain associated with significant morbidity due to their complexities and complications [1, 2]. Early and successful treatment, combined with careful postoperative care and rehabilitation, is crucial to maximize functional results and improve the quality of life of the involved patients. Continued research and innovation promise to improve the prognosis and management strategies for this challenging injury. These injuries are classified as type IV under the widely used Pipkin's classification for femur-head fractures [3, 4], and the same classification will be used throughout this chapter as a standard. This chapter delves into the intricacies of Pipkin IV fractures, encompassing their anatomy, classification, mechanisms, clinical presentation, diagnostic approaches, treatment strategies, potential complications, and prognostic factors.

9.2 Epidemiology and Pathophysiology

Femur-head fractures are quite rare forms of injury that occur with considerable force, such as in motor vehicle accidents (dashboard injuries), certain sports, or falling from a significant height. Such injuries have an estimated prevalence of two cases per one million people. However, the growing number of road traffic accidents

A. Kumar · V. Trikha (✉)
JPNATC, AIIMS, New Delhi, India

R. K. Sen, S. K. Tripathy (eds.), *A Practical Guide to Management of Femoral Head Fracture-Dislocation*, https://doi.org/10.1007/978-981-96-9852-3_9

is increasing the incidence of such injuries. Given the rarity of these femoral injuries, accurately estimating the prevalence of type IV Pipkins classification subtypes is nearly impossible. Reported rates of such injuries vary considerably. Enocson et al. [4] noted in their case series that 55% of all head femurs fractures were type IV. Scolaro et al. [5] reported even lesser proportion of type IV fractures in his series (15%). In a systematic review on type IV fractures, Giannoudis et al. [1] also reported a relatively low prevalence (30%).

Historically, the hypothesized mechanism resembles that of hip dislocation where the dashboard impact causes posterior dislocation. Nonetheless, some authors regard it as more related to axial impact to the hip as the driver executes a right foot brake with the hip flexed—adduction and internal rotated [6]. Fracture of the femur-head with hip dislocation fractures is said to result from the combination of shear force and axial force acting on the femur-head. The presence of these forces together with alignment of acetabulum contour determines the existence and site of femur-head fracture [7].

In most high-energy insults, the hip is flexed with some degree of aggressive adduction as well as pulling down along the axis of the body, particularly in dashboard collisions (Fig. 9.1). Generally speaking, in such circumstances, the compression force acts on the femur-head and is almost coincident with the posterior wall articular boundary. Therefore, it results in unobstructed posterior dislocation or a misalignment of compression on the femoral head and posterior wall. If the hip is flexed without adduction, the compressive force acting on the femur-head is perpendicular to the posterior wall. This directional mismatch can result in a variable-size head fragment fracture exiting suprafoveally (Fig. 9.2). Such a force can result in an acetabular fracture or femoral neck fracture as well. Axial stress in an intermediate adduction and variable hip flexion can result in the inferior surface of the femur-head coming in compression over the posterior wall, leading to an infrafoveal

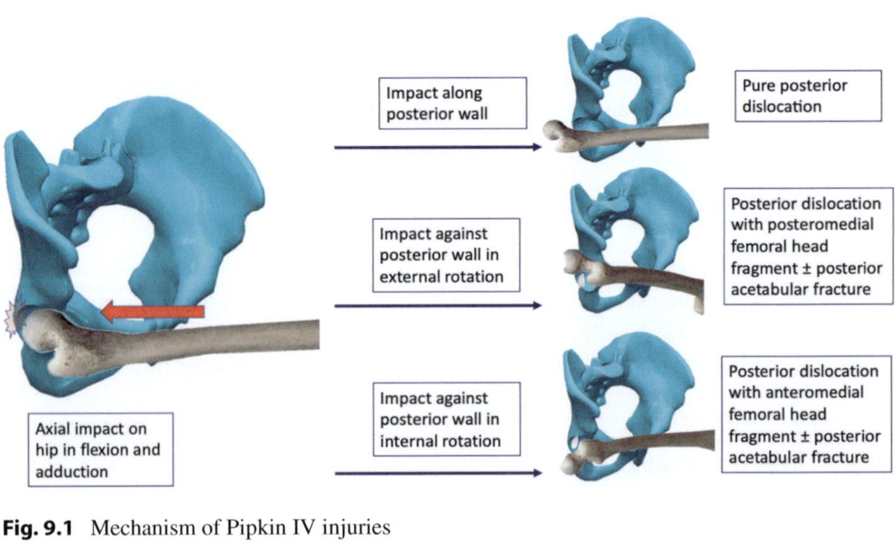

Fig. 9.1 Mechanism of Pipkin IV injuries

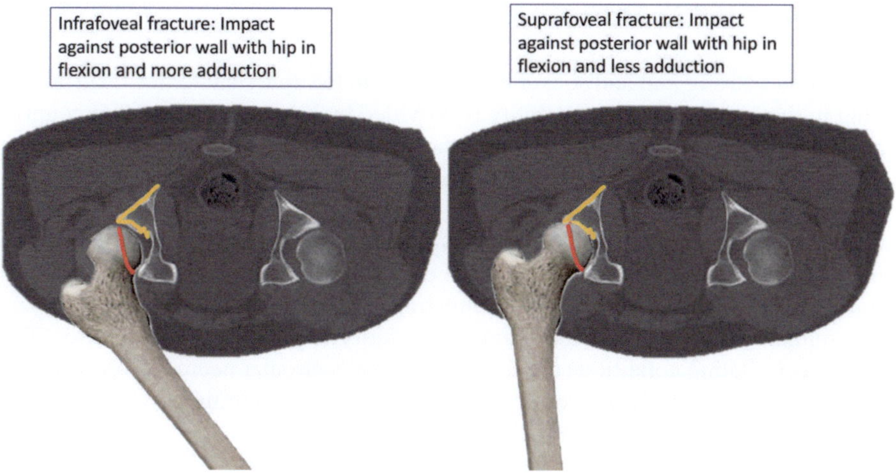

Fig. 9.2 Variation in adduction resulting in changing relation of femur-head fracture concerning the fovea capitis

fractured fragment (Fig. 9.2). In anterior dislocation, the compressive forces onto the femur-head are not likely to correspond with the acetabular lining, which means there is a greater incidence of femur-head fractures. There is also the anterior acetabular rim bearing down on the femur-head, which causes either a fracture or impact injury. Such injury could happen in both anterior and posterior locations depending upon the rotation of the femur-head at the time of impact. An internally rotated position favors anterior fracture, while posterior fracture occurs with external rotation (see Fig. 9.1).

Anterior dislocations make up a meager portion of 7–13% of all hip dislocations. Dislocations can also be iliac and obturator types based on the dislocated position of the femur-head in injury radiographs. The most important mechanism is forceful abduction with some external rotation for anterior dislocation. At high degrees of flexion, the femur-head dislocates under the pubofemoral ligament and settles on the obturator foramen causing an obturator dislocation. In extension, the femur-head dislocates anterosuperiorly between the pubofemoral ligament and iliofemoral ligament forming iliac type-dislocation. Iliac-type dislocations can also be accompanied by an avulsion fracture of the anterior inferior iliac spine from where the iliofemoral ligament originates. Dislocations of the anterior hip typically have a related femur-head fracture, the incidence ranging from 12% to 87% in various series [8, 9]. Nearly 90% of femur-head fractures of anterior dislocation are of obturator-type dislocations.

9.3 Applied Anatomy

Hip joint is a strong ball and socket type joint, with the spherical femur-head articulating in the acetabulum. The stability is provided by bony structures, joint congruency, ligaments, muscles, labrum, and the joint capsule. Although these remain constant for hip dislocations and most femur-head fractures, the important anatomical issue in Pipkin IV injuries is the femur-head blood supply which can be compromised due to energy impact and hip dislocation. This would require extra care keeping in mind the requirement of large exposure for acetabular and femur-head injuries which are often in opposite directions. It means the acetabular injury is predominantly posterior and the femur-head injury is predominantly anterior. The most incapacitating conditions of these injuries are avascular necrosis (AVN) of the femur-head, followed by heterotrophic ossification and posttraumatic arthritis. The clinical prognosis is poorer in Pipkin IV injuries [1, 2].

The critical blood supply to the femur-head, particularly the weight-bearing segment, comes from the medial femoral circumflex artery [10]. The medial epiphyseal artery and the lateral femoral circumflex artery provide insignificant femur-head blood supply. The medial femoral circumflex artery's deep branch typically arising from the profunda femoris provides numerous muscular branches, and the major vessel which supplies the femur-head passes posterior to obturator externus tendon. It enters the hip capsule slightly proximal to the insertion of superior gemellus and branches out into various end branches. These branches run beneath the synovium down the posterosuperior surface of the femoral neck and enter the femur-head lateral to the articular junction. It is quite simple to injure this vessel when working with the posterior capsule and making a capsular incision along the posterosuperior aspect of the femoral neck. Surgical dissection over the femur-head needs to be done taking care not to expose the key posterosuperior capsule where the dominant vascularity to the femur-head exists. Epstein et al. [11] conjectured that an anterior approach will compromise the critical femur-head vascularity as the posterior elements had already been weakened. But now, it has been determined that by approaching posteriorly, the femur-head AVN risk is higher. Therefore, respecting the vascular anatomy of the femur-head with meticulous capsulotomy regardless of the approach becomes necessary [1].

9.4 Clinical Evaluation

Pipkin Type IV fractures by are most complicated as these involve both acetabulum and femur-head and scarcely the femoral neck, hence demanding a complex approach to treatment. Femur-head fracture dislocations are an orthopedic emergency. Early clinical evaluation and reduction is a priority to minimize the risk of early and long-term complications. Life-threatening injuries should be addressed first. Patients with femur-head fracture dislocations, such as Pipkin IV fractures, would present with symptoms akin to the hip dislocation and other forms of femur-head fractures. These include:

- Severe Hip Pain: Frequently immediate and severe after trauma.
- Affected Limb Movements: Secondary to pain and mechanical disruption of the joint.
- Visible Deformity: Shortening of the limb, adducted-internal rotated limb in posterior dislocations. Extension and external rotation of the hip in iliac-type dislocation and flexed—abducted and external rotated hip in obturator-type dislocations.
- Neurovascular Compromise: Includes sciatic nerve damage, manifesting as numbness, weakness, or lower limb paralysis
- Associated Injuries: Because of the high-energy impact of the injury, there may be additional injuries present, and these need to be diagnosed early.

9.5 Radiologic Evaluation

These also involve initial imaging of anteroposterior and lateral views of the involved hip to detect dislocations and relevant fractures.

Findings on imaging of a Pipkin IV fracture are typically:

(a) Femur-Head Fracture: Fracture through the femur-head, usually in the region of the fovea (where ligament teres is attached), seen on anteroposterior (AP) and lateral hip radiographs as loss of femur-head sphericity. Displacement of fragments may be apparent, depending on severity. In some cases, there can be associated ipsilateral femoral neck fracture.
(b) Femoral Neck Fracture: Though uncommon in Pipkin type IV injuries, this may be possible where improper reduction methods have been employed.
(c) Acetabular Fracture: There is an acetabular fracture (most commonly the posterior wall) on radiographs. Special views (Judet views) may be requested to evaluate the acetabular fracture. The fracture is primarily a part of the posterior acetabular rim or extends into the weight-bearing zone of the acetabulum. Anterior acetabular rim involvement rarely occurs in anterior dislocations.
(d) Hip Dislocation: The dislocations in Pipkin IV fractures are primarily posterior hip dislocations and very infrequently the anterior ones. This is visible on radiographs as a protrusion of the femur-head out of the acetabulum on X-ray and broken Shenton's line.
(e) Joint Congruity: The joint congruity of the articular surface of the femur-head and acetabulum can be disturbed. X-rays will reveal the loss of congruity of a normal joint.

On post-reduction films of hip dislocation, we must evaluate the alignment of the femur-head, joint reduction, and the fracture fragment position.

Computed tomography (CT) scan allows for clear imaging of fracture patterns, particularly complex acetabular fractures, making surgical planning possible. The CT scan is most often done following the closed reduction. It may be requested ahead of the reduction in cases of irreducible dislocations or closed reduction avoidance (iatrogenic or associated ipsilateral femoral neck fracture), which necessitates an open reduction method [12, 13]. Three-dimensional reconstructions facilitate preoperative planning as well as a comprehension of spatial fracture relation. The dissociated femur-head fragment can displace anomalously within the hip joint and become incongruent even after reduction of the hip. Often, the posterior wall/acetabular rim fragments can be trapped within the joint space and are hard to detect on radiographs. Computed tomography aids in determining the direction and site of the femur-head fracture line, particularly regarding fovea capitis. The femur-head fragmentation is hard to diagnose on radiographs, and CT gives a clear picture. The CT scan reveals the location of any fragments of the femur-head or acetabular rim and their position in relation to the acetabulum, including the extent of displacement or impaction and secondary fracture lines which can be obscured on radiographs.

There can be damage to the cartilage of the acetabulum or femur-head, and chondral fractures can be present that are not apparent in radiographs or CT scans. In addition, labral tears associated with these injuries may be present and not visible on radiographs or CT scans. Magnetic Resonance Imaging (MRI) can diagnose these pathologies, but no such defined role exists in managing these injuries.

9.6 Treatment

After the life-threatening injuries have been treated and the patient is hemodynamically stable, clinical and radiological evaluation for the femur-head fracture-dislocation must be done. While in geriatric patients, such an injury should ideally be treated with an early joint replacement surgery, in young patients, immediate reduction in the emergency department must be done [4]. There is a straight correlation between delayed reduction and higher occurrence of osteonecrosis of the femur-head, particularly in case the delay exceeds 6 hours [14]. Axial traction is maintained along the femoral axis with the hip slowly flexed to 90 degrees and in adducted and internal rotated position in posterior dislocations with smooth rotatory movements (Fig. 9.3a) [14]. In the majority of anterior hip dislocation cases, traction along with deformity is generally required. For iliac-type anterior dislocations, inline traction on the femur, extension of the hip, and external rotation are necessary (Fig. 9.3b). For obturator-type dislocations, hyperextension is also necessary (Fig. 9.3c). Reduction is felt as a palpable pop at the hip joint with restoration of deformity and limb length. In case of failure of reduction, there is a possibility that the method might be improper. Particularly in the case of Pipkin IV injury, the reduction must correct two elements, i.e., the femur-head fracture and the hip dislocation. The closed reduction can only handle the hip dislocation element. The detached femur-head fragment can become reduced with hip reduction, rotate in the axial plane, and even flip upside down. The femur-head fracture component of the displaced position can be corrected only by open reduction. To maintain reduction of a posterior dislocation irrespective of associated fracture of the posterior column, any axial stress on the posterior structures must be avoided. Therefore, traction in extended position will be helpful and flexion must be avoided. In the case of anterior

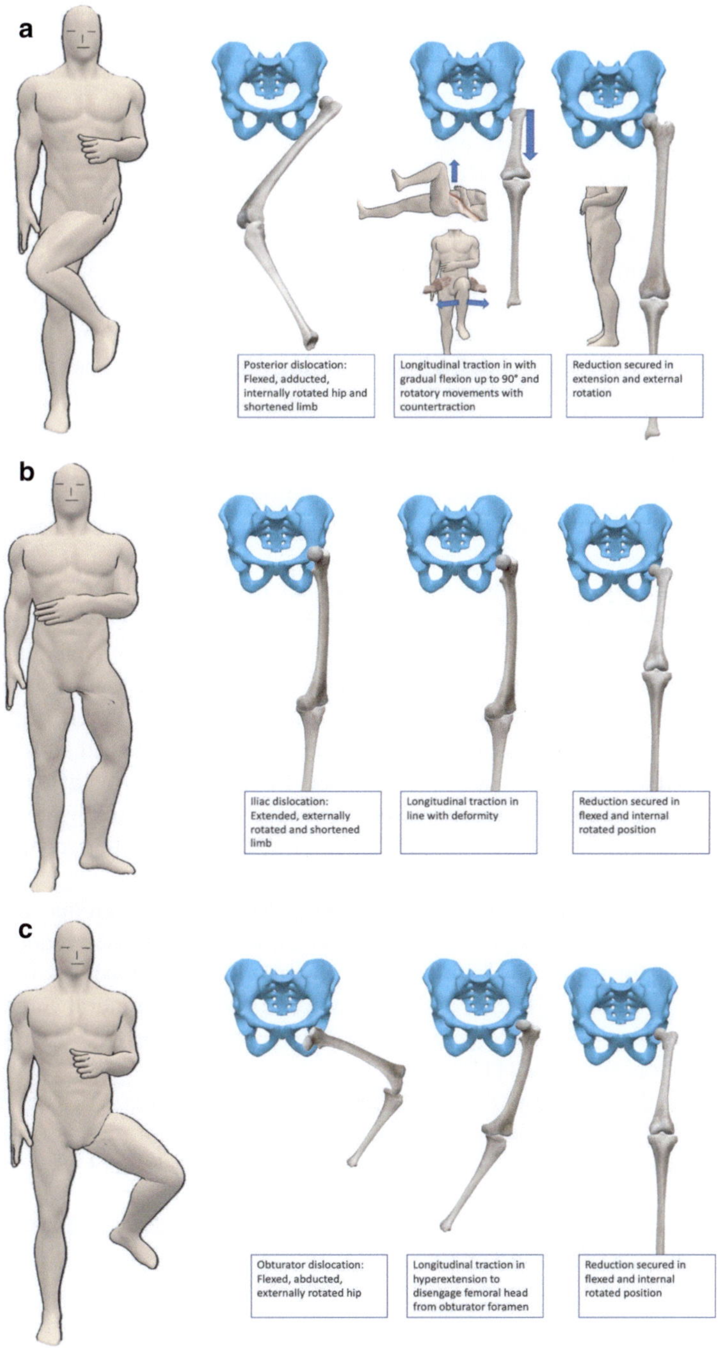

Fig. 9.3 (**a**) Posterior hip dislocation and its reduction maneuver. (**b**) Iliac-type anterior dislocation of the hip and its reduction maneuver. (**c**) Obturator-type anterior dislocation and its reduction maneuver

dislocations with or without fractures of the anterior column, stress must be avoided on the anterior structures, and hence, traction in flexion with the aid of a Bohler Braun splint must be continued.

Reduction should be done in emergency department under proper analgesia. In cases with facility, sedation or anesthesia may be employed to facilitate relaxation of muscles around the hip. Reduction is challenging when there is impaction between the posterior acetabular wall and the femur-head. Posterior acetabular wall notch may be produced by femur-head impact, thus making closed reduction challenging. Frequently, the proximal femur herinates into the superior-posterior gap between the acetabular rim and the labrum, and hence, closed reduction is not possible. Other reasons for irreducibility are interposition of piriformis, ligamentum teres, labrum, and, on occasion, buttonholing through the posterior capsule. Occasionally, rotation of the head fragment around the ligamentum teres and osteochondral fragment blocks the reduction. These patients are candidates for urgent open reduction and fracture fixation.

Also, one should be cautious about the femoral neck for any fracture (post-reduction or post-injury), and a computed tomography scan could be prescribed first if there is still doubt [13]. The cases with related neck femur fractures should be managed better by open reduction and internal fixation. Closed reduction could further displace the femoral neck fracture, which could further complicate the fracture and further increase the risk of osteonecrosis. Therefore, such patients are indicated for urgent open reduction. For those with unstable reduction with a high tendency to redislocate, temporary skeletal traction can be offered, followed by early open reduction and fixation. After reduction has been achieved, post-reduction radiographs, including the special views used for acetabular fracture assessment, can be obtained. The ultimate management of femur-head fracture dislocations is to have an anatomically reduced femur-head and acetabulum with a congruent and stable reduction.

This can be done either operatively or nonoperatively in certain instances [1, 2]. Nonoperative treatment can be undertaken when, following closed reduction, anatomic or near anatomic reduction (<2 mm step) of the femur-head fragment is obtained, the hip joint is stable, and no interposed bony or chondral fragments are present to interfere with a congruent reduction. About 10% of type IV injuries can be managed nonoperatively [1].

Still, given the precarious nature of Pipkin IV injuries, potential loss of reduction on follow-up and morbidities of being bedridden for a long duration, an operation is preferred. Indications for surgical intervention are listed in Table 9.1.

9.7 Surgical Approaches

Various surgical approaches have been suggested for the treatment of femur-head fractures, such as anterior (Smith-Petersen), posterior (Kocher-Langenbeck), anterolateral (Watson-Jones), and medial (Ludloff) [1]. The anterior and posterior approaches are the popular approaches used in such injuries. Alexander Gibson had

Table 9.1 Indications for surgical management in Pipkin IV injuries

1.	Nonanatomic reduction of the femur-head fragment
2.	Unstable hip joint
3.	Noncongruent joint
4.	Incarcerated bone/chondral fragments
5.	Fracture extending to weight-bearing zone

already described the posterior approach in hip fractures in 1950 which was almost like the Kocher-Langenbeck approach but through a more anterior interval [15]. Moed adapted the Gibson technique with a straight skin incision for improved exposure of the anterosuperior acetabulum, blood supply preservation to the anterior half of the gluteus maximus, and also minimizing the risk of iatrogenic injury to the sciatic nerve [8]. The anterior hip approach was originally described in 1881 by German surgeon Carl Hueter as a muscle-sparing internervous approach to treat hip pathology, including arthroplasty [16]. Marius N. Smith-Petersen was the first to describe the anterior approach in English literature in 1917 [17]. The superficial surgical plane of both these approaches is between the sartorius and tensor fascia lata, and the deep plane is between the rectus femoris and gluteus medius. This classic anterior approach originally described by Hueter has a high incidence of damage to the lateral cutaneous nerve of the thigh. Thus, a modified Hueter technique employing a more lateral incision has been created to minimize the risk of injury to this cutaneous nerve. The modified Hueter anterior approach employs the distal limit of the Smith-Peterson approach between the tensor fascia lata and the sartorius and does not involve the release of these muscles from their origin.

In Pipkin IV fractures involving the infrafoveal portion of the femur-head with a congruent hip joint, the acetabular posterior wall or rim fracture is treated operatively through a posterior approach, and the infrafoveal fragments are not disturbed. For suprafoveal femur-head fractures or where the infrafoveal fragment interferes with congruent reduction, both the femur-head and the acetabular fractures have to be addressed. Then, as the comminuted piece of the head of the femur is located predominantly anteromedially, it is challenging to stabilize it with the posterior (Kocher-Langenbeck) technique utilized for acetabular fracture fixation and dislocation reduction of the hip, and an anterior one would be required. And also in situations where infrafoveal fragments are impeding reduction or require fixation taking into account their size, the Kocher-Langenbeck will not offer adequate visualization.

The previous evidence did not favor the anterior approach for femur-head fracture-dislocation fixation. It was believed that as posterior structures were already compromised, further anterior exposure would further compromise the femur-head vascularity [11]. But now it has been established that it is essential to maintain the blood supply during surgical exposure regardless of the surgical approach [10]. As the vascular supply of importance to the critical femur-head passes beneath the posterosuperior capsule, published literature points to a nearly fourfold increased risk of AVN of the femur-head with the posterior approach compared to the anterior approach [1]. The anterior approach, however, had a higher rate of heterotopic ossification.

Anterior approach by itself with or without surgical dislocation of the femur-head is adequate for Pipkin IV injuries with accompanying anterior column fractures. The anterior approach (Smith-Petersen/Hueter or their modifications) offers adequate exposure of the anterior column up to the iliopectineal eminence and is adequate for most anterior column fractures not needing fixation past this bony landmark. But when more exposure and fixation is needed beyond iliopectineal eminence, the modified Stoppa's approach will be useful, which gives an extra medial working window for exposure beyond iliopectineal eminence. The same approach will be useful when more fixation of quadrilateral plate is needed. The lateral window incision can be taken distally to adequately expose the hip capsule. The anteromedial approach is useful for femur-head fractures' internal fixation since most of the femur-head fragments lie in the anteromedial position. The rectus femoris tendon can be let out to enhance exposure. Femur-head fracture exposure may be done with Z-shaped or T-shaped capsulotomy using available capsular tear. Beware not to impair the posterosuperior corner of the capsule and surrounding synovium as that contains the principal branches of the medial femoral circumflex artery (MFCA) supplying the femur-head. Femur-head dislocation is avoidable if the exposure is satisfactory. Despite these, there have been issues over the limited operative exposure for screw path needed if multidirectional screw fixation is necessitated by comminuted fragments of the femur-head. In these instances, anterior dislocation may be done.

The anterior approach would, however, not permit the fixation of posterior wall fractures and restore the posterior structures such as the capsule and labrum. Such treatment would require double approaches with management of injuries posterior structures, including acetabular fractures. The isolated anterior approach, however, can be appropriate in patients with small posterior wall fragments that are not suitable for fixation and do not jeopardize hip stability. Dynamic stress images under fluoroscopy constitute a well-established procedure to determine instability in posterior wall fractures [18]. In supine position and under anesthesia, the hip is slowly flexed beyond 90° with increasing manual force being applied along the longitudinal axis of the femur toward the hip separately in anteroposterior and the obturator oblique fluoroscopic views. If the hip joint remains congruent throughout this maneuver, the test is repeated with the addition of about 20° of adduction and about 20° of internal rotation. Frank redislocation is unnecessary; posterior subluxation of the femur-head (widening of medial clear space or loss of joint parallelism on fluoroscopic examination) is a marker for dynamic hip instability and a sign of need for posterior wall fixation. So, Pipkin IV fractures with minimal posterior wall fragment, in the absence of dynamic instability, can be managed by the anterior approach alone. In the presence of dynamic instability, Kocher-Langenbeck or Gibson's approach would be required for the management of posterior wall injury.

The current standard for the treatment of Pipkin IV fractures necessitating address of both posterior wall and femur-head fracture is surgical dislocation described by Reinhold Ganz [19, 20]. The trochanteric flip osteotomy enhances anterior exposure of the femur-head, and at the same time, posterior structures may also be addressed. Approach and intervals are the same as for normal Kocher-Langenbeck or Gibson's approach. The procedure details are outlined in the following sections.

Previous literature favored the removal of all fragments, as long as the fragments accounted for less than one third of the femur-head. But there are no explicit guidelines on fixation vs. removal of femur-head fragments. All fragments in the weight-bearing zone should always be fixed is the consensus [21]. Also, when a fragment is large enough to enable stable internal fixation, then fixation should be performed. Small or comminuted pieces or pieces outside the weight-bearing area of the femur-head can be removed without compromising the clinical outcome [22]. The reduction should be anatomical and direct and can be held temporarily by K-wires. Final fracture fixation is then done with interfragmentary lag screws. Various screw choices are available, such as 3.5- or 2.7-mm lag screws, headless cancellous screws, and bioabsorbable pins. No consensus has been established on the superiority of any single implant. For very severely compromised weight-bearing zones of the femur-head, particularly in the elderly population, hemiarthroplasty or total hip replacement can be a suitable option for early functional restitution. Nevertheless, for young patients, fixation must be the initial treatment, and joint replacement needs to be done or be undertaken as a second operation.

9.8 Author's Preference

The author's preferred method for Pipkin IV injuries fixation is the trochanteric flip osteotomy and safe hip surgical dislocation [23]. In most cases, we first address the femur-head and then the posterior wall/labrum injuries. But in a posterior column fracture case, we stabilize posterior column fracture first to obtain stable acetabular support and then femur-head fracture and subsequently any other posterior wall/labrum injury. We stabilize the column to obtain a stable platform on which the femur-head will lay. The labrum/posterior wall injuries are tackled only after femur-head fixation because capsulotomy is altered to incorporate the existing capsular/labral tears and their attached posterior wall fragments. By this, we avoid the devascularization of any wall fragments and their mobility increases the surgical exposure of femur-head. In addition, posterior capsule/wall repair without fixation of the femur-head may generate an excessive tension on the joint when compared to such repair after femur-head fixation. Column fixation on the other hand does not cause such problems as the column is anatomically fixed and supports femur-head in appropriate position.

Technique Lateral positioning of the patient (operative side upward) is done to permit convenient access to the hip joint. Ensure the contralateral limb is adequately padded and positioned to prevent pressure injuries. The Kocher-Langenbeck approach is employed without harming the external rotators and adjacent capsule. A curved incision is planned along the middle of the greater trochanter, going ~10 cm distally parallel to the femoral axis and posterosuperiorly toward posterior superior iliac spine. After making an incision through fascia lata, gluteus maximus is incised and trochanteric bursa is dissected. A greater trochanteric osteotomy is done using an oscillating saw beginning inferiorly from the posterosuperior border of the vastus ridge and extending proximally to the posterior border of the posterosuperior edge of the greater trochanter while leaving the mobile bone fragment measuring 1.5 cm thickness attached to proximal gluteus medius and distally to vastus lateralis. The MFCA's deep branch is guarded by remaining lateral to the insertion of short external rotators and maintaining the innermost part of the fibers of the gluteus medius, which were sharply cut after osteotomy completion. The trochanteric fragment with muscles attachments preserved is rotated anteriorly. Next, the zone between the posteroinferior border of gluteus minimus and superior border of piriformis is entered and dissected to expose the capsule of the hip. The posterior column if fractured is now fixed. A Z-shaped capsulotomy is then carried out. If posterior dislocation occurs along with capsule rupture, capsulotomy may be adapted to include traumatic capsulotomy not to devascularize posterior wall fragments that are capsularly attached. Transection of ligamentum teres is done if it is traumatically disrupted. Through manipulation of the leg into adduction and external rotation, the hip is anteriorly dislocated. To maximize the exposure of the retro acetabular region, short external rotators are transected, taking at least 2 cm away from the posterior trochanteric crest to avoid jeopardizing the deep branch of the MFCA. After anterior dislocation, visually and with the help of fluoroscopy, evaluate the femur-head fracture. In some instances, ligamentum teres must be transected in order to dislocate the femur-head. All attempts must be made to maintain the soft tissue attachments of the inferior femur-head fragment. Reduce fracture fragments anatomically. For small fragments, reduction may involve the use of fine instruments such as reduction clamps. Stabilize the femur-head fracture with small screws (e.g., 2.4 mm headless compression screws). Place screws countersunk so that they do not create incongruity of the joint. Verify reduction of the fracture and accurate placement of the screws with intraoperative fluoroscopy. Following fixation, place the femur-head gently into the acetabulum by reversing the dislocation maneuver (adduction, internal rotation, and extension). Reduce the joint capsule to its anatomic position. Repair of the hip capsule was accomplished with a 2-0 absorbable suture. Avoid tightened closure so that retinacular vessels do not get damaged. The posterior wall fractures can then be stabilized by lag screws/plates or both as per fragment size. Reattach the osteotomized greater trochanter with 3.5/4 mm lag screws or a trochanteric plate. Fix the short external rotators (piriformis and obturator internus) to their anatomical sites. Muscle fiber damage, if present, can be debrided. Post the wound wash, close deep fascia, subcutaneous tissue, and skin in layers. Use a drain if needed to avoid hematoma formation.

Weight-Bearing Restrictions The patient must be kept non-weight-bearing or partially weight-bearing for 3–4 weeks, depending upon the stability of fixation.

Deep Vein Thrombosis (DVT) Prophylaxis We permit continuation of anticoagulation therapy as warranted. In the majority of patients, we employ aspirin prophylaxis and mechanical control of DVT.

Heterotrophic Ossification (HO) Prophylaxis Present evidence does not form consensus of HO prophylaxis in Pipkin fractures. The guidelines are those of HO formation in acetabular surgeries. In the past, indomethacin or external beam irradiation therapy (XRT) in single dose has been employed as HO prophylaxis. The XRT is associated with issues of cost and radiation-related hazards such as malignancy and infertility. Indomethacin is associated with NSAID-related risk and possible risk factor of non-union. Additionally, NSAIDs can be contraindicated in patients with existing comorbidities. In all patients treated surgically, we prefer to resect gluteus minimus, the operation which has been proven to decrease HO rates. In patients with no risk factors and contraindications, we prescribed a 3-week regimen of indomethacin 75 mg daily.

Physical Therapy: Start early passive range-of-motion exercises, advancing to active exercises as healing permits.

Follow-Up Imaging: Have X-rays or CT scans on a periodic basis to gauge healing and to recognize early complications such as avascular necrosis or failure of the hardware. Monitor for the following complications:

- Avascular Necrosis: Especially with damaged retinacular blood supply. Risk for AVN after trochanteric flip osteotomy and secure dislocation is minimal, as has been observed in our series.
- Nonunion of the Trochanteric Osteotomy: This can be reduced by stable fixation and protected weight-bearing.
- Infection: Prevented by prophylactic antibiotics and meticulous surgical technique.
- Sciatic Nerve Injury: Prevented by gentle handling and protection of the nerve during dissection.
- Heterotrophic ossification: This possible risk may be associated with vigorous muscular stripping from the ilium with the approach. Excision is a treatment for symptomatic heterotopic ossification.

These steps, when done very carefully, may minimize the chance of complications and enhance the prospects of a good outcome for femur-head fractures. Two case scenarios have been presented for better clarification.

9.9 Case Example 1

A 29-year-old male was involved in a road traffic accident. He presented with severe pain in the right hip, inability to move the leg, and an internally rotated, shortened right lower limb. Physical examination revealed signs of a posterior hip dislocation. Radiographs showed a posterior dislocation of the right hip with a fracture of the femur-head inferior to the fovea capitis and a displaced posterior wall fracture (Fig. 9.4).

Closed reduction was achieved in the emergency. Although the closed reduction was confirmed, the medial clear space was widened, and the joint space was non-congruent. CT scan established the fracture pattern and classified it as a Pipkin IV injury. Given the displaced nature of the fracture, its large size, nonanatomic reduction of the femur-head fragment, noncongruent joint, and unstable nature of injury considering comminuted posterior wall fracture, operative treatment was chosen. The trochanteric flip osteotomy-based safe surgical dislocation was performed, and anatomical reduction of infrafoveal femur-head fracture was performed under direct vision and was confirmed in fluoroscopy. The posterior wall was fixed with a lag screw and neutralization plate. Early physical therapy with emphasis on range of motion and strengthening exercises was started in the early postoperative period. The patient had a good clinical and radiological result at a 2-year follow-up without any evidence of AVN or posttraumatic arthritis.

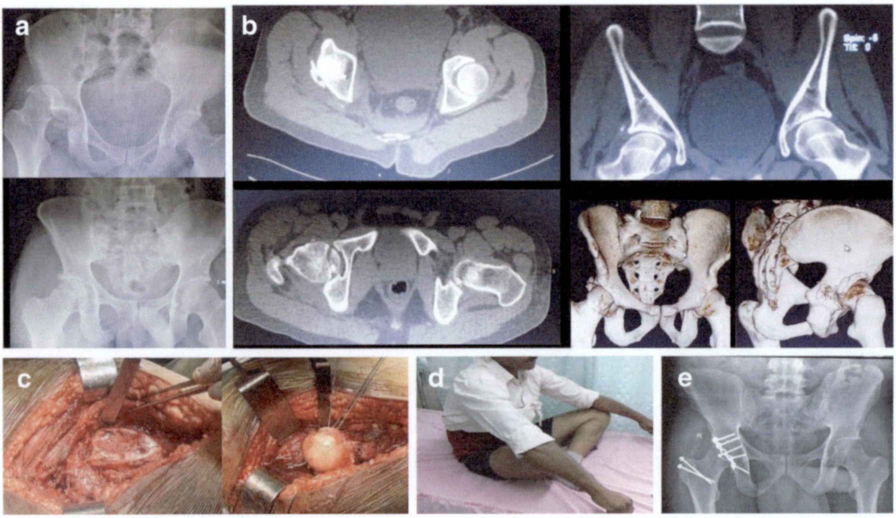

Fig. 9.4 (**a**) Pre-reduction and post-reduction radiographs of a Pipkin IV injury. (**b**) Computed tomography images confirming infrafoveal femur-head fracture and displaced posterior wall fragment and a noncongruent reduction. (**c**) Intraoperative images showing trochanteric flip osteotomy and anatomical reduction of femur-head through safe surgical dislocation of the hip. (**d**) The patient had good functional outcomes. (**e**) Two-year follow-up radiograph showing maintained femur-head shape with no signs of avascular necrosis

9.10 Case Example 2

A 26-year-old male in a road traffic accident incurred numerous injuries such as a fracture at the region of the hip, which is represented in Fig. 9.5. There was pain on the right side of the hip, loss of movement at the leg, and an internally rotated, shortened lower limb at the right. During physical examination, we have observed signs of a posterior hip dislocation. Upon radiography, we visibly see the infrafoveolar femur-head fracture. There is also comminuted acetabular fracture with ilioischial line and iliopectineal lines disrupted, with some portion of the dome remaining in continuity with the axial skeleton. Other views on the radiograph indicate the acetabular fracture to be a comminuted T-type fracture according to the Letournel and Judet classification. The closed reduction was tried but was not successful. Additional reduction was not carried out, keeping in mind the complexity of the injury and likely impaction of the femur-head against the posterior wall causing notching and absence of stable acetabular support for closed reduction. CT scan was requested and established infrafoveal femur-head fracture, T-type acetabular fracture with comminution, and Pipkin's type IV fracture dislocation of the femur-head.

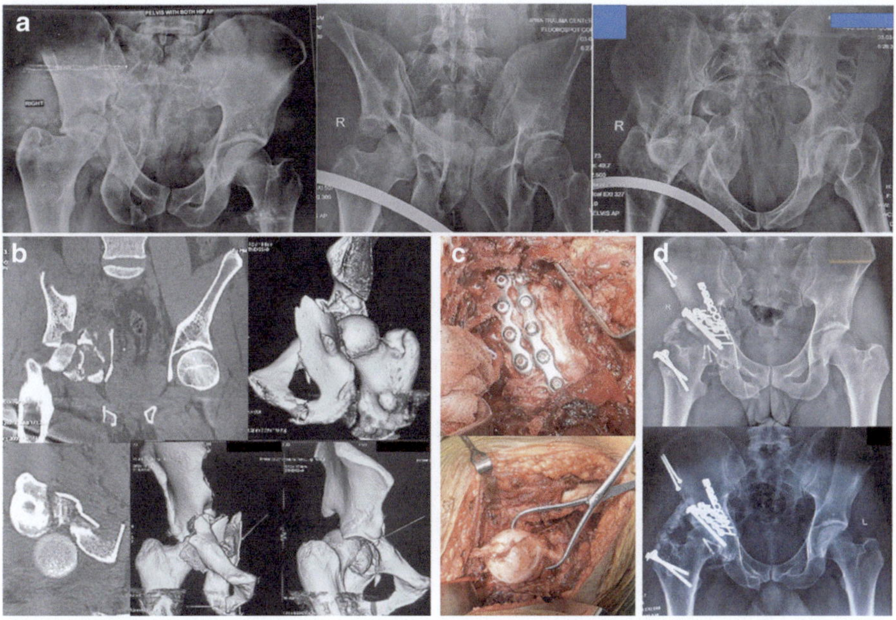

Fig. 9.5 (**a**) Radiographs showing T-type acetabular fracture with infrafoveal femoral fracture. (**b**) Computed tomography images showing displacement and comminution of acetabular fracture and infrafoveolar fracture of the femur-head. (**c**) Intraoperative images showing fixation of the posterior column through the Kocher-Langenbeck approach and direct anatomical reduction of the femur-head through trochanteric flip osteotomy combined with safe surgical dislocation. (**d**) Follow-up radiographs at 6 months and 2 years suggestive of no signs of AVN or posttraumatic arthritis, but with radiological evidence of heterotrophic ossification

Now, while planning the management, we should realize what components have to be managed. The dislocation is the first component. The dislocation was reduced under the assistance of trochanteric traction with a bone hook. As the dislocation was posterior, a stable posterior support would avoid further dislocation. Keeping in mind that it would not be possible to fix the posterior column and anterior column together, we did the Kocher-Langenbeck first and anatomically fixed the posterior column with the assistance of various reduction instruments. There were no isolated posterior wall fragments. With the same approach, the trochanteric flip osteotomy and safe surgical dislocation can be used to fix the femur-head. The same was done, and the femur-head was anatomically reduced and stabilized with three headless cancellous screws. The femur-head was reduced once more, the capsule was repaired, and the wound was closed in layers. The patient was then placed supine for the anterior column fixation. In this case, the anterior approach to the hip joint is not required since the femur-head has already been taken care of. We employed a modified iliofemoral approach with anterior superior iliac spine osteotomy to manage the anterior column. Early physical therapy with range of motion was started. Although the patient had satisfactory overall clinical results at 6 months and 2-year follow-ups without any evidence of AVN or posttraumatic arthritis, there was radiological proof of heterotrophic ossification. As the heterotrophic ossification was not disrupting function, nothing else was performed.

9.11 Complications/Prognosis

Complications and poor functional results are commonly seen in Pipkin IV fractures, and risk is greater than in other Pipkins [1]. The greater severity of injury involving three components, i.e., femoral fracture, acetabular fracture, and related dislocation, is likely to be the contributing factor. The primary complications were traumatic sciatic nerve injury, posttraumatic osteoarthritis, avascular necrosis of the femur-head, and heterotrophic ossification formation. Engel et al. [24] found in a study that 87.5% of the patients developed posttraumatic arthritis and 57.1% needed conversion to total hip arthroplasty at an average of 20.5 months from the time of injury. HO is estimated to develop in Pipkin IV injury at a rate of approximately 19%, but little evidence exists as these injuries are rare [21]. The HO, however, seldom needs any surgical procedure, and patients' hip function is maintained to some degree. The use of anterior approach to hip has been implicated as possible risk factor heterotrophic ossification.

The majority of literature has employed the radiographic and functional outcome based on Thompson and Epstein's criteria for evaluating the outcomes for femur-head fracture dislocations. The criteria were derived from radiographic results based on the severity of joint arthropathy and clinical results based on normal to disabling function. The results were graded as excellent, good, fair, and poor, with priority being given to the lower grade of the clinical or radiographic criteria. Already mentioned above, the Pipkin IV injuries have the poorest results since they include both the acetabulum and the femur-head. In general, nearly half of Pipkin IV injuries achieve excellent or good outcomes, and nearly one-third experience poor outcomes. There can be an improvement with improved knowledge of surgical methods and femur-head vascularity. For instance, Wang et al. [21] had excellent results in 47.6% and good in 28.5% of Pipkin IV fractures. Therefore, it is critical to realize that such fractures necessitate anatomical reduction and stable fixation of femur-head and acetabular lesions with emphasis on restoration of stable and congruent hip joint and cautious management of femur-head vascularity.

9.12 Summary

The current chapter discusses the management of Pipkin IV fractures, which involve both femur-head and acetabular injuries associated with hip dislocation, typically resulting from high-energy trauma. The understanding of hip anatomy and the vascular supply is crucial, particularly the medial femoral circumflex artery, to prevent complications such as avascular necrosis during surgical procedures. The author outlines a preferred surgical approach, which includes a trochanteric flip osteotomy and safe dislocation of the hip, prioritizing the fixation of the femur-head first, followed by addressing any posterior wall or labrum injuries. It is important to intervene early, with a focus on anatomical reduction and fixation, to improve functional outcomes and minimize complications like joint stiffness and heterotopic ossification. The role of imaging, particularly CT scans, is equally important in accurately assessing the extent of fractures and guiding treatment decisions. Postoperative care is crucial, with recommendations for early physical therapy and monitoring for potential complications such as deep vein thrombosis and heterotopic ossification.

9.13 Key Points

- Pipkin IV fractures are rare and complex injuries involving both femur-head and acetabular injuries associated with hip dislocation.
- The closed reduction should be performed as early as possible.
- Most of these fractures require surgery, considering their unstable nature.
- While several surgical approaches have been described, the trochanteric flip osteotomy and safe dislocation of the hip with the Kocher-Langenbeck approach is the standard approach for the fixation of these fractures.
- The prognosis is usually guarded in these injuries, and outcomes are poor compared to other Pipkins.
- Safe surgical dislocation with delicate handling of the hip joint capsule and anatomical congruity gives better outcomes.

References

1. Giannoudis PV, Kontakis G, Christoforakis Z, Akula M, Tosounidis T, Koutras C. Management, complications and clinical results of femur-head fractures. Injury. 2009;40(12):1245–51.
2. Marshall SC, Li J, Leary EV, Crist BD. Femur-head fractures systematic review and meta-analysis. Ann Surg Case Rep. 2024;7(1):1085.
3. Pipkin G. Treatment of grade IV fracture dislocation of the hip. J Bone Joint Surg Am. 1957;39:1027–42.
4. Enocson A, Wolf O. Pipkin fractures: epidemiology and outcome. Eur J Trauma Emerg Surg. 2022;48(5):4113–8. https://doi.org/10.1007/s00068-022-01951-w. Epub 2022 Mar 25.
5. Scolaro JA, Marecek G, Firoozabadi R, Krieg JC, Routt ML. Management and radiographic outcomes of femur-head fractures. J Orthop Traumatol. 2017;18:235–41.
6. Monma H, Sugita T. Is the mechanism of traumatic posterior dislocation of the hip a brake pedal injury rather than a dashboard injury? Injury. 2001;32(3):221–2. https://doi.org/10.1016/s0020-1383(00)00183-2.
7. Chiron P, Lafontan V, Reina N. Fracture-dislocations of the femur-head. Orthop Traumatol Surg Res. 2013;99(1):S53–66.
8. Lima LC, do Nascimento RA, de Almeida VM, Façanha Filho FA. Epidemiology of traumatic hip dislocation in patients treated in Ceará, Brazil. Acta Ortop Bras. 2014;22(3):151–4. https://doi.org/10.1590/1413-78522014220300883.
9. Yu JS. Easily missed fractures in the lower extremity. Radiol Clin North Am. 2015;53(4):737–55, viii. https://doi.org/10.1016/j.rcl.2015.02.003. Epub 2015 Mar 18. PMID: 26046508.
10. Kalhor M, Horowitz K, Gharehdaghi J, Beck M, Ganz R. Anatomic variations in femur-head circulation. Hip Int. 2012;22(3):307–12. https://doi.org/10.5301/HIP.2012.9242.
11. Epstein HC, Wiss DA, Cozen L. Posterior fracture dislocation of the hip with fractures of the femur-head. Clin Orthop Relat Res. 1985;201:9–17.
12. Li QW, Zhou CS, Li YP. Case report of a delayed iatrogenic Pipkin III femur-head fracture-dislocation. Medicine (Baltimore). 2022;101(4):e28773. https://doi.org/10.1097/MD.0000000000028773.
13. Foulk DM, Mullis BH. Hip dislocation: evaluation and management. J Am Acad Orthop Surg. 2010;18(4):199–209. https://doi.org/10.5435/00124635-201004000-00003.
14. Dawson-Amoah K, Raszewski J, Duplantier N, Waddell BS. Dislocation of the hip: a review of types, causes, and treatment. Ochsner J. 2018;18(3):242–52. https://doi.org/10.31486/toj.17.0079.
15. Gibson A. Posterior exposure of the hip joint. J Bone Joint Surg Br. 1950;32:183–758.
16. Rachbauer F, Kain MSH, Leunig M. The history of the anterior approach to the hip. Orthop Clin North Am. 2009;40:311–20.
17. Smith-Petersen MN. A new supra-articular subperiosteal approach to the hip joint. J Bone Joint Surg Am. 1917;s2–15:592–5.
18. Grimshaw CS, Moed BR. Outcomes of posterior wall fractures of the acetabulum treated non-operatively after diagnostic screening with dynamic stress examination under anesthesia. J Bone Joint Surg Am. 2010;92(17):2792–800. https://doi.org/10.2106/JBJS.J.00112.
19. Siebenrock KA, Gautier E, Woo AKH, Ganz R. Surgical dislocation of the femur-head for joint debridement and accurate reduction of fractures of the acetabulum. J Orthop Trauma. 2002;16(8):543–52.
20. Ganz R, Gill TJ, Gautier E, Ganz K, Krügel N, Berlemann U. Surgical dislocation of the adult hip a technique with full access to the femur-head and acetabulum without the risk of avascular necrosis. J Bone Joint Surg Br. 2001;83(8):1119–24. https://doi.org/10.1302/0301-620x.83b8.11964.
21. Wang SX, Li BH, Li J, Huang FG, Xiang Z, Zhong G, Fang Y, Yi M, Zhao XD, Liu L. Middle-term follow-up results of Pipkin IV femur-head fracture patients treated by reconstruction plate and bioabsorbable screws. Chin J Traumatol. 2018;21(3):170–5. https://doi.org/10.1016/j.cjtee.2017.12.004. Epub 2018 Apr 26. PMID: 29793730; PMCID: PMC6033733.

22. Menger MM, Braun BJ, Herath SC, Küper MA, Rollmann MF, Histing T. Fractures of the femur-head: a narrative review. EFORT Open Rev. 2021;6(11):1122–31. https://doi.org/10.1302/2058-5241.6.210034.
23. Trikha V, Das S, Madegowda A, Agrawal P. Midterm results of trochanteric flip osteotomy technique for management of fractures around the hip. Hip Int. 2018;28(2):148–55. https://doi.org/10.5301/hipint.5000539. Epub 2017 Sept 10.
24. Engel JL, Johnsen P, Patel NK, Satpathy J, Mounasamy V. Pipkin IV femur-head fractures: a case series and review of literature. Eur J Orthop Surg Traumatol. 2021;31(4):791–5. https://doi.org/10.1007/s00590-020-02838-5. Epub 2020 Nov 19. PMID: 33211232.

Transchondral and Impaction Injury of the Femoral Head

10

Manish Sharma, Sujit Kumar Tripathy, and Ramesh Kumar Sen

10.1 Introduction

The hip joint is formed by the femoral head articulating with the acetabulum. It is inherently a stable joint where the femoral head is concentrically surrounded by the bony acetabular cavity, further deepened by the peripheral labrum. It offers dual function by having sufficient range of movement at the hip joint along with even distribution of weight transfer from the torso down to the lower limb. Therefore, any traumatic condition affecting the articular surfaces on either side, disrupting the congruency of the joint like hip dislocations, compromises the hip function. In excessive axial loading during trauma, significant energy is transferred through the opposing joint surfaces that may result in osteochondral injury and subchondral impactions [1, 2]. The incidence of impaction injuries of the femoral head is historically estimated to be around 7–16% and most commonly seen in association with dislocation of the hip joint. These injuries range from small isolated cartilaginous defects (transchondral injury) to large osteochondral impaction fractures of the femoral head [2–6]. The isolated chondral defects are difficult to detect on plain radiographs [7, 8]. Though most of these injuries are small and remain asymptomatic, significant injuries may have serious long-term complications like posttraumatic osteoarthritis of the joint and osteonecrosis of the femoral head leading to poorer outcome [14, 15]. In a study by Poletti et al. in 2018, they found that femoral head

M. Sharma
Indira Gandhi Medical College, Shimla, India

S. K. Tripathy
Department of Orthopedics, All India Institute of Medical Sciences, Bhubaneswar, Odisha, India
e-mail: ortho_sujit@aiimsbhubaneswar.edu.in

R. K. Sen (✉)
Institute of Orthopedic Surgery, Max Super Speciality Hospital, Mohali, Punjab, India

R. K. Sen, S. K. Tripathy (eds.), *A Practical Guide to Management of Femoral Head Fracture-Dislocation*, https://doi.org/10.1007/978-981-96-9852-3_10

impactions seen with acetabular fractures are itself an independent predictive factor for the need of delayed total hip arthroplasty [18]. Studies have shown that isolated chondral impaction injuries of the femoral head are probably far more common than what the literature reports, as X-rays and sometimes even CT scans tend to miss these injuries when there is minimal or no subchondral bone damage [9].

10.2 Mechanism of Injury

Femoral impaction injuries affecting the cartilage and subchondral region are uncommon injuries which are caused by high-energy trauma as seen in road traffic accidents, fall from significant height, and sports injuries [5, 10]. These fractures mostly occur when there is direct impact and torsional forces loading the hip joint as seen in dashboard-type injuries with dislocation of the hip joint. Study by Poletti et al. showed that such fractures can also arise without dislocation of the hip joint as seen commonly with transverse fractures of the acetabulum. The damage may be either limited to the chondral part alone or affect the subchondral bone also [11]. Epstein et al. in a study in 1985 mentioned about slice fractures of the femoral head seen during posterior dislocation of the hip as a result of dashboard type of injuries. These split depression or slice fractures of the femur head occur due to additional shear forces acting on the femoral head by the posterior acetabular rim during dashboard injuries [9]. Tehranzadeh et al. found that all the impaction fractures of the femoral head had a history of dislocation. They were associated with posterior dislocation of the hip in around 63% and with anterior dislocation in around 100% cases. In posterior dislocation of the hip, the impaction on the femoral head is seen on the anterior aspect as it presses against the posterior rim of the acetabulum. Similarly, in anterior dislocation, the impaction on the head is often seen on the posterior aspect. [7, 9]. Similar findings were noted by Patrice Richardson et al. (1990), as they showed that the impaction injuries of the femoral head were seen mostly in the posterior dislocation of hip and were akin to Hill-Sach's lesion of the humeral head [23].

10.3 Classification

It was Birkett, in 1869, who first described about the fractures of the femoral head and postulated that during posterior dislocation, violent axial forces through the femoral shaft were driven upward and backward toward the hip joint [12]. This force was responsible for either dislocation of the joint alone or associated fractures about the hip joint [11, 22]. The work by Garrett Pipkins in 1957 gave a detailed insight on femoral head fractures with posterior dislocation of the hip. He classified these injuries into four types which were based on the location of the fracture line on the head of the femur and associated fractures of the ipsilateral neck of the femur or acetabulum with posterior dislocation [13]. This universally accepted classification system fails to classify chondral and osteochondral impaction injuries of the femoral head as a separate entity. Countering the issue, in 1987, Brumback et al. gave a classification system for femoral head fractures (Table 10.1). The impaction injuries of the femoral head were classified as Brumback type 4A and 4B injuries which were indentation type and transchondral shear type, respectively [21] (Figs. 10.1 and 10.2).

Buckwalter in a study in 1998 stated that it is the direct impact along with torsional joint loading that leads to chondral and subchondral injuries and classified such injuries broadly into three types (Table 10.2). In type 1, there is internal chondral injury with intact articular surface and a possible injury to the subchondral bone, type 2 is with mechanical disruption of the articular surface limited to the cartilage, and type 3 is with mechanical disruption of both the articular cartilage and the subchondral bone [19].

In the AO/OTA classification system, the depression type of femoral head fractures is referred to as 31C2 type (Table 10.3). They further classified these injuries

Table 10.1 Brumback classification system of hip dislocations and femoral head fractures [21]

Type	Description
Type 1A	Posterior dislocation with fracture of the inferomedial aspect of the femoral head with minimal or no acetabular rim fracture: stable hip
Type 1B	Type 1A with significant acetabular rim fracture: unstable hip
Type 2A	Posterior dislocation with fracture of the superomedial aspect of the femoral head with minimal or no acetabular rim fracture: stable hip
Type 2B	Type 2A with significant acetabular rim fracture: unstable hip
Type 3A	Dislocation of the hip joint (unspecified direction) with femoral neck fracture
Type 3B	Type 3A with associated femoral head fracture
Type 4A	Hip dislocation with femoral head fracture: indentation type; depression of the superolateral weight-bearing surface of the femoral head
Type 4B	Hip dislocation and femoral head fracture: transchondral shear type; osteo-cartilaginous shear fracture of the weight-bearing surface of femoral head
Type 5	Central fracture dislocation with femoral head fracture

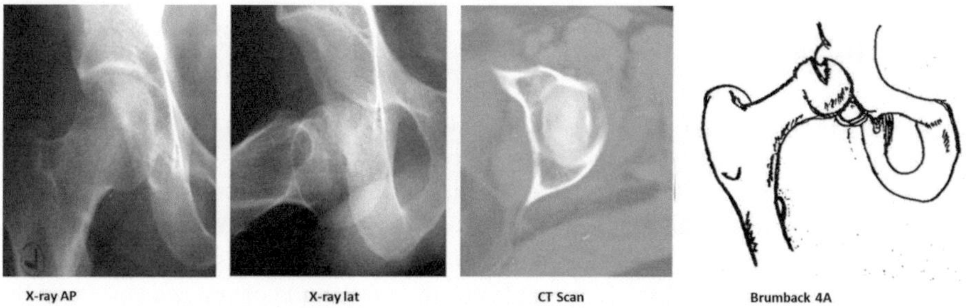

Fig. 10.1 Brumback type 4A injury

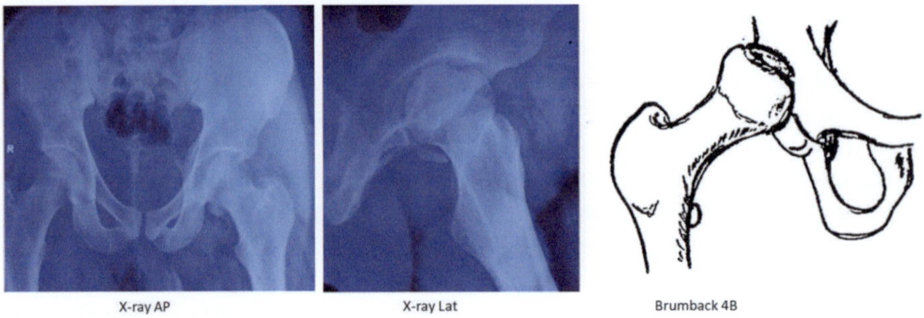

Fig. 10.2 Brumback type 4B injury

Table 10.2 Buckwalter classification of chondral/osteochondral

Type	Description
Type 1	Damage to chondral matrix or subchondral bone without visible disruption of the articular surface
Type 2	Chondral fractures or ruptures
Type 3	Osteochondral fractures

Table 10.3 AO/OTA classification

Type	Description
31C2 depression type	
31C2.1	Chondral lesion
31C2.2	Depression impaction fracture
31C2.3	Split depression fracture

into three subtypes depending upon fracture depression of the femoral head with chondral lesion alone, with impaction, and with a split depression fracture [17]. Impaction fractures of the femoral head are often associated with hip dislocation and acetabulum fractures; therefore, all such patients need careful assessment [16, 18].

10.4 Clinical Assessment

10.4.1 History

Every patient with major trauma around the hip joint is suspected to have impaction fractures of the femoral head as stressed upon by the study by Poletti et al. [18]. Careful evaluation of patient is needed, which should start with a detailed history. Information regarding the mechanism of injury, ability of the patient to stand and bear weight after trauma, presence of associated fractures, or dislocation of the hip joint is documented. All this gives an idea of the magnitude of trauma sustained by the patient. Fracture dislocations are the most common cause for impaction injuries to the femur head as observed by Tehranzadeh et al. in their study. They stated that it was even possible to predict the area of involvement of the femoral head just by knowing the type of hip dislocation, thus highlighting the importance [9]. It is vital to document the time taken from injury to reduction of joint which may be detrimental for future outcome of hip function.

10.4.2 Examination

On inspection, look for signs of swelling, contusions, and trauma marks around the knee joint indicating dashboard injury. The *attitude* of the lower limb post reduction of the hip joint is often unremarkable. The patient may guard the hip joint due to *pain* which is the most common complaint and is present in the groin region that may radiate to the knee joint. *Movements* of the lower limb are reduced and rotations are often painful. *Limp* is associated with pain and is severe when the weight-bearing zone is involved. Application of axial force along the femur and pelvic compression tests may elicit pain in the hip joint. At the end of examination, always assess and document the distal neurological and vascular status of the limb.

10.4.3 Radiologic Evaluation

Femoral head impaction injuries pose a diagnostic challenge as there may be either very small chondral/subchondral impaction fractures that are generally asymptomatic or they are associated with other major injuries and often overlooked. A high degree of suspicion is therefore required for diagnosing these injuries. Plain AP radiographs of the pelvis and frog leg lateral views of the proximal femur are the first line of imaging. Most of the AO/OTA C2 sub-type 1 injuries are likely to be missed on plain X-rays. Even the CT scans tend to miss these subtle isolated chondral impaction injuries. Often, they appear as small flattened area of the femoral head, suggesting an antecedent impaction injury [9]. A high-resolution CT scan is the investigation of choice for diagnosing Brumback 4B or AO/OTA C2 sub-type 2 and type 3 injuries (Fig. 10.3). CT scan gives important insight to the size of lesion, location, and associated comminution of fracture fragments [2, 18]. They are also helpful for planning a surgical intervention by 3D mapping of the femur important before transplantation. MRI arthrogram is the gold standard modality in diagnosing AO/OTA C2 sub-type 1 isolated chondral injuries. On MRI, the osteochondral lesions are typically characterized by cartilage surface irregularities with abnormal bone marrow signals in the subchondral bone [20]. In the setting of trauma and underlying edema, its superiority over CT scan is questionable for detecting AO/OTA sub-type 2 and type 3 injuries. MRI is useful for both the evaluation of defects and during the follow-up to assess signs of developing osteonecrosis. Recently, there has been an increasing interest in arthroscopic evaluation of the osteochondral

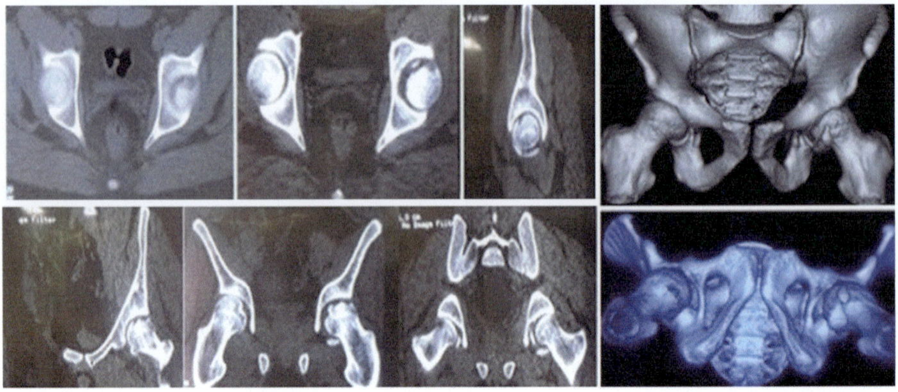

Fig. 10.3 Brumback type 4B CT images

defects of the femoral head. Despite considerable initial challenges, arthroscopy has proven diagnostic as well as treatment potential.

10.5 Treatment

Once diagnosed with impaction injuries of the femoral head, a bigger challenge is the management. The treatment of these injuries depends upon the size of lesion, site, area of involvement, age, and any pre-existing arthrosis of the joint. It aims to reduce symptoms, promote the healing process, and improve the joint function.

10.5.1 Conservative

Nonoperative management of the impaction injuries of the femoral head is advised to patients having minimal symptoms, with small lesion and stable joint, not involving the weight-bearing area and no mechanical hindrance to function. A patient not willing to undergo surgical procedure is also an important factor deciding to continue conservative treatment. Such chondral/osteochondral impaction injuries can be managed conservatively by non-weight-bearing for around 6–12 weeks [24, 32]. Results are often favorable with patient education about their condition, judicious use of anti-inflammatory medicines, lifestyle modification toward aggravating activities, and dedicated physiotherapy practices. Patient evaluation is necessary for decision-making, and we prefer conservative management for impaction as well as split depression fractures that involve non-weight-bearing zone with stable hip joint and preserved hip function (Figs. 10.4 and 10.5).

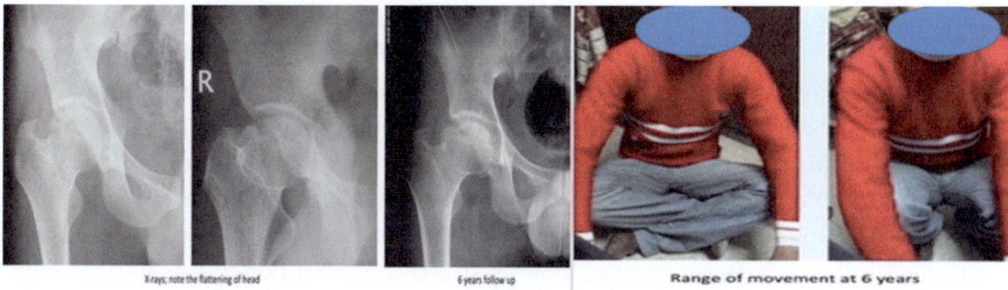

Fig. 10.4 Brumback type 4A injury of the non-weight-bearing area

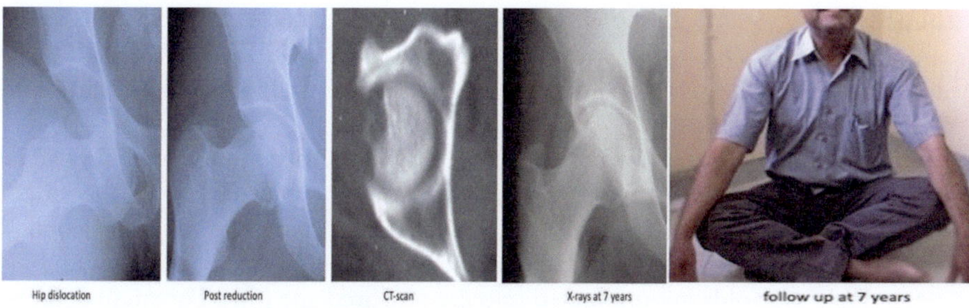

Fig. 10.5 Brumback type 4B injury of the non-weight-bearing area

10.5.2 Joint Preservation Surgery

Surgery is offered to the patients in the event of worsening of symptoms or failure to achieve desired relief with conservative treatment. Joint preservation surgery aims at addressing the lesion and offering appropriate surgical procedure to restore the native anatomy and improve joint function.

1. *Chondroplasty*: When there is low-grade, partial thickness chondral tears, debridement of the lesion is done, and the edges are smoothened. It aims at reducing the unstable loose chondral fragment edges, thereby preventing formation of loose bodies and removing mechanical blocks in the joint [26]. In a retrospective study by Bedard and Pugely, they found that chondroplasty was the most commonly performed procedure during hip arthroscopy and was done in around 49% cases [25, 33]. Yen and Kocher found that in all patients under 50 years, if chondroplasty is done during hip arthroscopy, there is increased risk of conversion to total hip arthroplasty. In contrast, they observed good clinical outcomes with chondroplasty done during hip arthroscopy for low-grade partial tears only. It should also be avoided in patients with advanced arthritis who require total hip arthroplasty [26]. The decision of offering this procedure should be based on the age of the patient, size and extent of lesion, severity of injury, and existing condition of the joint for a better outcome.

2. *Microfracture*: In this procedure, damaged cartilage is debrided and removed exposing the subchondral bone, and then drill holes are made around 3 mm wide at 3 mm distance apart into the bone to a depth of 6 mm. It allows extrusion of bone marrow and formation of clots rich in mesenchymal stem cells and growth factors that promote healing of the defect by formation of fibrocartilage [34]. The fibrocartilage formed as repair tissue has inferior properties when compared to the native hyaline cartilage putting concerns of long-term outcome. Mardones et al. found that lesions smaller than 2–4 cm^2 respond better to this treatment [27]. Observations by Philippon and Schenker have shown that this procedure, done with good patient selection, offers good clinical outcome [35]. In contrast, McGill et al. stated that microfracture is not suitable when there is involvement of underlying subchondral bone and hip joint with advanced arthritis [28]. There are few complications seen with microfracture like ossification, fragility, failure to fill the gap, and poor quality of new cartilage formation which is prone to breakdown [29].
3. *Autologous chondrocyte implantation (ACI):* This procedure is used for larger chondral lesions that are not amenable to treatment by microfracture. The procedure is carried in two stages. First, the damaged cartilage is debrided and removed, and next, autologous harvested chondrocytes alone or mixed with biodegradable scaffolds are implanted into the prepared site [30]. For small defects, scaffolds can be introduced via arthroscope, whereas in larger defects, hip dislocation is needed which has its own complications. Lee et al. reported that ACI using biodegradable scaffolds had a better stabilization of the bone marrow clots and filling of the chondral defects. The percentage of hyaline cartilage formation was higher as compared to microfracture. They found a significant improvement in the hip function of their patients after ACI [31].
4. *Osteochondral autograft transplantation (OAT) and mosaicplasty*: These are single-stage procedures, where the damaged chondral lesion is removed and the floor is prepared by drilling hole into the lesion. A same size osteochondral plug is then harvested from the non-weight-bearing surface of the femoral head or the ipsilateral knee joint of the patient. This plug is then inserted into the prepared site. OAT technique is used to treat lesion that is large for microfracture, with subchondral damage or when chondroplasty or microfracture has failed. Mosaicplasty is a similar technique where multiple small osteochondral plugs are used to fill the defect [36]. OAT may be performed arthroscopically; on the other hand, hip dislocation is needed for mosaicplasty which has its own side effects [30]. Petit et al. harvested the osteochondral plugs from the peripheral anterior non-weight-bearing zones of the femoral head or ipsilateral knee [37]. Girard et al. had promising results with increased functional scores of the hip joint after mosaicplasty of the femoral head cartilage. Both OAT and mosaicplasty are economical, single-stage surgeries using native hyaline osteochondral graft [43].
5. *Osteochondral allograft transplant (OCA):* Osteochondral allograft transplant surgery is a well-established procedure for the treatment of full-thickness chondral lesion with promising results especially in the young patients. In this proce-

Table 10.4 Proposed algorithm by El Bitar et al. for femoral head chondral/osteochondral lesion

Size of lesion	Femoral head
<2 cm^2	1st line: microfracture, chondral defect repair
	2nd line: mosaicplasty/osteochondral autograft transplantation (OAT), osteochondral allograft transplantation (OCA)
2–6 cm^2	Microfracture, osteochondral allograft transplantation (OCA)
6–8 cm^2	Osteochondral allograft transplantation (OCA), total hip arthroplasty
>8cm^2	Total hip arthroplasty

dure, osteochondral allograft plugs are harvested from the cadaveric donors. The chondral damage is debrided, and the site is prepared by making drill holes; finally, the allograft plugs are then inserted into the defects. Meyers et al. reported high success rate of around 80% with OCA in young patients with AVN and segmental collapse of the femoral head [38]. Similar results were found by Oladeji et al., who concluded that OCA is effective in young and healthy patients. History of smoking, steroid intake, acetabular fractures, and concomitant AVN are few risk factors for failure of OCA [39]. There is no donor site morbidity, and 3D-CT mapping can be done to match the recipient defect. Few challenges with OCA procedure are as follows: there is potential of graft non-union and failure to transform into live tissue, and time from harvest to implantation should be less than 28 days for better incorporation [40, 42]. De Lee et al. in their study postulated that large osteochondral impaction fractures with depths greater than 4 mm after dislocation of the hip joint are often associated with poor outcomes and progress to severe arthritis of the hip joint [41]. El Bitar et al. developed an algorithm to assist in decision-making in patients with full-thickness femoral head chondral/osteochondral lesions (Table 10.4).

6. *Open reduction and internal fixation:* Large osteochondral sleeve or split depression fragments, classified as Brumback type 4B and AO/OTA 31C2.3, can be managed with open reduction and internal fixation. Ganz et al. described a posterior-based approach with greater trochanteric flip osteotomy for the safe surgical dislocation of the hip joint [44]. This approach aimed at preserving the major blood supply to the head of the femur. In 213 cases of femur head fracture operated using this approach, they did not report any osteonecrosis of the head. Patient counselling with guarded prognosis regarding the development of osteonecrosis of head or secondary osteo-arthritis after open reduction and internal fixation is recommended. We prefer the Ganz osteotomy for safe surgical dislocation to expose the femoral head and osteosynthesis for these fracture dislocations, with good post-op hip function (Fig. 10.6).

10.5.3 Rehabilitation Protocol After Hip Preservation Surgeries

For desired outcome of the hip preservation surgeries, the patient needs to follow appropriate postoperative protocol [44]. Patients undergoing chondroplasty do not

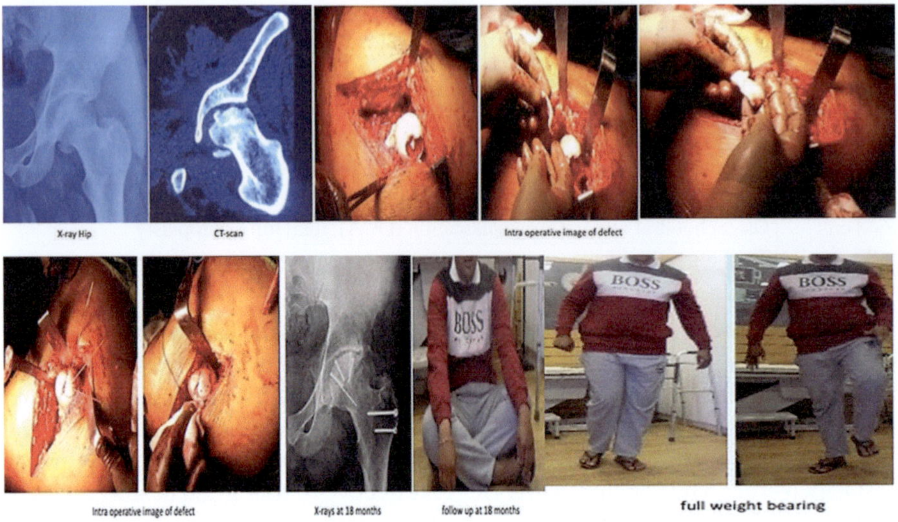

Fig. 10.6 Brumback type 4B injury of the weight-bearing area (repaired with depressed bone fragment elevation with underlying bone grafting, fixing with headless Herbert screw, and suturing the associated chondral flap with suture anchor/nonabsorbable sutures)

need any strict postoperative restrictions of activities. Adler et al. suggested that after microfracture procedure, the patient is required to abstain from weight-bearing activities for a period ranging from 2 to 8 weeks. In contrast, systemic reviews have found that after microfracture surgery, early rehabilitation may be beneficial [44, 45]. After autologous chondrocyte implantation and mosaicplasty, Rolf et al. started the patients on toes touch-down weight-bearing for first 6 weeks followed by partial weight-bearing for the next 6 weeks [44, 46]. Open reduction and internal fixation require protection from weight-bearing till there is sign of bone-to-bone union on postoperative radiographs. The rehabilitation protocol may vary as per discretion of the treating surgeon and depends on patient-specific conditions.

10.5.4 Total Hip Arthroplasty

Chondral/osteochondral impaction injuries of the femoral head can worsen after hip preservation surgery. They may result in damage to the protective chondral/subchondral layer leading to advanced arthrosis of the hip joint or osteonecrosis of the subchondral bone. In such patients, total hip arthroplasty is the standard procedure with the aim to relieve symptoms, alleviate pain, improve hip function, and the quality of life of the patient. Primary THA in impaction fracture of the femoral head is reserved for elderly patients and in those with pre-existing advanced joint arthritis. It is also considered in the patients having large defects that are not amenable to any hip preservation surgeries. Despite all efforts, the disease may continue and lead on to end-stage arthritis of the joint. Delayed total hip arthroplasty is the treatment of choice in osteonecrosis and advanced arthritis caused secondary to impaction fractures. Observations made by Poletti et al. stated that dislocations, impaction fractures of the femoral head, and transverse fractures of the acetabulum are independent factors predictive of need for delayed THA in such patients [18].

10.6 Author's Preferred Treatment

Author's preference of management is conservative treatment for impaction fractures that involve the non-weight-bearing area of the femur head, with stable hip and preserved joint function. A trial of hip preservation surgery is attempted for impaction or transchondral injury in the young patients when the lesion is in the weight-bearing zone. However, they are explained about the risk of hip arthrosis with subsequent need of delayed THA (Figs. 10.4, 10.5, and 10.6). In contrast, primary THA is the preferred management in the elderly and in patients with underlying joint arthritis.

10.7 Summary

The impaction fractures of the femoral head are inconspicuous injuries and often go undiagnosed. High degree of suspicion is recommended for detecting these injuries in all patients with hip dislocations and fractures of the acetabulum. High-resolution CT scans and MRI are helpful in classifying the lesions and planning a treatment. Appropriate management in the form of conservative, hip preservation surgery or THA is planned depending upon the injury and patient-specific conditions. It should be aimed at reducing symptoms and restoring hip joint function to improve the quality of life. Newer hip preservation techniques, which are more standardized, have less morbidity, are easily available, have low complication rate, and have more predictable outcomes, are desired.

10.8 Key Points

Impaction injuries of the femoral head are more prevalent than reported. These fractures mostly occur when there is direct impact and torsional forces loading the hip joint as seen in dashboard-type injuries. Most of these injuries remain asymptomatic, whereas significant injuries may have serious long-term complications like osteonecrosis of the femoral head and posttraumatic osteoarthritis of the joint. Therefore, every patient with major trauma around the hip joint is suspected to have impaction fractures of the femoral head, and a high degree of suspicion is required for diagnosing these injuries.

References

1. Stewart MJ, Milford LW. Fracture-dislocation of the hip: an end result study. J Bone Joint Surg Am. 1954;36-A:998.
2. Hougaard K, Lindquist S, Nielsen LB. Computerized tomography after posterior dislocation of the hip. J Bone Joint Surg (Br). 1987;69(4):556–7.
3. Ordway CB, Xeller CF. Transverse computerized axial tomography of patients with posterior dislocation of the hip. J Trauma. 1984;24(1):76–794.
4. Epstein H. Posterior fracture-dislocation of the hip: long-term follow-up. J Bone Joint Surg Am. 1974;56-A:1103–11275.
5. Larson CB. Fracture dislocations of the hip. Clin Orthop. 1973;92:147–1546.
6. Pipkin G. Treatment of grade IV fracture-dislocations of the hip. J Bone Joint Surg Am. 1957;39-A(5):1027–42.
7. Stein H. Computerized tomography for ascertaining osteo cartilaginous intra-articular (slice) fracture of the femoral head. Isr J Med Sci. 1983;19(2):180–4.
8. Urist MR. Fracture dislocation of the hip joint. J Bone Joint Surg Am. 1984;30A(3):699–727.
9. Tehranzadeh J, et al. Osteochondral impaction of the hip associated with hip dislocation: CT study. AJR Am J Roentgenol. 1990;155(5):1049–52.
10. Epstein HC. Traumatic dislocations of the hip. Clin Orthop. 1973;92:116.
11. Rogers LF. The hip and femoral shaft; radiology of skeletal trauma, vol. 2. 1st ed. New York: Churchill-Livingstone; 1982.
12. Birkett J. Description of a dislocation of the head of the femur, complicated with its fracture; with remarks by John Birkett (1815–1904). 1869. Clin Orthop Relat Res. 2000;377:4–6.
13. Pipkin G. Treatment of grade IV fracture dislocation of the hip. J Bone Joint Surg Am. 1957;39:1027–42.
14. Murray P, McGee HM, Mulvihill N. Fixation of femoral head fractures using the Herbert screw. Injury. 1988;19:220–1.
15. Gardner MJ, et al. Surgical dislocation of the hip for fractures of the femoral head. J Orthop Trauma. 2005;19:334–42.
16. Tonetti J, et al. Is femoral head fracture-dislocation management improvable: a retrospective study in 110 cases. Orthop Traumatol Surg Res. 2010;96(6):623–31.
17. Marsh JL, et al. Fracture and dislocation classification compendium –2007: orthopaedic trauma association classification, database and outcomes committee. J Orthop Trauma. 2007;21(suppl):S1–133.
18. Poletti PA, et al. Femoral head subchondral impaction on CT; what does it mean in patients with acetabular fracture? Skeletal Radiol. 2019;48(6):939–48.
19. Buckwalter JA. Articular cartilage injuries. Clin Orthop Relat Res. 2002;402:21–37. https://doi.org/10.1097/00003086-200209000-00004.
20. Brittberg M, Winalski CS. Evaluation of cartilage injuries and repair. J Bone Joint Surg Am. 2003;85-A(Suppl 2):58–69.
21. Brumback RJ, Kenzora JE, Levitt LE, Burgess AR, Poka A. Fractures of the femoral head. Hip. 1987:181–206.
22. Epstein HC, Wiss DA, Cozen L. Posterior fracture dislocation of the hip with fractures of the femoral head. Clin Orthop Rel. 1985;201:9–17.
23. Richardson P, et al. CT detection of cortical fracture of the femoral head associated with posterior hip dislocation. AJR. 1990;155:93–4.
24. Ly PN, Fallat LM. Trans-chondral fractures of the talus: a review of 64 surgical cases. J Foot Ankle Surg. 1993;32:352–74.
25. Bedard NA, Pugely AJ, Duchman KR, et al. When hip scopes fail, they do so quickly. J Arthroplast. 2016;31:1183–7.
26. Yen YM, Kocher MS. Chondral lesions of the hip: microfracture and chondroplasty. Sports Med Arthrosc. 2010;18:83–9.

27. Mardones R, Larrain C. Cartilage restoration technique of the hip. J Hip Preserv Surg. 2016;3:30–6.
28. McGill KC, Bush-Joseph CA, Nho SJ. Hip microfracture: indications, technique, and outcomes. Cartilage. 2010;1:127–36.
29. Steadman JR, Rodkey WG, Briggs KK. Microfracture to treat full-thickness chondral defects: surgical technique, rehabilitation, and outcomes. J Knee Surg. 2002;15:170–6.
30. Fortun CM, Streit J, Patel SH, Salata MJ. Cartilage defects in the hip. Oper Tech Sports Med. 2012;20:287–94.
31. Lee YH, et al. Autologous matrix-induced chondrogenesis in the knee: a review. Cartilage. 2014;5(3):145–53.
32. McGovern RP, Martin RL, Kivlan BR, Christoforetti JJ. Non-operative management of individuals with non-arthritic hip pain: a literature review. Int J Sports Phys Ther. 2019;14(1):135–47.
33. Sampson TG. Arthroscopic treatment for chondral lesions of the hip. Clin Sports Med. 2011;30(2):331–48.
34. Chen H, Sun J, Hoemann CD, Lascau-Coman V, Ouyang W, McKee MD, Shive MS, Buschmann MD. Drilling and microfracture lead to different bone structure and necrosis during bone-marrow stimulation for cartilage repair. J Orthop Res. 2009;27(11):1432–8.
35. Philippon MJ, Schenker ML, Briggs KK, Maxwell RB. Can microfracture produce repair tissue in acetabular chondral defects? Arthroscopy. 2008;24(1):46–50.
36. Viamont-Guerra MR, Bonin N, May O, Le Viguel-Loux A, Saffarini M, Laude F. Promising outcomes of hip mosaicplasty by minimally invasive anterior approach using osteochondral autografts from the ipsilateral femoral head. Knee Surg Sports Traumatol Arthrosc. 2020;28(3):767–76.
37. Petit CJ, Philippon MJ. Arthroscopic management of osteochondral defects of the hip. Oper Tech Sports Med. 2008;16:194–200.
38. Meyers MH. Resurfacing of the femoral head with fresh osteochondral allografts. Long-term results. Clin Orthop Relat Res. 1985;197:111–4.
39. Oladeji LO, Cook JL, Stannard JP, Crist BD. Large fresh osteochondral allografts for the hip: growing the evidence. Hip Int. 2018;28:284–90.
40. Stuhlman CR, Krych AJ, Levy BA, Kelly BT. Cartilage restoration of the hip. Oper Tech Sports Med. 2015;23:175–83.
41. DeLee JC, Evans JA, Thomas J. Anterior dislocation of the hip and associated femoral-head fractures. J Bone Joint Surg Am. 1980;62:960–4.
42. Garcia-Mansilla I, Jones KJ, Sassoon AA. Surgical hip dislocation and fresh osteochondral allograft transplantation for femoroacetabular impingement and concomitant chondral lesion. Arthrosc Tech. 2020;9(12):e1857–63.
43. Girard J, Roumazeille T, Sakr M, Migaud H. Osteochondral mosaicplasty of the femoral head. Hip Int. 2011;21(5):542–8.
44. Ganz R, Gill TJ, Gautier E, Ganz K, Krugel N, Berlemann U. Surgical dislocation of the adult hip a technique with full access to the femoral head and acetabulum without the risk of avascular necrosis. J Bone Joint Surg Br. 2001;83(8):1119–24.
45. Orth P, Gao L, Madry H. Microfracture for cartilage repair in the knee: a systematic review of the contemporary literature. Knee Surg Sports Traumatol Arthrosc. 2020;28(3):670–706. https://doi.org/10.1007/s00167-019-05359-9. Epub 2019 Jan 18. PMID: 30659314.
46. Rolf S, Kwan CK, Stoddart M, Li Y, Fu SC. Timing of postoperative weightbearing in the treatment of traumatic chondral injuries of the knee in athletes - A systematic review of current concepts in clinical practice. Asia Pac J Sports Med Arthrosc Rehabil Technol. 2022;27:1–8. https://doi.org/10.1016/j.asmart.2022.01.001. PMID: 35155127; PMCID: PMC8803964.

Atypical Femur Head Fracture Pattern: Management Issues

11

Ramesh Kumar Sen, Shahnawaz Khan,
and Sujit Kumar Tripathy

11.1 Introduction

Femoral head fractures are uncommon injuries, with the majority of available literature comprising case reports or small case series. Multicentric studies and comprehensive review papers that define the epidemiology of these fractures remain limited. Due to subtle findings on conventional radiographic imaging, Pipkin first described the classical fracture patterns, providing a foundation for diagnosis and management [1]. Over time, additional classifications, including the AO, Brumback, and Chiron classifications, each encompassing various fracture characteristics, have been introduced. Despite having so many classification systems, Pipkin's classification remains the most favored due to its simplicity. However, this classification system also has many shortcomings. It is based on fracture morphology, including significant bone fragments and associated injuries, such as acetabular wall fractures or femoral neck fractures. However, the classification does not account for specific variations, such as osteochondral fragments, impacted fractures, or the variability in acetabular wall involvement. This can lead to challenges in management, as these variations may require distinct treatment strategies despite being grouped under Pipkin type IV fractures. A recent study by Giannoudis et al. revealed that around 2.4% of femoral head fractures were not classified as per Pipkin's classification [2]. This calls for modification in the current classification systems. A well-defined classification system with protocol-based treatment strategies is essential to optimize the management of these fractures.

R. K. Sen (✉)
Institute of Orthopedic Surgery, Max Super Speciality Hospital, Mohali, Punjab, India

S. Khan · S. K. Tripathy
Department of Orthopedics, All India Institute of Medical Sciences, Bhubaneswar, Odisha, India
e-mail: ortho_sujit@aiimsbhubaneswar.edu.in

R. K. Sen, S. K. Tripathy (eds.), *A Practical Guide to Management of Femoral Head Fracture-Dislocation*, https://doi.org/10.1007/978-981-96-9852-3_11

The advent of computed tomography (CT) imaging has become routine in evaluating femoral head fractures, allowing for more accurate characterization and validation of classification systems. CT imaging facilitates the identification of subtle fracture details, including osteochondral fragments and impacted fractures, which are often overlooked in conventional radiographs.

In this chapter, we discuss some of these atypical femoral head fractures, which are not included in any of the classification systems but have a significant bearing on the outcomes of the patient.

11.2 Types of Atypical Fractures

Several uncommon patterns of femoral head fractures, often documented in isolated case reports, are beyond the scope of the Pipkin classification and its standard management protocols. These patterns include:

1. Femoral head fracture without hip dislocation
2. Combined femoral head and neck fractures (and may be trochanteric fracture) without hip dislocation
3. Femoral head fractures associated with anterior hip dislocation
4. Fracture of the superior part of the femur head
5. Multi-fragment, impacted, or sleeve fractures of the femoral head, with or without hip dislocation

Due to the rarity of these fracture patterns and combinations, standardized management guidelines remain poorly understood. Further studies are needed to clarify the mechanism of injury, develop appropriate treatment protocols, and improve patient outcomes for unclassified femoral head fractures. A better understanding of such atypical patterns will contribute to refining classification systems and optimizing surgical strategies.

11.3 Femur Head Fracture Without Hip Dislocation

A femoral head fracture is most commonly associated with posterior hip dislocation [1, 2]. This injury pattern is typically caused by a posteriorly directed force applied to the knee with the hip flexed [1]. However, femoral head fractures without accompanying hip dislocation are a rare entity. These fracture patterns have recently gained importance owing to sporadic case reports [3–5] (Fig. 11.1). These atypical injuries are not included in any of the existing classification systems.

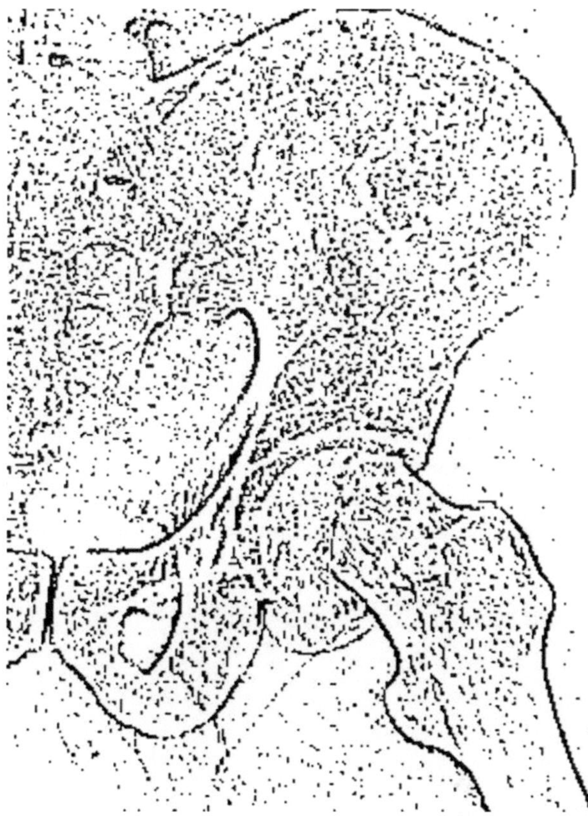

Fig. 11.1 Fracture of the femur head and neck without dislocation of the hip joint

11.3.1 Mechanism of Injury

The proposed mechanism for these injuries involves high-energy trauma in which the force is transmitted directly to the femoral head (may be lateral impaction along with vertical shear) without causing hip dislocation [3–5]. Two additional reports describe cases of femoral head fractures without dislocation, where the mechanism appears to involve spontaneous reduction of the dislocation. In one case, ligament avulsion of the femoral head was reported [6], while another involved a classical Pipkin II fracture accompanied by an ipsilateral knee injury [7].

Management: These fracture patterns need a high index of suspicion to diagnose, and the inability to diagnose the same leads to total hip arthroplasty [3, 4]. Some authors have managed these fractures conservatively as well [5]. In younger patients with such injuries, timely diagnosis is crucial, as open reduction and internal fixation (ORIF) can provide favorable outcomes, especially if the fracture fragment is extensive and involves the weight-bearing region (Pipkin II). Subarticular fixation is essential, necessitating the use of techniques such as headless compression screws, countersinking screws, or suture anchor repair. When these injuries are diagnosed late, a planned total hip arthroplasty is typically the most appropriate treatment strategy.

11.4 Femur Head and Neck Fracture (/Trochanter) Without Hip Dislocation

Another pattern not described by the existing classification systems is a Pipkin's fracture with a sub-capital neck fracture without hip dislocation [8, 9] (Fig. 11.2).

11.4.1 Mechanism of Injury

The hip does not dislocate, suggesting that the fracture of the femoral neck extended into the femoral head rather than the opposite [9].

A case report proposed the mechanism of shear stress acting on the femoral neck, followed by lateral impaction in a motorbike injury [8]. This report further

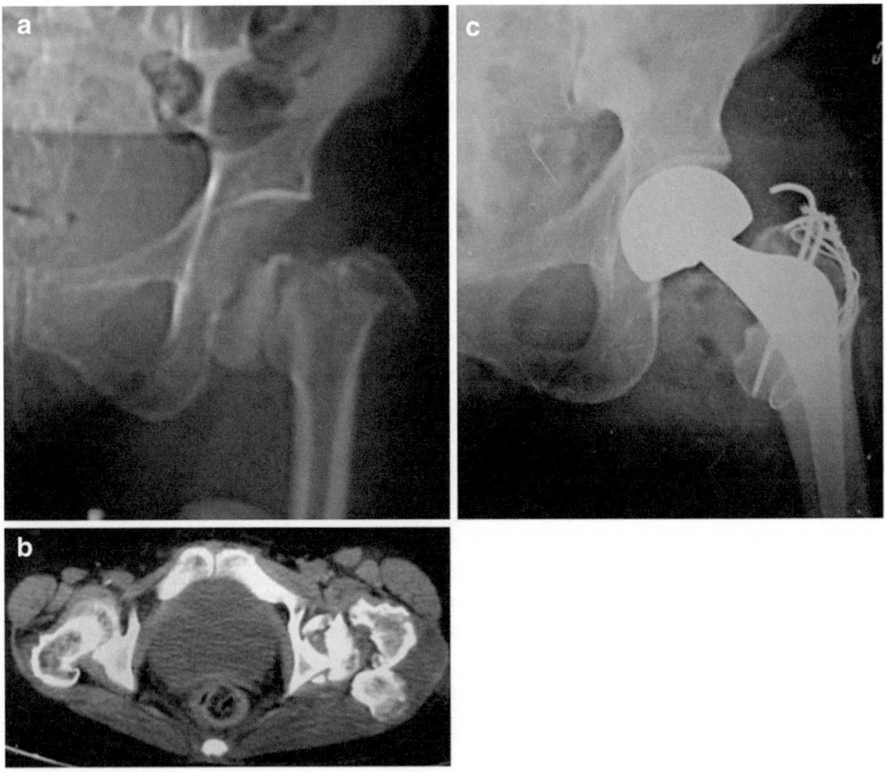

Fig. 11.2 (**a**) Femur head and neck fracture with trochanteric fracture in an elderly male patient, (**b**) axial cut of CT scan, and (**c**) trochanteric reconstruction along with bipolar hemiarthroplasty

emphasized that the continued momentum of the falling bike caused the patient's hip to move into extension, adduction, and external rotation, followed by lateral impaction during the fall. This sequence resulted in a sub-capital femoral neck fracture and additional impaction against the femoral head fragment, creating another fracture of the femoral head with an inferior femoral head fragment.

11.4.2 Prognosis

This type of injury involves extensive damage to the cancellous bone and vascularity of the femoral head. Osteosynthesis in such cases is associated with a high risk of avascular necrosis, subchondral collapse, secondary osteoarthritis, and fixation failure. Consequently, the patient may require a total hip arthroplasty after fixation.

11.5 Femur Head Fractures with Anterior Hip Dislocation

Obvious femoral head fractures in a case of anterior hip dislocation are a rare entity, and these are often indentation or impaction injuries. There are very few case reports on femur head fracture and anterior hip dislocation [10–12]. The proposed mechanism of injury involves the hip being in external rotation, abduction and extension in motor vehicle accident, or fall from height [10]. When a sudden brake is applied, the force transmitted across the knee reaches the femoral head, causing the upper and outer portion of the femoral head to impact the acetabulum (Fig. 11.3).

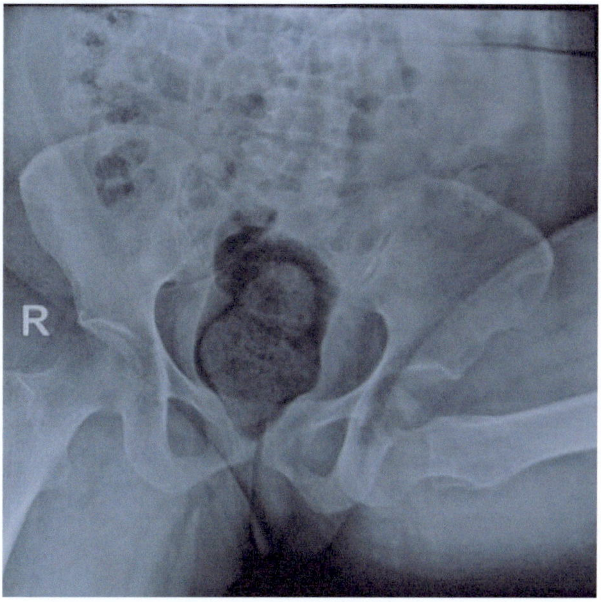

Fig. 11.3 Femur head fracture with anterior hip dislocation

Simultaneously, the femoral neck experiences significant shear stress, resulting in a vertical shear fracture.

A similar case was reported by Hu et al. in which there was an obturator type of anterior hip dislocation, femoral head and neck fractures, and pubic fractures [13]. Treatment included open reduction, internal fixation with cannulated screws, a medial support plate, and artificial bone grafting to support the femoral head defect. The patient showed good hip function and fracture healing at the 6-month follow-up without displacement, implant loosening, valgus deformity, or signs of femoral head necrosis. Prompt partial weight-bearing and hip abductors strengthening exercises were suggested to prevent muscular atrophy.

11.6 Fracture of the Superior Part of the Femur Head

A classical Pipkin fracture typically involves the anterior-inferior aspect of the femoral head, occurring due to a posterior hip dislocation. However, in some cases, only the superior part of the femoral head is fractured, while the lower portion remains intact (Fig. 11.4). Reconstruction in such cases is usually less complex, as part of the femoral neck remains uninjured.

The Ganz approach is often employed to access the affected part of the femoral head for fragment reconstruction. Despite successful reconstruction, the risk of avascular necrosis (AVN) remains high. As a result, these cases frequently progress to requiring hip arthroplasty.

11.7 Multi-fragment, Impacted, or Sleeve Fractures of the Femoral Head, with or Without Hip Dislocation

A Pipkin's fracture is typically a simple split fracture. However, there are reports of more complex cases involving significant comminution of proximal femoral fractures (Fig. 11.2). Such fractures are often observed in older individuals with osteoporotic bones, while they are rare in younger individuals. Due to their comminuted nature, these fractures are commonly managed with arthroplasty.

These cases stand out due to their extreme rarity and the complexity of the management strategies they require. Achieving proper anatomical reduction and stable fixation of all components is essential, along with careful postoperative rehabilitation to ensure optimal outcomes. Hip preservation procedures in young adults may include techniques such as fresh frozen osteochondral graft implantation, autologous chondrocyte implantation, and cartilage repair using suture anchors after debridement of small comminuted fragments. In cases deemed unreconstructable, total hip arthroplasty is performed.

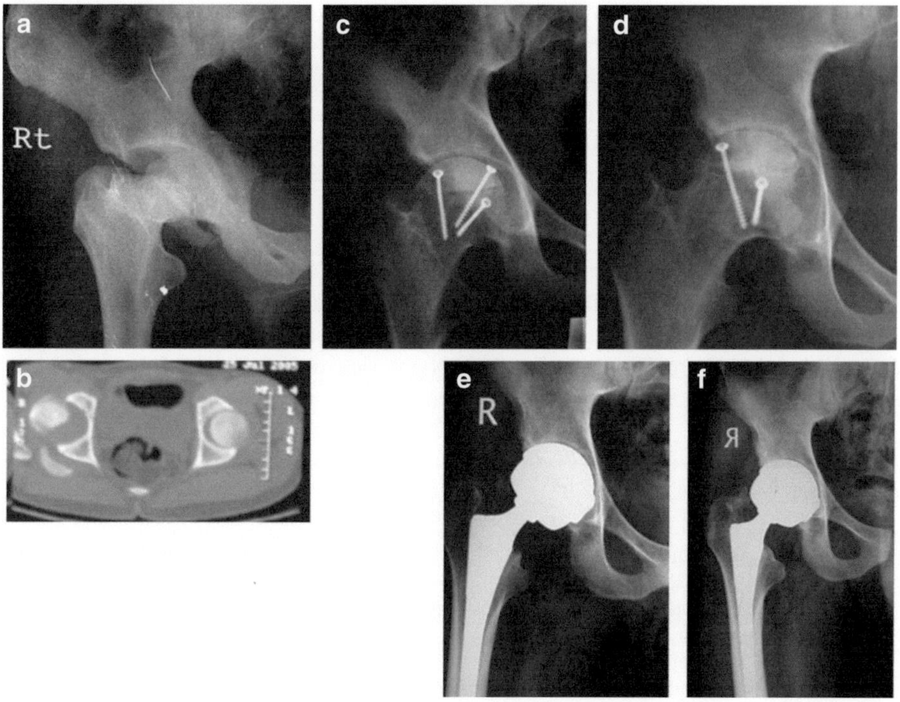

Fig. 11.4 (**a**) Fracture in the superior aspect of the femur head without dislocation; (**b**) axial cut section of the CT scan shows the displacement of the femoral head fragment with reduced hip joint; (**c**) surgical reduction and fixation of the fragment; (**d**) after 1 year, there is AVN of the femur head with decreased joint space; and (**e, f**) 1-year and 4-year follow-up following THR

11.8 Modified Brumback Classification

Wani et al. modified Brumback classification to involve cases involving femoral head fractures associated with femoral neck fractures and both anterior and posterior hip dislocations [14]. They subdivided the type III fracture pattern of the Brumback classification system into four types (Table 11.1). These modifications aim to address the broader spectrum of injury patterns and provide a more comprehensive framework for classification and management.

11.9 Summary

While most femoral head fractures can be categorized using the Pipkin classification, many unique patterns exist involving the femoral head in combination with various other injuries. Each specific fracture pattern often corresponds to a distinct mechanism of injury, requiring tailored reduction steps and fixation techniques.

Table 11.1 Wani's modification of type III Brumback classification

Types	Description
3A1	Posterior dislocation without femoral head fracture
3A2	Anterior dislocation without femoral head fracture
3A3	Posterior dislocation with femoral head fracture
3A4	Anterior dislocation with femoral head fracture

As the incidence of trauma continues to rise in the developing world, it becomes increasingly essential to define and refine management protocols for these injuries. Specific fracture patterns, such as femoral neck fractures with hip dislocation or femoral head fractures combined with trochanteric fractures, are not as rare as previously thought and warrant particular attention in clinical practice.

References

1. Pipkin G. Treatment of grade IV fracture-dislocation of the hip. J Bone Joint Surg Am. 1957;39-A:1027–42. passim
2. Giannoudis PV, Kontakis G, Christoforakis Z, Akula M, Tosounidis T, Koutras C. Management, complications and clinical results of femoral head fractures. Injury. 2009;40:1245–51. https://doi.org/10.1016/j.injury.2009.10.024.
3. Mody BS, Wainwright AM. Fracture of the femoral head without associated hip dislocation following low-energy trauma. A report of two cases. Arch Orthop Trauma Surg. 1996;115:300–2. https://doi.org/10.1007/BF00439059.
4. Aggarwal AK, Soni A, Singh D. Femoral head fracture without hip dislocation. Chin J Traumatol Zhonghua Chuang Shang Za Zhi. 2013;16:304–7.
5. Yoon PW, Jeong HS, Yoo JJ, Koo K-H, Yoon KS, Kim HJ. Femoral head fracture without dislocation by low-energy trauma in a young adult. Clin Orthop Surg. 2011;3:336–41. https://doi.org/10.4055/cios.2011.3.4.336.
6. Kumar P, Agarwal S, Rajnish RK, Aggarwal S, Kumar V, Jindal K. Ipsilateral posterior cruciate ligament insertion avulsion and femoral head fracture without dislocation: a rarest of rare dashboard injury and principles of management: a case report. JBJS Case Connect. 2019;9:e0245. https://doi.org/10.2106/JBJS.CC.18.00245.
7. Lee Y-K, Min JJ, Koo K-H. Pipkin type IV femoral head fracture without dislocation. Ann Surg Case Rep. 2019;2
8. Pawar K, Kandhari VK. A rare medley: concurrent ipsilateral femur head and neck fracture without hip dislocation. J Surg Case Rep. 2016;2016:rjv177. https://doi.org/10.1093/jscr/rjv177.
9. Kim KI, Koo KH, Sharma R, Park HB, Hwang SC. Concomitant fractures of the femoral head and neck without hip dislocation. Clin Orthop. 2001:247–50. https://doi.org/10.1097/00003086-200110000-00028.
10. DeLee JC, Evans JA, Thomas J. Anterior dislocation of the hip and associated femoral-head fractures. J Bone Joint Surg Am. 1980;62:960–4.
11. Dussault RG, Beauregard G, Fauteaux P, Laurin C, Boisjoly A. Femoral head defect following anterior hip dislocation. Radiology. 1980;135:627–9. https://doi.org/10.1148/radiology.135.3.7384446.

12. Jithin CR, Vincent A, Thamby R, Sajil Krishna K, Kumar NS. Anterior dislocation of the hip with femoral head fracture and osteochondral fracture of contralateral patella – a case report. J Orthop Rep. 2022;1:100070. https://doi.org/10.1016/j.jorep.2022.100070.
13. Hu Y, Gao F, Liu H, Chen L, Li Y, Li Z, Huang C, Wang Y, Piao C. Obturator dislocation of the femoral head combined with ipsilateral femoral neck and pubic fractures. Medicine (Baltimore). 2019;98:e17150. https://doi.org/10.1097/MD.0000000000017150.
14. Wani MM, Hussain A, Bashir A, Wani I, Moosa M, Wani MM, Mir BA, Halwai MA. Anterior dislocation of hip with ipsilateral femoral neck and head fracture. Eur J Orthop Surg Traumatol. 2010;3:245–9. https://doi.org/10.1007/s00590-009-0545-4.

Complications of Femoral Head Fracture-Dislocations

12

Rahul Vaidya, and Daniel Jonathan Joiner

12.1 Introduction

Femoral head fracture-dislocations are severe orthopedic injuries that often result from high-energy trauma, such as motor vehicle accidents or falls from height. Due to the complex anatomy and biomechanical environment of the hip joint, these injuries can lead to a variety of complications. Prompt recognition and management are crucial to minimize long-term morbidity and optimize patient outcomes. This chapter will discuss the various complications associated with femoral head fracture-dislocations, exploring both acute and chronic issues. It should be noted that the incidence of femoral head fractures is low, making studies difficult through a single institution. The majority of literature regarding femoral head fractures/femoral head fracture dislocations is through meta-analysis and retrospective studies. For the purposes of this chapter, we will use the Pipkin classification to describe the injury pattern, determine treatment, and guide prognostic evaluation [1]. The complexity of these fractures lies not only in their classification but also in the nature of the injuries sustained by surrounding structures, particularly the soft tissues, nerves, cartilage, and the vascular supply to the femoral head.

12.2 Failed Closed Reduction

With fracture dislocations of the femoral head, closed reduction may be easy (Fig. 12.1) or hard due to a locked dislocation (Fig. 12.2). This is due to the remaining head having a flat surface on its inferior border and being button holed through the posterior capsule. In these situations, an open reduction is the best option to avoid repeated attempts and a femoral neck fracture (Fig. 12.2b) turning a Pipkin II

R. Vaidya (✉) · D. Jonathan Joiner
Detroit Medical Center, Wayne State University, Detroit, MI, USA

R. K. Sen, S. K. Tripathy (eds.), *A Practical Guide to Management of Femoral Head Fracture-Dislocation*, https://doi.org/10.1007/978-981-96-9852-3_12

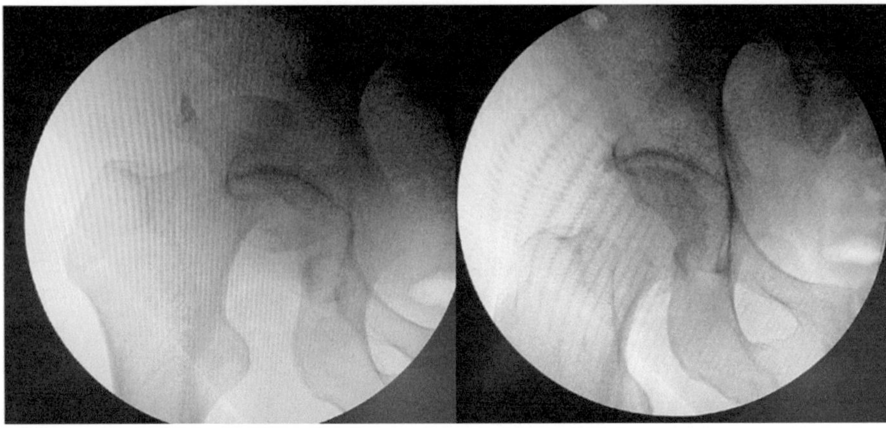

Fig. 12.1 Pipkin type II fracture successfully managed with closed reduction

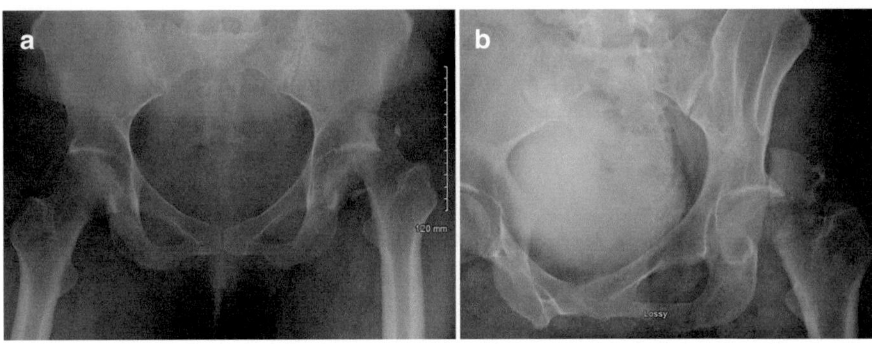

Fig. 12.2 (**a**) Irreducible Pipkin type II fracture-dislocation. (**b**) Multiple failed closed reduction attempts resulted in iatrogenic femoral neck fracture, converting it to a Pipkin type III injury

fracture into III, which has a high rate of avascular necrosis and nonunion (Fig. 12.2b).

12.3 Hemorrhage

Significant hemorrhage may occur at the time of injury, especially in cases involving fractures of the femoral head or neck which are associated with pelvic or acetabular injury. Algorithms for acute bleeding are usually related to pelvic injury and should follow ATLS Stop the Bleed protocols [2], including massive transfusion availability, pelvic binders, packing, and angiography [3]. Bleeding during surgery can be avoided by avoiding the quadratus femoris muscle to not disrupt the medial femoral circumflex vessel or dissecting and retracting carefully along the sciatic notch to prevent injury to the superior gluteal artery. Maintaining the vascularity of the femoral head is paramount in avoiding later avascular necrosis. Sudden bursts of bleeding can be packed and placed under pressure, followed by getting control of the vessel more proximally with a clamp. If the bleeding cannot be controlled due to vessel retraction, 10–20 min of pressure may alleviate serious hemorrhage. This can be followed by angiography and embolization when it is available (Fig. 12.3) [3]. Bone bleeding can be dealt with reduction of fractures or placing bone wax into arterial entry points that bleed after disruption of the periosteum. The prevention of postoperative hematoma can be aided by the use of tranexamic acid which can be administered through IV, topically, or combining both methods (which may be most effective) [4, 5].

12.4 Neurologic Injury

The reported incidence of a sciatic nerve injury following a femoral head fracture is 4–10%, and it is implied to be higher in a fracture-dislocation [6–10]. It can be caused by the injury or be iatrogenic during the surgery from stretching, compression, or laceration by surgical instruments. Late compression can occur by the formation of heterotopic ossification [11]. Patients may present with neurological deficits which include complete sciatic nerve palsy, just a peroneal nerve palsy, or partial nerve injuries which can be sensory, motor, or both. Emergent relocation of the hip should be attempted either closed or open to release pressure. A thorough physical exam and vigilant follow-up exams are warranted to document injury to the sciatic nerve and its changing status to ensure the best outcome [10–13]. Timing of intervention for sciatic nerve injury is controversial; however, it can be divided into early, mid-term, or late. Typically observation in the early phase is performed, because contusion and neuropraxia are the most likely mechanisms of injury in this setting [10]. Magnetic resonance imaging can help diagnose a laceration [12]. Acute rupture or laceration of the sciatic nerve is rare. If a laceration is considered in this

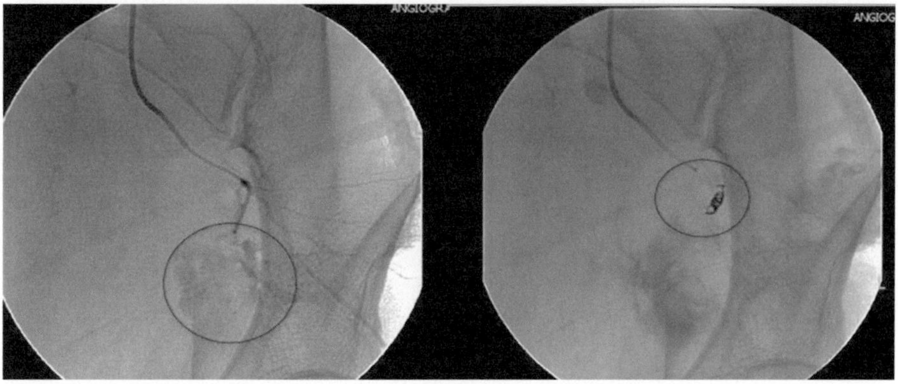

Fig. 12.3 Intraoperative control of bleeding from the sciatic notch during a Kocher-Langenbeck approach using packing, followed by embolization of the superior gluteal artery via angiography

interval, acute repair is warranted—despite poor results of repair or grafting [10, 11]. Mid-term intervention includes nerve conduction studies after 3 months of observation with neurodiagnostic testing to evaluate progression of recovery. Approximately 65% recover when caused by the injury and about 75% when it is iatrogenic because they are neuropraxia or axonotmesis [12–15]. It can take 2–3 years to fully recover in the case of axonotmesis. Rehabilitation should start right away to prevent equinus deformity of the foot [12]. Late intervention can include tendon transfers if one branch is spared or ankle arthrodesis [10–12]. Postoperative gradual onset of sciatic nerve palsy can be caused by the formation of heterotopic ossification and can be progressive. Identification and decompression can solve this issue.

12.5 Infection

The rate of postoperative infection after treatment of fracture dislocation of the femoral head is 1–3.2% [16]. Due to the paucity of cases in most series, there was no general consensus of treatment of infection when it occurs after surgery in this situation. Even when taking care of infection after acetabular fractures, it is important to prevent a destructive septic arthritis of the hip or osteomyelitis by early recognition, irrigation, careful debridement, and culture-specific antibiotics for 6 weeks minimum. The problem with infection is that it may render the hip unsuitable for total hip arthroplasty [17, 18] (Fig. 12.4a, b). In those instances, a hip fusion or girdle stone hip resection may be the only options to allow ambulation.

12.6 Joint Dislocation/Recurrent Instability

Recurrent instability after the treatment of Pipkin fracture dislocations is sparsely mentioned in the literature but may be one of the causes of early failure resulting in posttraumatic osteoarthritis. There are few articles that mention recurrent instability or escape of the hip [19–21]. Recurrent dislocation may be caused by the loss of capsular or muscular constraints [19, 21]. This can be treated by varus derotation osteotomy [19] or total hip replacement that may also need to be constrained [21]. Varus derotation osteotomy has also been used in cases where the hip starts to sublux or escape, in hips with a high femoral neck shaft angle [20] with success in two cases. Hips that have some ongoing instability may go on to osteoarthritis [21] which is usually treated with a total hip arthroplasty.

12.7 Avascular Necrosis (AVN)

Avascular necrosis of the femoral head is one of the most common complications of femoral head fractures [16]. The disruption of the medial and lateral circumflex arteries can lead to ischemic necrosis of the femoral head, osteochondral fractures,

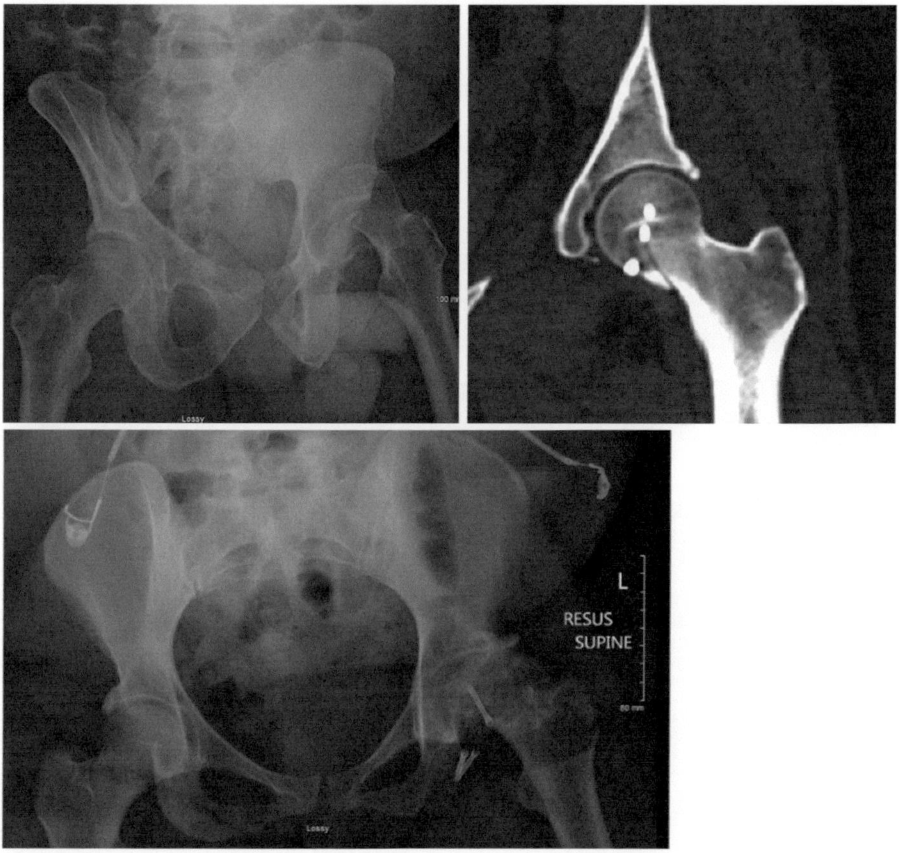

Fig. 12.4 (**a**) A Pipkin II fracture dislocation was reduced and (**b**) fixed using screws. (**c**) Subsequent joint infection rendered the hip unsuitable for arthroplasty

collapse of the femoral head, and osteoarthritis. The incidence of AVN varies, but recent meta-analysis describes a rate of 8.8% of all Pipkin cases [22]. Pipkin type III fractures have the highest rate of AVN with almost 65% due to fracture of the femoral neck disrupting the femoral circumflex vessels, and many advocate immediate total hip arthroplasty (THA) for this condition [22] (Fig. 12.5). The approach used for open treatment also makes a difference in the rate of AVN with a trochanteric flip surgery having 2.8 times less incidence of AVN than an anterior approach and 2.1 times less incidence of AVN than a Kocher-Langenbeck approach for treatment [22]. Not all cases of AVN go on to pain and collapse [8] (Fig. 12.6). The treatment options for AVN depend on the age of the patient. In young patients, attempts at salvage with core decompression may be beneficial for some. If there is collapse of the head, there are rotational osteotomies which have success rates of anywhere from 50% to 80% [23, 24], as well as impaction grafting of the AVN segment using a surgical dislocation approach [24–26]. Both of these techniques

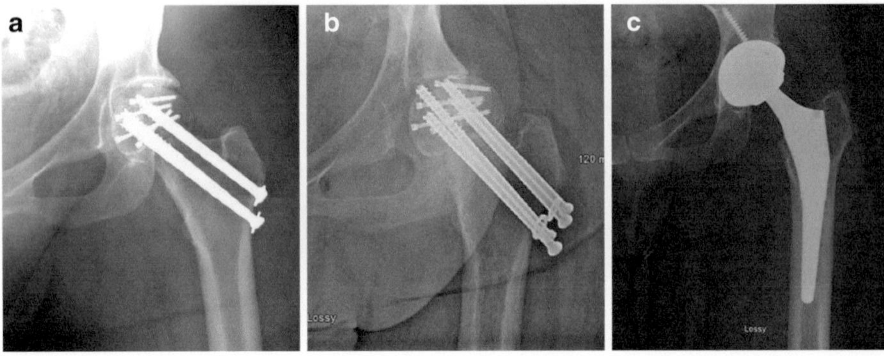

Fig. 12.5 (**a**) Pipkin type III fracture treated with open reduction and internal fixation (ORIF). (**b**) Developed avascular necrosis (AVN) and nonunion. (**c**) Managed with conversion to total hip arthroplasty (THA)

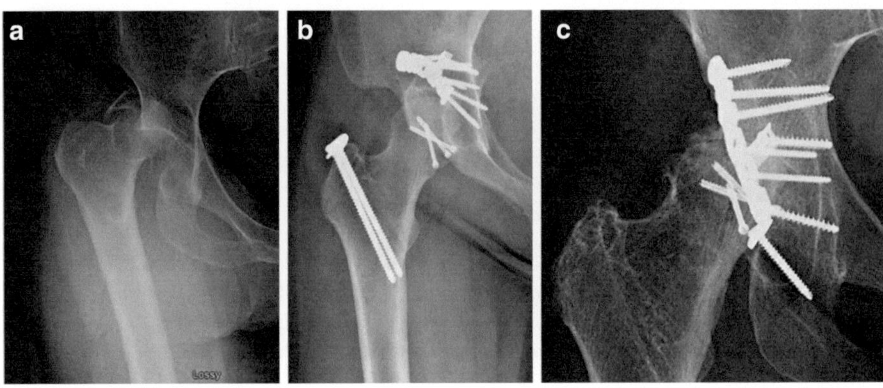

Fig. 12.6 (**a**) Pipkin type II fracture-dislocation. (**b**) Treated with surgical hip dislocation and ORIF. (**c**) Progressed to femoral head subluxation, AVN, and collapse, although THA has not yet been performed

attempt to preserve the hip in young patients up to 50 years of age. In older patients, THA is the best solution [27].

12.8 Posttraumatic Osteoarthritis

Posttraumatic osteoarthritis may develop due to the incongruence of the joint surfaces following fracture-dislocations, as a secondary consequence of traumatic cartilage damage to the femoral head, avascular necrosis, or instability [8, 9, 22, 27]. The altered biomechanics and prolonged immobility can contribute to degenerative changes in the articular cartilage, subsequently leading to chronic pain, stiffness, and a decrease in functional mobility over time. While posttraumatic arthritis is a commonly seen midterm complication within 6–12 months or late, the degree of symptoms, onset of symptoms, and disability are variable [9, 22, 27, 28]. The initial injury in the intra-articular fracture leads to immediate chondrocyte death and the release of metal metalloprotease in an inflammatory cascade within the synovial fluid that propagates further chondrocyte injury; therefore, time to reduction and fixation has proven to be the best indicator of functional outcome [22]. Pipkin III fractures in individuals >35 yrs should be treated with primary THA due to the high incidence of failure of treatment with ORIF (almost 100% in some studies) [22]. Pipkin IV fractures also have a 28.5% conversion to THA at 12 months especially cases of suprafoveal and head impaction or patients of older age and should be considered for immediate THA as well [29].

Total hip arthroplasty for posttraumatic osteoarthritis whether from Pipkin or acetabular fractures is more difficult. The treating surgeon has to deal with soft tissue scarring, which may include the sciatic nerve, existing hardware, and increased risk of complications. These include infection reported as high as 16%, implant loosening 1–24%, and heterotopic ossification 28–63% with 5-year survival rates of the implant reported to be 70–100% [29]. Outcomes with arthroplasty have proven to be good after posttraumatic osteoarthritis and allow for immediate weight bearing and resumption of daily activities and significant improvement in pain and function even at 10-year follow-up [29, 30] (Fig. 12.7).

12.9 Heterotopic Ossification

Heterotopic ossification (HO) is the most common complication after fracture dislocation of the femoral head reported to occur in 15.4% of cases [22]. It is characterized by the formation of bone in non-osseous tissues, occurring in response to trauma or surgical intervention. It can restrict mobility, compress the sciatic nerve, and cause discomfort. HO is graded using the Brooker grading system that ranges from I to IV with IV being complete synostosis of the joint [31]. Symptoms include pain, stiffness, or decreased range of motion of the hip joint (more prevalent with higher grades of HO) and nerve compression of the sciatic or less commonly the

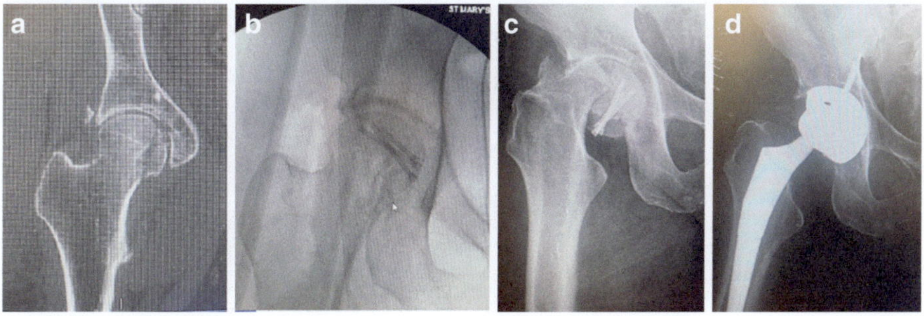

Fig. 12.7 (**a**) Pipkin type II fracture. (**b**) Post-ORIF radiograph. (**c**) A second femoral neck fracture was noted 12 months later. (**d**) Managed with primary THA

femoral nerve. The risk may be increased in individuals with higher energy injuries, traumatic brain injury/spinal cord injury, burns, and injured soft tissues enveloping the hip joint [32–34]. HO prevention after pelvic and acetabular surgery has been extensively investigated with most studies using either post-op radiation (800 cGy local within 72 h) or oral indomethacin (25 mg TID start within 24 h—6 weeks post-op). A systematic review by Blokhuis et al. in 2009 found that RDT was more effective than indomethacin in preventing HO [32]. A more recent systematic review by Bueno et al. [33] found there was insufficient evidence to show that either was effective in the prevention of HO after acetabular and pelvic surgery, but indomethacin had more reported complications [33]. Once HO is present and symptomatic, the treatment consists of resection. Of the few reports of HO resection, some advocate waiting until the HO is mature with cold bone scans or a normalization of serum alkaline phosphatase [34, 35]. Meanwhile, others advocate early resection as early as 3 months to preserve the patient's range of motion, to facilitate rehab, and to be able to delineate the new bone from native bone [36]. Post-op radiation plus indomethacin for 6 weeks may be employed for recurrence which happens in 30–40% of cases to some degree. Repeat excision may be necessary when resection is done early, but advocates mention the ability to maintain range of motion throughout recovery is a benefit. When the HO is posterior to the hip joint (Fig. 12.8), the sciatic nerve may need to be decompressed as occasionally it is pushed laterally or encased within the bone leading to symptoms of compression which include pain, weakness, and altered or absent sensation. The easiest way to protect it is to locate it distally and follow it back and then often unroof the tunnel it is encased in with Kerrison Rongeurs. Anterior HO can be hard to excise, and when large, a dissection of the femoral artery and control of the profunda artery prior to excision can prevent uncontrolled bleeding (Fig. 12.9). Heterotopic ossification above the joint is less common, and as long as you stay away from the neurovascular structures, you should be fine (Fig. 12.10). Outcomes are good with resection but also depend on the original injury [36].

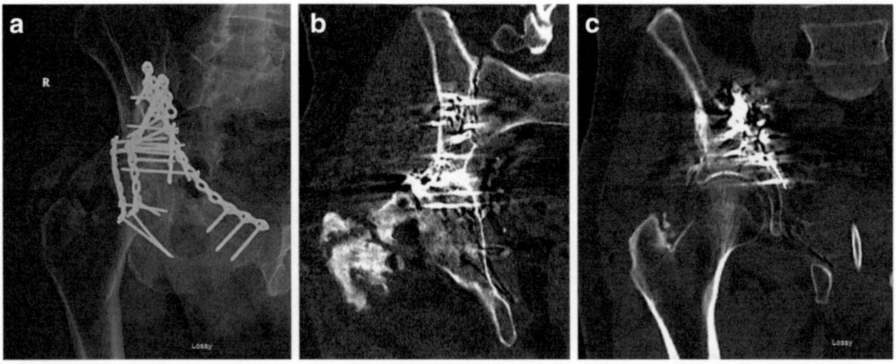

Fig. 12.8 (**a**) Extensive posterior heterotopic ossification causing hip synostosis. (**b**) CT imaging. (**c**) Post-resection, full range of motion restored

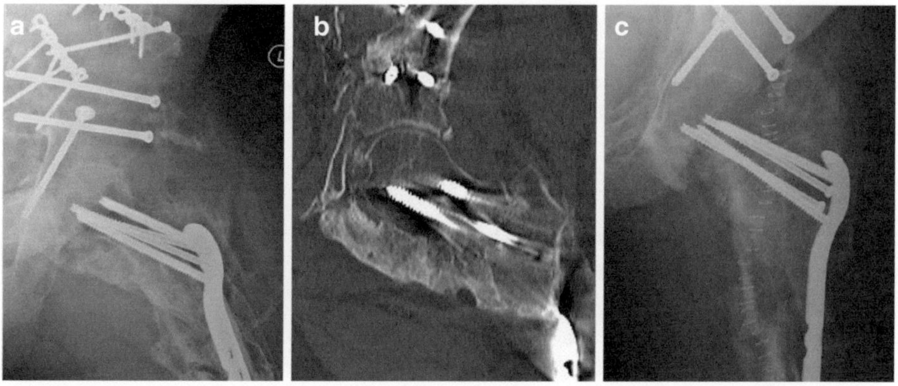

Fig. 12.9 (**a**) Anterior heterotopic ossification. (**b**) CT confirmation. (**c**) Post-resection status. Dissection of femoral and profunda vessels facilitates safe bone resection and hemorrhage control

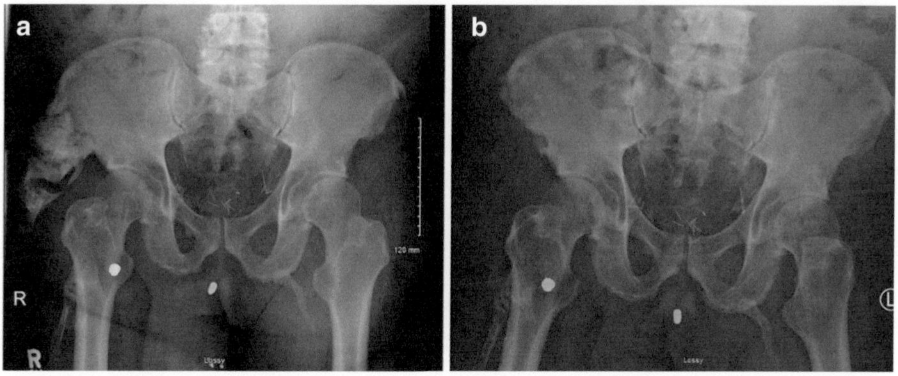

Fig. 12.10 (**a**) Superior heterotopic ossification of the hip joint. (**b**) Status post-surgical resection

12.10 Malunion Nonunion

Malunion of the femoral head is a relatively rare occurrence with only a few reports of correction within the literature. Femoral head fractures (Pipkin fractures) involve the articular surface of the hip joint, which makes restoration of a congruous joint surface a primary goal in most surgical interventions. Failure to restore this congruity can result in bony mechanical block and/or hip pain, femoroacetabular impingement, osteoarthritis, and osteonecrosis. Small boney fragments can be excised [37], while larger fragments have been osteotomized and re-fixed open [38] or by arthroscope [39] with moderate success reported in two cases. Total hip arthroplasty is a good alternative in older patients.

Nonunion of bony fragments leads to resorption and progression to joint incongruency, instability, pain, and discomfort. Early treatment of fragment excision and hardware removal may help, but eventually joint incongruency will lead to posttraumatic osteoarthritis and THA. Nonunion of the trochanteric flip osteotomy (TFO) occurs in 3.4% of cases in a recent metanalysis [40] which is treated by repeat surgery and fixation. Trochanteric bursitis due to hardware for the TFO is commonly reported and may benefit from hardware removal once the osteotomy has healed [40].

12.11 Chronic Pain and Disability with Generalized Deconditioning

Patients who experience femoral head fracture-dislocations may undergo prolonged periods of immobility due to pain and restriction of movement, leading to muscle atrophy, decreased bone density, and generalized deconditioning. Addressing physical health holistically through rehabilitation programs is important to minimize these implications and enhance recovery.

Chronic pain is frequently reported among patients who suffer from femoral head fracture-dislocations, even after successful surgical intervention. This pain may result from arthritis, avascular necrosis, instability, or capsular stiffness. Persistent disability can significantly impact the quality of life, requiring long-term rehabilitation and possibly additional procedures for pain management. It is essential to provide immediate and midterm follow-up with imaging and clinical evaluation to provide recommendations for additional treatments. The incidence of arthroplasty is significant for these types of injuries despite early intervention, anatomic reduction, and successful rehabilitation.

12.12 Conclusion

Femoral head fracture-dislocations pose significant risks of complications that can have lasting impacts on patients' physical health and overall quality of life. The main posttraumatic complications include osteoarthritis, heterotopic ossification, AVN, and neurovascular injury [8, 9, 22, 27]. Proper acute management, early reduction of dislocations, and careful monitoring for vascular injuries can help identify and perhaps mitigate the risk of these complications. Long-term follow-up and a comprehensive rehabilitation approach are vital in addressing chronic pain and disability while fostering recovery and optimizing functional outcomes. As our understanding of these injuries evolves, ongoing research is necessary to improve surgical techniques and postoperative care to reduce complication rates and enhance patient outcomes.

References

1. Pipkin G. Treatment of grade IV fracture-dislocation of the hip. J Bone Joint Surg Am. 1957;39-A:1027–42, passim.

2. American College of Surgeons. ATLS advanced trauma life support: student course manual. 10th ed. Chicago: American College of Surgeons; 2018. Electronic Resource.
3. Vaidya R, Waldron J, Scott A, Nasr K. Angiography and embolization in the management of bleeding pelvic fractures. J Am Acad Orthop Surg. 2018;26(4):e68–76. https://doi.org/10.5435/JAAOS-D-16-00600. PMID: 29351135; PMCID: PMC5794236.
4. Shu HT, Mikula JD, Yu AT, Shafiq B. Tranexamic acid use in pelvic and/or acetabular fracture surgery: a systematic review and meta-analysis. J Orthop. 2021;28:112–6. https://doi.org/10.1016/j.jor.2021.11.018.
5. Sun Y, Jiang C, Li Q. A systematic review and meta-analysis comparing combined intravenous and topical tranexamic acid with intravenous administration alone in THA. Hills RK, ed. PLoS One. 2017;12(10):e0186174. https://doi.org/10.1371/journal.pone.0186174.
6. Hougaard K, Thomsen PB. Traumatic posterior fracture-dislocation of the hip with fracture of the femoral head or neck, or both. J Bone Joint Surg. Am. 1988;70(2):233–9.
7. DeLee JC, Evans JA, Thomas J. Anterior dislocation of the hip and associated femoral-head fractures. J Bone Joint Surg Am. 1980;62(6):960–4.
8. Sen RK, Tripathy SK, Goyal T, Aggarwal S, Kashyap S, Purudappa PP, Chandrappa MH. Complications and functional outcome of femoral head fracture-dislocation in delayed and neglected cases. Indian J Orthop. 2021;55(3):595–605.
9. Giannoudis PV, Kontakis G, Christoforakis Z, Akula M, Tosounidis T, Koutras C. Management, complications and clinical results of femoral head fractures. Injury. 2009;40(1):36–44.
10. Stavrakakis IM, Kritsotakis EI, Giannoudis PV, Kapsetakis P, Dimitriou R, Bastian JD, Tosounidis TH. Sciatic nerve injury after acetabular fractures: a meta-analysis of incidence and outcomes. Eur J Trauma Emerg Surg. 2022;48(4):2639–54.
11. Hillyard RF, Fox J. Sciatic nerve injuries associated with traumatic posterior hip dislocations. Am J Emerg Med. 2003;21(7):545–8.
12. Cornwall R, Radomisli TE. Nerve injury in traumatic dislocation of the hip. Clin Orthop Relat Res. 2000;377:84–91.
13. Liu Z, Fu B, Xu W, Liu F, Dong J, Li L, Zhou D, Hao Z, Lu S. Incidence of traumatic sciatic nerve injury in association with acetabular fracture: a retrospective observational single-center study. Int J Gen Med. 2022;15:7417–25.
14. Klifto KM, et al. Treatment approach to isolated common peroneal nerve palsy by mechanism of injury: systematic review and meta-analysis of individual participants' data. J Plast Reconstr Aesthet Surg. 2022;75(2):683–702.
15. Birkett J. Description of a dislocation of the head of the femur, complicated with its fracture; with remarks by John Birkett (1815–1904). Clin Orthop Relat Res. 2000;377:4–6.
16. Menger MM, Braun BJ, Herath SC, Küper MA, Rollmann MF, Histing T. Fractures of the femoral head: a narrative review. EFORT Open Rev. 2021;6(11):1122–31. https://doi.org/10.1302/2058-5241.6.210034. PMID: 34909230; PMCID: PMC8631236.
17. Li Q, Liu P, Wang G, et al. Risk factors of surgical site infection after acetabular fracture surgery. Surg Infect. 2015;16(5):577–82. https://doi.org/10.1089/sur.2014.134.
18. Mardanpour K, Rahbar M, Mardanpour S, Rezaei M. Risk factors for surgical site infections after open reduction and internal fixation of acetabulum fracture in the west of Iran. Int J Surg Open. 2020;27:119–22. https://doi.org/10.1016/j.ijso.2020.11.006.
19. Marti RK, Kloen P. Chronic recurrent posterior dislocation of the hip after a Pipkin fracture treated with intertrochanteric osteotomy and acetabuloplasty. A case report. J Bone Joint Surg Am. 2000;82(6):867–72.
20. Miyamoto S, Nakamura J, Iida S, Suzuki C, Ohtori S, Orita S, Takahashi K. Femoral varus osteotomy for hip instability after traumatic fracture dislocations of the hip associated with femoral head fractures: a report of two cases. Case Rep Orthop. 2016;2016:1450842. https://doi.org/10.1155/2016/1450842. Epub 2016 May 16. PMID: 27293934; PMCID: PMC4884837.
21. Zuelzer DA, Ryan L, Mayer R, Pease T, Warner S, Eastman J, Wright RD, Routt MLC. Using an intraoperative stress examination to direct treatment in posterior femoral head fracture-dislocations. J Orthop Trauma. 2024;38(12):641–7. https://doi.org/10.1097/BOT.0000000000002912. PMID: 39213419.

22. Kloub M, Látal P, Giannoudis P. Techniques and results of reconstruction of femoral head fractures: an update. Injury. 2024;55(6):111473. https://doi.org/10.1016/j.injury.2024.111473. Epub 2024 Mar 5. PMID: 38538488.
23. Atsumi T, Nakanishi R, Yoshikawa Y, Watanabe M, Nishi M, Inagaki K. High-degree posterior rotational osteotomy for extensive collapsed femoral head osteonecrosis in teenagers: remodeling and results with a mean of 10-year follow-up. Arch Orthop Trauma Surg. 2023;143(10):6039–48. https://doi.org/10.1007/s00402-023-04864-4. Epub 2023 Apr 27. PMID: 37106100.
24. Xia T, Liu J, Shi L, Zhang C, Yao C, Shen J. Comparison of surgical dislocation and impacting bone graft and surgical dislocation and rotational osteotomy for the treatment of ARCO III femoral head necrosis. Medicine (Baltimore). 2020;99(20):e20215. https://doi.org/10.1097/MD.0000000000020215. PMID: 32443350; PMCID: PMC7253930.
25. Hanke MS, Keel MJB, Cullmann JL, Siebenrock KA, Bastian JD. Transfer of osteochondral shell autografts to salvage femoral head impaction injuries in hip trauma patients. Injury. 2020;51(3):711–8. https://doi.org/10.1016/j.injury.2020.01.037. Epub 2020 Jan 28. PMID: 32033805.
26. Shon HC, Lim EJ, Yang JY, Jeon SJ. Femoral head fracture with large crushed defect in weight-bearing area treated with autologous osteochondral transplantation (repositionplasty): a case report. Medicine (Baltimore). 2022;101(52):e32569. https://doi.org/10.1097/MD.0000000000032569. PMID: 36595972; PMCID: PMC9803454.
27. Beebe MJ, Bauer JM, Mir HR. Treatment of hip dislocations and associated injuries: current state of care. J Bone Joint Surg Am. 2016;99(14):1234–42.
28. Tornetta P III, Ricci WM, Ostrum RF, McQueen MM, McKee MD, Court-Brown CM. Rockwood and Green's fractures in adults. 9th ed. Philadelphia: Lippincott Williams & Wilkins, a Wolters Kluwer Business; 2019. p. 2224–5.
29. Cichos KH, White PA, Bergin PF, Ghanem ES, McGwin G Jr, Hawkins J, Spitler CA. Risk factors for early conversion total hip arthroplasty after Pipkin IV femoral head fracture. J Orthop Trauma. 2023;37(4):181–8. https://doi.org/10.1097/BOT.0000000000002512. PMID: 36730828.
30. Stibolt RD Jr, Patel HA, Huntley SR, Lehtonen EJ, Shah AB, Naranje SM. Total hip arthroplasty for posttraumatic osteoarthritis following acetabular fracture: a systematic review of characteristics, outcomes, and complications. Chin J Traumatol. 2018;21(3):176–81. https://doi.org/10.1016/j.cjtee.2018.02.004. Epub 2018 Apr 26. PMID: 29773451; PMCID: PMC6033725.
31. Brooker A, Bowerman J, Robinson R, Riley L. Ectopic ossification following total hip replacement incidence and a method of classification. J Bone Joint Surg. 1973;55(8):1629–32.
32. Blokhuis TJ, Frölke JPM. Is radiation superior to indomethacin to prevent heterotopic ossification in acetabular fractures?: a systematic review. Clin Orthop Relat Res. 2009;467(2):526–30. https://doi.org/10.1007/s11999-008-0532-9.
33. Bueno TSP, Godoy GP, Furukava RB, Gaggioli NT, Tamaoki MJS, Matsunaga FT, Belloti JC. Heterotopic Ossification In Acetabular Fractures: Systematic Review And Meta-Analysis Of Prophylaxis. Acta Ortop Bras. 2021;29(6):331–40. https://doi.org/10.1590/1413-785220212906244689. PMID: 34849100; PMCID: PMC8601386
34. Biering-Sørensen F, Tøndevold E. Indomethacin and disodium etidronate for the prevention of recurrence of heterotopic ossification after surgical resection. Two case reports. Spinal Cord. 1993;31(8):513–5. https://doi.org/10.1038/sc.1993.83.
35. Tibone JE, Sakimura IT, Nickel VL, Hsu JD. Heterotopic ossification around the hip in spinal cord-injured patients. A long-term follow-up study. J Bone Joint Surg. 1978;60(6):769–75. **https://pubmed.ncbi.nlm.nih.gov/100499/**. Accessed 12 July 2024.
36. Wu XB, Yang MH, Zhu SW, et al. Surgical resection of severe heterotopic ossification after open reduction and internal fixation of acetabular fractures: a case series of 18 patients. Injury. 2014;45(10):1604–10. https://doi.org/10.1016/j.injury.2014.05.018.
37. Yoon TR, Chung JY, Jung ST, Seo HY. Malunion of femoral head fractures treated by partial ostectomy: three case reports. J Orthop Trauma. 2003;17:447–50.

38. Ross JR, Clohisy JC. Correction of a femoral head fracture malunion with surgical dislocation of the hip: a case report. JBJS Case Connect. 2012;2:e71.
39. Matsuda DK. Arthroscopic osteosynthesis of femoral head malunion. Arthrosc Tech. 2014;3:e31–4.
40. Khalifa AA, Haridy MA, Fergany A. Safety and efficacy of surgical hip dislocation in managing femoral head fractures: a systematic review and meta-analysis. World J Orthop. 2021;12(8):604–19. https://doi.org/10.5312/wjo.v12.i8.604. PMID: 34485106; PMCID: PMC8384609.

Recent Advances in the Management of Femoral Head Fracture

13

Robert Cooke, Asim Rajpura, and Nikhil Shah

13.1 Introduction

Femoral head fractures are rare injuries typically resulting from high-energy trauma, often occurring in conjunction with acetabular fractures. Due to their infrequent occurrence, most available evidence on their management is derived from small case series and case reports, limiting comprehensive understanding and consensus on treatment strategies.

Giannoudis et al. [1] emphasized several challenges in establishing standardized management guidelines for femoral head fractures. These challenges include the absence of a classification system with clear prognostic value, variability in treatment approaches, and the lack of a validated outcome assessment tool.

Given the scarcity of significant advancements in the diagnosis, assessment, and management of femoral head fractures, it remains crucial to revisit the fundamental principles of their evaluation and treatment. This chapter aims to provide a detailed review of the evolution of femoral head fracture management over time while highlighting recent developments in this field.

The key aspects covered in this chapter include:

- Classification systems
- Femoral head blood supply
- Surgical approaches
- Surgical treatment options
- Minimally invasive treatment strategies

R. Cooke · A. Rajpura · N. Shah (✉)
Wrightington Hospital, Wigan, UK
e-mail: Robert.cooke@doctors.org.uk; Nikhil.shah@wwl.nhs.uk

R. K. Sen, S. K. Tripathy (eds.), *A Practical Guide to Management of Femoral Head Fracture-Dislocation*, https://doi.org/10.1007/978-981-96-9852-3_13

13.2 Classification Systems

Over the years, multiple classification systems have been introduced to enhance the understanding and prognostication of femoral head fractures. These include the **Pipkin, Brumback, AO, Chiron, and New** classification systems.

The **Pipkin classification**, first described in 1957, was an extension of **Stewart and Milford's** grade IV hip dislocation classification [2, 3]. Despite the development of several alternative systems, the **Pipkin classification remains the most widely utilized** in both clinical practice and research.

A study by **Wu et al.** [4] evaluated the universality, reliability, and reproducibility of various classification systems by assessing **231 femoral head fractures** with four independent observers. Their findings suggested that the **Pipkin and Chiron classifications** were the most applicable for clinical and research use due to their superior interobserver and intraobserver agreement.

In a **systematic review by Giannoudis et al.** [1], which analyzed **350 femoral head fractures**, the Pipkin classification emerged as the most frequently used system, applied in **301 cases**.

Pipkin's original study [2] suggested a **progressive decline in clinical outcomes as the classification advanced from type I to type IV**. However, Giannoudis' review [1] did not find a statistically significant difference in outcomes between individual **Pipkin subtypes**. Instead, statistical significance was only noted when **types I and II were grouped together and compared to types III and IV**, with the latter showing **poorer outcomes (Fig. 13.1)**.

Additionally, the systematic review highlighted that **coexisting acetabular fractures and joint instability** were key factors associated with **less favorable prognoses** in femoral head fractures.

13.3 Femoral Head Blood Supply

Our understanding of the vascular impact of femoral head dislocation and subsequent relocation has evolved significantly over time. The potential disruption of the arterial supply to the femoral head and the associated risk of avascular necrosis (AVN) remain key concerns, reinforcing the urgent need for emergency reduction in cases of hip dislocation.

The primary arterial supply to the femoral head is derived from three key sources:

- Deep branch of the medial femoral circumflex artery (MFCA)
- Posterior inferior nutrient artery (arising from the MFCA)
- Piriformis branch of the inferior gluteal artery

Among these, multiple studies have identified the deep branch of the MFCA as the most critical, with its terminal nutrient arteries supplying nearly the entire femoral head [5].

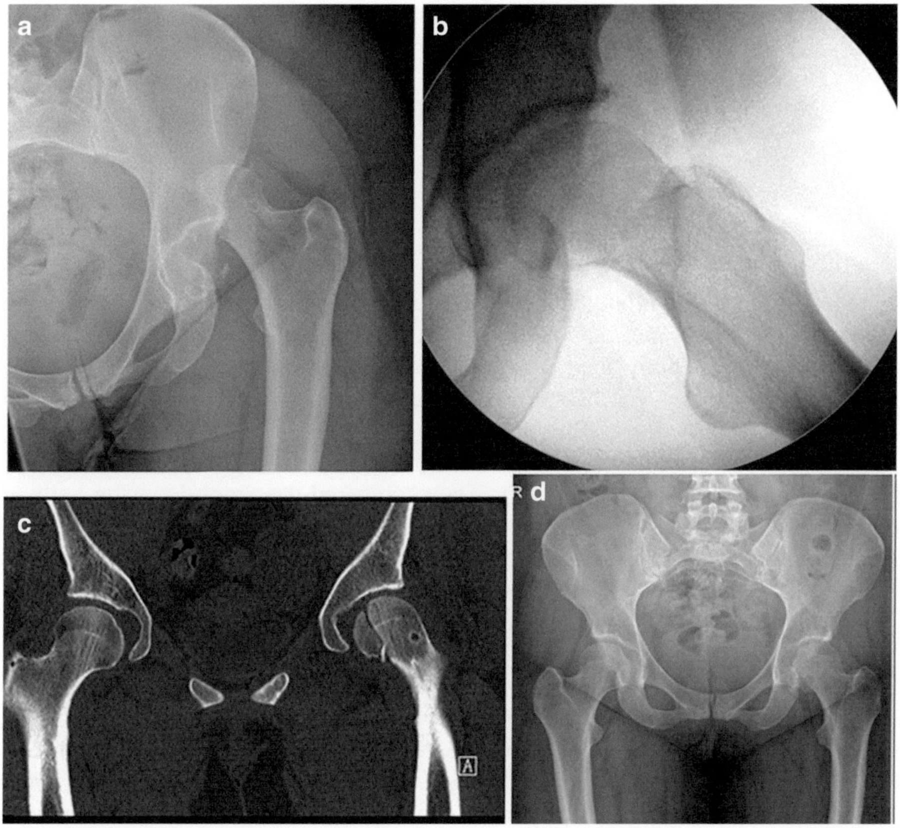

Fig. 13.1 (**a**) Pipkin type I fracture dislocation in a young male. (**b**) After closed reduction under general anesthesia. (**c**) Post-reduction CT scan shows reduced hip and well-aligned femoral head fracture. (**d**) After 6 weeks of conservative management, the fracture united with good functional outcome

A study by Złotorowicz et al. [6] reviewed 35 computed tomography (CT) angiographies of patients who had undergone hip reduction for posterior dislocation with an acetabular fracture. These findings were compared to a control group from their 2012 study [5]. While they initially hypothesized that the deep branch of the MFCA would be significantly compromised after dislocation and reduction, they found that 91% of cases demonstrated an enhancing deep branch of the MFCA on post-reduction CTA. However, they were unable to assess real-time perfusion changes during dislocation.

Among the three patients who showed no enhancement of the deep branch of the MFCA post-reduction, two developed AVN, whereas the third did not—possibly due to a well-developed posteroinferior nutrient artery compensating for the blood supply deficit.

Interestingly, their study also suggested that ischemia during the dislocated state, rather than post-reduction vascular compromise, was the primary trigger for AVN. Notably, no patient who underwent reduction within 12 hours developed AVN, underscoring the critical importance of early hip reduction in preserving femoral head viability.

13.4 Surgical Approaches

Giannoudis et al. [1] highlighted the wide variety of approaches used to access the femoral head in managing femoral head fractures and the variation in surgical procedures which were performed. The low incidence of these injuries is a key component to this variance seen. This leads to multiple crossovers in approaches and management strategies in the published data [3, 7–9].

Singh et al. [10] attempted to answer the question as to which is the best approach for exposure in their cadaveric study. They compared the Smith-Peterson without rectus release, Smith-Peterson with rectus release, surgical hip dislocation, and Hueter approach to the femoral head. They concluded that the surgical hip dislocation provided not only the best visualization of the femoral head but also the best access to the anatomical areas. In contrast, the Hueter approach led to both the worst visualization and access.

This study was limited as these approaches were performed on a bloodless cadaveric field so application into a clinical scenario may be different.

Furthermore, they chose not to include the Kocher-Langenbeck approach which is a widely utilized approach in managing femoral head fractures. They chose not to include this based on "lack of any known biologic advantages in conjunction with the anatomic disadvantages of a posterior approach for anteromedial located fracture fragments." Pipkin type IV fractures often involve posterior wall acetabular fractures which a posterior approach would have the benefit of being able to access both through a single approach.

Wang et al. [11] have described using pre-op 3D models to plan the surgical operation using a Ganz approach (Fig. 13.2). They used 3D models recreated from CT scans which both improved operative planning and allowed a preoperative trial of the planned procedure on the model. This enabled them to decide to trial and develop the ideal osteotomy, fixation method, and implant needed to achieve the desired outcome. The model was then sterilized so that it could be referenced intra-operatively.

13.5 Surgical Options: Fixation Versus Arthroplasty

The management of Pipkin type I and II femoral head fractures that achieve anatomical or near-anatomical reduction (<1 mm displacement) following closed hip reduction or minimally invasive reduction techniques has been explored by Kloub et al. [12]. In their series, minimally invasive screw osteosynthesis was performed

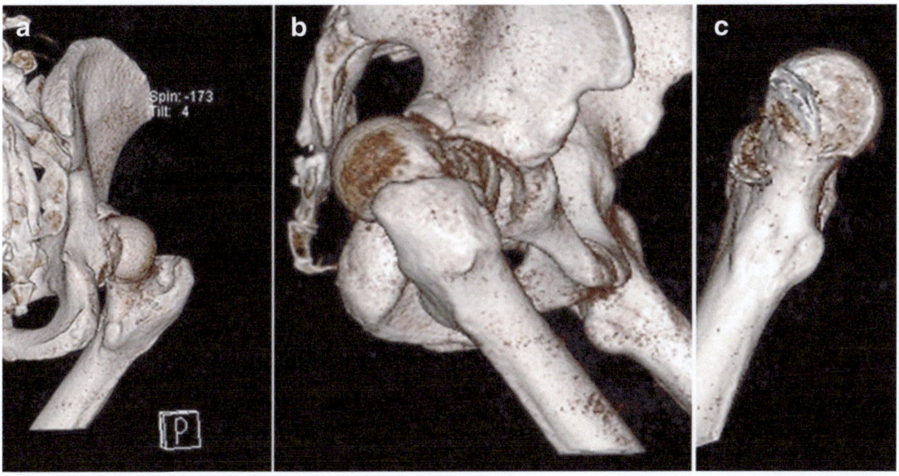

Fig. 13.2 3D CT images of Pipkin type I fracture-dislocation (**a, b**, posterior hip dislocation and infra-foveal femur head fracture). (**c**) Pelvis subtraction 3D CT images clearly delineates the femoral head fracture location

via the lateral femoral neck approach in seven patients. All fractures successfully united, with only one patient developing partial avascular necrosis (AVN) of the femoral head. Notably, none of the patients required further surgical intervention.

Their results were compared to those from the systematic review by Giannoudis et al. [1]. Kloub et al. [12] reported that 58% of their patients achieved an excellent outcome based on the Thompson and Epstein score, whereas only 13% of conservatively treated cases in the Giannoudis review had similar results. Additionally, none of their patients had a poor outcome, in contrast to the 27% poor outcome rate observed in the review.

Although this study represents a small case series with short-term follow-up, it highlights a potential approach for improving patient outcomes in selected Pipkin I and II fractures and warrants further investigation through larger studies with long-term follow-up.

Solberg et al. [13] presented a case series of 12 patients over a 6-year period with Pipkin type IV fractures, where a trochanteric flip osteotomy was utilized to provide access to both the femoral head and acetabulum for open reduction and internal fixation (ORIF). Their findings demonstrated an 80% good or excellent outcome with an average follow-up of 4 years. A key technical aspect of their approach was fixing the femoral head before addressing the acetabular fracture, as this allowed for better joint congruency and more anatomical acetabular reconstruction. However, they noted challenges in assessing hip stability, as both the osteotomy and acetabular fracture made intraoperative evaluation difficult. Despite these promising results, the study was limited by its small sample size and high loss to follow-up rate (20%).

Pipkin type III fractures present a significant management dilemma, given their high risk of avascular necrosis (AVN) yet frequent occurrence in younger patients mainly. The decision between fixation or hip replacement remains complex, as these fractures often lead to poor long-term outcomes.

A study by Wang et al. [14], which included 12 patients with Pipkin type III fractures who underwent ORIF, reflects this challenge. With a mean patient age of 34.2 years, their findings showed that 50% eventually required total hip arthroplasty (THA)—five cases due to AVN and one due to fracture non-union.

These findings emphasize the difficulty in preserving the native hip joint in Pipkin type III fractures and highlight the need for individualized treatment planning, balancing joint preservation efforts against the high likelihood of AVN and secondary procedures (Fig. 13.3).

Based on these findings, it is recommended that both total hip arthroplasty (THA) and open reduction internal fixation (ORIF) remain viable treatment options for Pipkin type III fractures. However, patients must be thoroughly counseled on the risks and expected outcomes and require close follow-up to monitor for complications.

In contrast, Tosounidis et al. [15], in their editorial, expressed reluctance regarding ORIF for these fractures. They advocated for primary THA as the preferred approach (Fig. 13.3), citing concerns over poor functional outcomes and the higher complication rates associated with salvage THA following failed ORIF. Their argument parallels observations seen in femoral neck fractures, where initial fixation followed by salvage THA often results in inferior outcomes compared to primary THA.

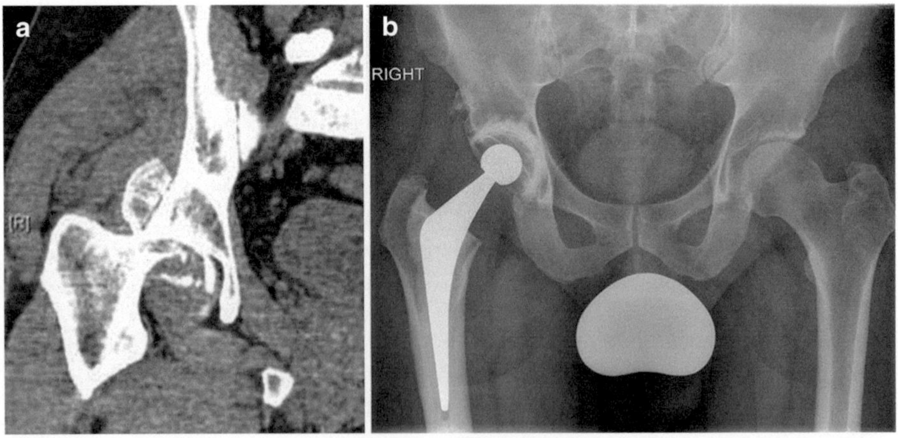

Fig. 13.3 (**a**) Pipkin type III fracture in a 28-year-old young male was managed with cemented THR. (**b**) Follow-up at 15 years shows good functioning THR

13.6 Surgical Options: Screw Choice

Traditionally, countersunk or headless compression screws have been used for open reduction and internal fixation (ORIF) of femur head fracture [3]. These screws are placed subchondrally, minimizing the impact on the remaining articular cartilage. However, retained metal implants carry the risk of implant-related complications, including stress shielding and the potential need for surgical removal.

To address these concerns, Prokop et al. [16] and Hermus et al. [17] have reported cases utilizing biodegradable screws made from polylactide as an alternative to traditional metal screws. In a small case series by Prokop et al. [16], most patients achieved satisfactory outcomes with an average follow-up of 54.2 months. These findings suggest that biodegradable screws may serve as a viable alternative by eliminating the need for implant removal and reducing MRI interference, potentially improving long-term patient outcomes.

13.7 Less Invasive Surgical Options

As previously mentioned, Kloub et al. [12] demonstrated that anatomically or near-anatomically reduced femoral head fractures can be successfully managed using minimally invasive screw fixation from the lateral femoral neck.

In addition, a small number of case reports have described arthroscopically assisted reduction and internal fixation for Pipkin type I and II fractures. Rojas-Sayol et al. [18], in their case report, outlined key "pearls and pitfalls" to consider when utilizing this technique.

A thorough preoperative CT evaluation is essential to assess fragment position and fracture pattern to determine whether the fracture is amenable to arthroscopic reduction and to identify the optimal portal placement for adequate access.

While the use of a traction table can enhance fluoroscopic visualization, it also poses risks such as fracture displacement and vascular injury to the femoral head. Additionally, accurate screw length measurement is crucial to prevent intra-articular screw protrusion or insufficient fixation.

Given these challenges, arthroscopically assisted reduction and fixation remains a selective approach that is best suited for carefully chosen cases where its advantages outweigh potential risks.

13.8 Arthroscopic Fracture Fragment Excision Surgical Technique

An arthroscopic approach may be used to remove loose bodies or unfixable fragments associated with femoral head fractures. The patient is positioned supine on a traction table with a padded perineal post. Gentle traction is applied to distract the hip. As most femoral head fractures are associated with hip dislocation, the capsuloligamentous injury would mean minimal force is generally required. Continual

X-ray screening of the joint during application of traction is advised to prevent overdistraction of the joint. Any associated pelvic injuries must also be monitored with X-ray to identify any displacement [19].

Once adequate distraction is achieved, central compartment access is established using a Seldinger technique, starting with the anterolateral portal. Further anterior and mid anterior portals are established under direct vision, and paraportal capsulotomies are made using a blade to allow mobility of the instruments. The joint is washed out and any hematoma evacuated. Low pump pressures and flow rates must be used to prevent significant fluid extravasation due to the capsular incompetence. The thigh and abdomen must be continuously monitored for signs of excessive swelling and compartment syndrome [20].

Arthroscopic cannulae are then placed in the working portals to allow easier removal of the loose fragments. A combination of graspers and shavers can then be used to remove the fracture fragments. Any associated labral injuries can also be repaired using sutures and bone anchors, and the remaining articular cartilage can also be assessed [21]. If larger capsulotomies are required, then capsular closure is advised to prevent further iatrogenic instability of the joint.

13.9 Miscellaneous Aspects

Femoral head fragment excision (Pipkin I) may be a surgical option in selected cases. An anterior approach can be used for fragment excision or fixation using mini-fragment screws. Fragment excision can be performed through both anterior and posterior (Kocher-Langenbeck) approaches based on the location of the free fracture fragment. Fragment excision is stated to have a better functional outcome in smaller series compared to conservative management.

One type of fracture that does not fit into the available Pipkin classification system is a femoral head impaction fracture. When this is located in the weight-bearing zone, then total hip replacement remains the most reliable option to treat the fracture.

13.10 Summary

The advances within femoral head fractures are small within the literature, and due to the nature and incidence of the injury, they lack significant evidence to recommend operative techniques over others. It therefore remains an area of controversy within orthopedics and without any large-scale studies is likely to continue to be the case.

From a practical point of view, the surgeon should focus on an early prompt relocation of the dislocated femoral head, followed by appropriate imaging to understand the morphology and location of the fracture before planning the surgical management.

References

1. Giannoudis P, Kontakis G, Christoforakis Z, Akula M, Tosounidis T, Koutras C. Management, complications and clinical results of femoral head fractures. Injury. 2009;40(12):1245–51.
2. Pipkin G. Treatment of grade IV fracture-dislocation of the hip. J Bone Joint Surg Am. 1957;39(A):1027–42.
3. Menger M, Braun B, Herath S, Küper M, Rollmann M, Histing T. Fractures of the femoral head: a narrative review. EFORT Open Rev. 2021;6:1122–31.
4. Wu S, Qian G, Huang Q, Dou B, Zheng Q, Wang W, Zhu X, Mei J. Clinical evaluation of femoral head fractures: which classification systems have the best universality, reliability, and reproducibility? Clin Orthop Relat Res. 2024;482:76–86.
5. Zlotorowicz M, Czubak J, Kozinski P, Boguslawska-Walecka R. Imaging the vascularisation of the femoral head by CT angiography. J Bone Joint Surg Br. 2012;94-B:1176–9.
6. Zlotorowicz M, Czubak J, Caban A, Kozinski P, Boguslawska-Walecka R. The blood supply to the femoral head after posterior fracture/dislocation of the hip, assessed by CT angiography. Bone Joint J. 2013;95-B(11):1453–7.
7. Chiron P, Reina N. Dislocation fracture of the femoral head in adult. EFORT Open Rev. 2022;7:375–83.
8. Chiron P, Lafontan V, Reina N. Fracture-dislocations of the femoral head. Orthop Traumatol Surg Res. 2013;99:53–66.
9. Asghar F, Karunakar M. Femoral head fractures: diagnosis, management, and complications. Orthop Clin N Am. 2004;35:463–72.
10. Singh K, Weitlich J, Zitsch B, Schweser K, Cook J, Crist B. Which surgical approach provides maximum visualization and access for open reduction and internal fixation of femoral head fractures? J Orthop Trauma. 2022;36:S12–6.
11. Wang J, Cai L, Xie L, Chen H, Guo X, Yu K. 3D printing-based Ganz approach for treatment of femoral head fractures: a prospective analysis. J Orthop Surg Res. 2019;14(1):338.
12. Kloub M, Holub K, Peml M, Urban J, Látel P. Closed reduction and minimally invasive screw osteosynthesis of Pipkin femoral head fractures. J Appl Biomed. 2023;21(1):1–6.
13. Solberg B, Moon C, Franco D. Use of a trochanteric flip osteotomy improves outcomes in Pipkin IV fractures. Clin Orthop Relat Res. 2009;467:929–33.
14. Wang S, Yu X, Li B, Ding Q, Wang T, Li Q, Liu L, Wu H. Pipkin type III femoral head fracture: which treatment strategy can be recommended? J Orthop Traumatol. 2023;24(28):1–7.
15. Tosunidis T, Aderinto J, Giannoudis P. Pipkin type-III fractures of the femoral head: fix it or replace it? Injury. 2017;48:2375–8.
16. Prokop A, Helling H, Hahn U, Udomkaewkanjana C, Rehm K. Biodegradable implants for Pipkin fractures. Clin Orthop Relat Res. 2005;432:226–33.
17. Hermus J, Laan C, Hogervorst M, Rhemrev S. Fixation of a Pipkin fracture with bio-absorbable screws – case report and a review of the Litera. Injury. 2005;36(3):458–61.
18. Rojas-Soyal R, De Caso J, Valera M. Arthroscopic-assisted percutaneous fixation of a femoral head fracture (Pipkin II) a case report. JBJS Case Connect. 2022;12(3):1–7.
19. Gaeda NG, Dantas P, Mascarenhas V, Campos V, Goncalves S. Is it safe to perform an early arthroscopy after a traumatic hip dislocation with an associated pelvic ring injury? Report of our technique. Arthrosc Tech. 2018;7(6):e679–e84.
20. Bartlett CS, DiFelice GS, Buly RL, Quinn TJ, Green DS, Helfet DL. Cardiac arrest as a result of intraabdominal extravasation of fluid during arthroscopic removal of a loose body from the hip joint of a patient with an acetabular fracture. J Orthop Trauma. 1998;12(4):294–9.
21. Park MS, Yoon SJ, Choi SM. Hip arthroscopic management for femoral head fractures and posterior acetabular wall fractures (Pipkin type IV). Arthosc Tech. 2013;2(3):e221–5.

Recent Advances, Hip Arthroscopy, and Orthobiologics in Femoral Head Fracture

14

Axel Gänsslen, Jan Lindahl, Dietmar Krappinger, Stephan Sehmisch, Tilman Graulich, and Ramesh Kumar Sen

14.1 Introduction

Pipkin fractures represent traumatic fracture-dislocations of the hip joint characterized by intra-articular fractures of the femoral head, which may occur in isolation or in association with femoral neck or acetabular fractures. The earliest surgical intervention for a femoral head fracture was reported by Riedel, who employed a lateral approach with greater trochanteric osteotomy following failed closed reduction in a 15-year-old boy. Although the femoral head fragments were anatomically repositioned into the acetabulum, the patient ultimately developed hip ankylosis [54].

Subsequently, Thompson and Epstein introduced a classification system for traumatic hip dislocations, identifying posterior fracture-dislocations involving the femoral head as grade V injuries, which were notably associated with poorer clinical outcomes [67]. Epstein later advocated for primary open reduction to improve treatment success in such cases [16].

A. Gänsslen (✉) · S. Sehmisch · T. Graulich
Department of Trauma Surgery, Hannover Medical School, Hannover, Germany
e-mail: sehmisch.stephan@mh-hannover.de; graulich.tilman@mh-hannover.de

J. Lindahl
Department of Orthopaedics and Traumatology, Helsinki University Hospital, University of Helsinki, Helsinki, Finland
e-mail: Jan.Lindahl@hus.fi

D. Krappinger
Department of Orthopaedics and Traumatology, Medical University of Innsbruck, Innsbruck, Austria
e-mail: dietmar.krappinger@tirol-kliniken.at

R. K. Sen
Institute of Orthopaedic Surgery, Max Super Speciality Hospital, Mohali, Punjab, India

R. K. Sen, S. K. Tripathy (eds.), *A Practical Guide to Management of Femoral Head Fracture-Dislocation*, https://doi.org/10.1007/978-981-96-9852-3_14

Stewart and Milford further contributed by proposing a classification system for hip dislocations, notably excluding central dislocations from their schema [64]. However, it was Garrett Pipkin in 1957 who provided the first comprehensive categorization of femoral head fracture patterns, establishing a classification system that remains widely utilized in clinical practice today [51].

14.2 Epidemiological Data

Epidemiological data on Pipkin fractures remain limited due to the rarity of these injuries and the correspondingly low case volumes encountered by individual surgeons or institutions. Nonetheless, several studies comprising cohorts of more than 30–40 patients have been published [15, 31, 38, 57, 59, 60, 68]. These investigations consistently report a similar incidence of Pipkin types I, II, and IV fractures, whereas type III injuries continue to be exceptionally uncommon [Table 14.1].

An apparent increase in the incidence of Pipkin fractures has been noted over the past two decades, likely attributable to a rise in high-energy trauma mechanisms. This trend is summarized in Table 14.2.

Pipkin fractures predominantly affect male patients, typically around the age of 40 years and are most commonly the result of high-energy trauma (Table 14.2).

Table 14.1 Distribution of Pipkin fractures based on larger patient series

Author	Year	Treatment period	No.	No./year	P I	P II	P III	P IV	Unknown
Kloen	2002	1970–1990	33	1,57	10	8	1	14	
Sahin	2003	1980–1994	57	3,8	19	26	9	3	
Lederer	2007	1982–2005	46	1,92	13	14	2	17	
Tonetti	2010	1972–2008	110	3,06	37	16	4	45	8
Scolaro	2017	2000–2013	147	10,5	40	62	7	23	15
Enocson	2022	2013–2022	47	4,7	7	13	1	26	
Shakya	2023	2011–2018	50	6,25	18	10	8	14	
Sum			5490		144	149	32	142	23

Table 14.2 Demographic data on Pipkin fractures based on larger patient series

Author	Year	No.	m/f	Age	MVA	MC	Fall from height	HE	Sport	Other
Kloen	2002	33	20/12	39	22	7	1	1	0	
Lederer	2007	46	32/14	42						
Tonetti	2010	110	89/21	37,1	52	18	0	20	11	9
Scolaro	2017	147	99/48	39,2						
Enocson	2022	47	35/12	48	17		19			11
Shakya	2023	50	37/13	40	31	2	14		2	1

14.3 Common Treatment modalities

In a meta-analysis by Giannoudis et al. involving 450 patients, fragment excision demonstrated superior outcomes compared to open reduction and internal fixation (ORIF) for Pipkin type I fractures, while ORIF was favored for type II fractures. However, when outcomes were assessed using the Thompson and Epstein criteria alone, no statistically significant differences were observed across the different Pipkin types [23].

Data from large patient series indicate that the majority of femoral head fractures are managed with ORIF. However, there is a lack of definitive evidence regarding the necessity and outcomes of concomitant acetabular stabilization (Table 14.3).

In an analysis of 110 patients encompassing all Pipkin fracture types, no specific treatment modality was found to be clearly superior. Notably, nearly 20% of patients required secondary total hip replacement (THR) within an average follow-up period of 6 months [68].

A more recent study evaluating 24 cases of Pipkin type I fractures demonstrated superior outcomes with fragment excision compared to closed reduction alone [10]. Similarly, an analysis involving 37 patients across all fracture types reported good to excellent outcomes in 67% of cases [29]. Interestingly, Giannoudis et al. observed that fragment size influenced outcomes, with smaller fragments—typical of Pipkin type I fractures—associated with poorer results compared to larger fragments seen in type II injuries [23].

In the meta-analysis by Giannoudis et al., long-term outcomes were not significantly influenced by treatment modality. Good to excellent results were reported in 63.1% of patients treated nonoperatively, 65% following fragment excision, 61.6% after ORIF, and 60% after primary THR [23].

More recently, surgical intervention has been increasingly favored over conservative management, with ORIF demonstrating superior outcomes compared to fragment excision in displaced Pipkin type I and II fractures [7].

Table 14.3 Data on type of treatment of Pipkin fractures based on larger patient series

Author	Year	No.	Cons	Excision	ORIF	pTHR	ORIF AC only	Other
Kloen	2002	33	7	5	21	0	0	0
Lederer	2007	46	4	10	26	6	0	0
Tonetti	2010	110	32	40	30	5	3	0
Scolaro	2017	147	28	37	78	3	0	1
Enocson	2022	47	4	7	21	13	0	2
Shakya	2023	50	8	0	37	5	0	0
Sum		433	83	99	213	32	3	3

14.4 Other Treatment Options

In addition to open reduction and internal fixation (ORIF), a limited number of case reports and series have documented successful management of femoral head fractures using arthroscopic techniques. These minimally invasive approaches offer the advantage of addressing associated intra-articular pathology with reduced soft tissue disruption.

To manage concomitant cartilage injuries—particularly impaction or focal defects of the femoral head—emerging techniques such as osteochondral allograft transplantation have been explored. In some cases, defects are managed by filling them with cancellous bone harvested from the greater trochanter, followed by coverage with a collagen membrane secured using fibrin glue.

Given the frequent presence of significant cartilage damage, especially in younger patients, joint-preserving strategies are often pursued, although their long-term outcomes remain largely undefined (Tables 14.4, 14.5, 14.6, and 14.7).

14.4.1 Osteochondral Transplantation

Osteochondral injuries of the femoral head (FH) commonly result from posterior hip dislocations, where the femoral head impacts the acetabular cavity or is injured by associated acetabular fracture fragments. Transverse components of acetabular fractures, particularly when centrally displaced, may cause both primary and secondary damage to the femoral head, as the sharp fracture margins exert shearing forces during joint motion.

While most literature on hip chondral lesions has focused on acetabular cartilage damage associated with femoroacetabular impingement, labral tears, avascular necrosis of the femoral head, developmental dysplasia of the hip, and osteochondritis dissecans of the acetabulum [13]; posttraumatic chondral lesions following dislocation, acetabular fracture, or femoral head fracture have also been described [1, 6, 26, 35].

As early as 1953, Jörg Böhler conducted experimental studies on femoral head morphology under axial loads ranging from 300 to 1400 kg [8]. His work demonstrated the occurrence of reversible, radiographically occult microfractures—referred to as the "table tennis ball effect"—alongside cartilage injury that may predispose to avascular necrosis of the femoral head. Similar findings were confirmed by Gay et al. [21, 22], who reported superficial abrasions, focal impactions, and full-thickness cartilage fractures in post-mortem analyses of polytrauma patients with acetabular fractures.

Marginal impaction injuries of the femoral head were not associated with elevated peak pressures on the femoral surface itself; however, they significantly increased load transmission to the acetabular dome, depending on the extent of the impaction defect [33]. Letournel reported superolateral femoral head impaction (5–15 mm) in approximately 2.1% of cases [41], while historical data indicate post-dislocation femoral head impaction rates of 7–16% [17, 37, 47, 51].

Table 14.4 Case descriptions of patients with FH fractures, treated with osteochondral autografts: demographic data

Author	Year	Age	Sex	MI	Pipkin	FH disl.	Reduction	i.a.	Impaction	OC # (cm)	FTCD (mm)	Labrum	AC#
Nam	2010	21	m	Ski	IV (II)	Posterior	2 h	Multiple	None	Superior 3 × 3	Ant-sup. 10x10	Anterior	sPW
Gagala	2014	34	m	Fall	IV (I)	Posterior	n.e.	n.e.	n.e.	None	None	None	PW
Gagala	2014	43	m	MVA	IV (II)	Posterior	1 h	n.e.	n.e.	None	None	n.e.	sPW
Won	2016	31	m	Fall	IV(II)	Posterior	1d	Multiple	None	None	Superior 25x10	n.e.	PW

MI mechanism of injury, *MVA* motor vehicle accident, *disl.* Dislocation, *i.a.* intra-articular/loose fragments, *OC #* osteochondral fracture, *FTCD* full-thickness cartilage defect, *Spw* small posterior wall avulsion

Table 14.5 Case descriptions of patients with FH fractures, treated with osteochondral autografts: surgical details and follow-up results

Author	Year	Age	Sex	Approach	Treatment	Ips. GHL	After-treatment	f/u	Clinical result
Nam	2010	21	m	KL/SHD	FOF (bPAs), sFR, OCP	FH	6w non-WB	>5y	VAS = 0, good
								13y	VAS = 0, good, III° degeneration
Gagala	2014	34	m	KL/SHD	FHFF (3 OCP (press-fit)), PW fixation (screw)	Knee	n.e.	80	VAS = 0, excellent
Gagala	2014	43	m	KL/SHD	FHFF (3 OCP (press-fit)), 2 OCP (press-fit)	Knee	n.e.	24	VAS = mild, good
Won	2016	31	m	KL/SHD	FHFF (screws), sFR, OCP (screws)	FH	12w partial WB	12	Good, capsulitis

KL/SHD Kocher-Langenbeck+ surgical hip dislocation, *CD* cartilage debridement, *FOF* fixation osteochondral fracture, *OCP* osteochondral plugs, *bPAp* bioabsorbable polylactic acid pins, *bPAs* bioabsorbable polylactic acid screws, *MF* microfracture procedures, *sFR* small fragment removal, *FHFF* FH fracture fixation, *ORIF AC* open reduction internal fixation acetabular fracture, *GHL* graft harvesting location, *ips.* Ipsilateral, *WB* weight bearing, *f/u* follow-up, *VAS* Visual Analog Pain Scale, *HO* heterotopic bone formation

Importantly, these impaction injuries are often missed on conventional radiographs [63] and may remain subtle even on computed tomography (CT) scans [66]. A CT study from 1990 identified femoral head lesions in 62.5% of posterior dislocations [66], with lesions typically located in the anterosuperior quadrant (11–1 o'clock position). Conversely, anterior dislocations tended to produce posterolateral femoral head damage (4–5 o'clock), analogous to Hill-Sachs lesions in the shoulder [53]. More recent data by Ferguson et al. found a 19.6% incidence of femoral head impaction among patients over 60 years of age, based on an analysis of 173 radiographs [18].

Hidden et al. described a case involving a superolateral femoral head impaction associated with a medially displaced anterior column-posterior hemitransverse (ACPHT) acetabular fracture [27]. Closed reduction was achieved through initial medialization of the femoral head followed by axial traction to relocate it beneath the acetabular roof. However, no specific treatment was provided for the femoral head impaction in that case.

While several classification systems exist for chondral pathology in general—such as the Outerbridge classification and the International Cartilage Repair Society

Table 14.6 Case descriptions of patients with superior femoral head lesions, treated with osteochondral autografts: demographic data

Author	Year	Age	Sex	MI	Chiron	FH disl.	Reduction	i.a.	Impaction	OC # (cm)	FTCD (mm)	Labrum	AC#
Nam	2010	15	m	MVA	V	Posterior	2 h	Multiple	Superior	Superior 3 × 3	Ant-sup. 20 × 5–8	0	None
Krych	2012	15	m	MVA	V	Posterior	1 h	Multiple	Superior	Superior 3 × 3	Superior 20 × 5–8	0	None
Krych	2012	29	f	Equestrian	V	Posterior	1 h	Multiple	Superior	Ant-sup. 2 × 2	Ant.-sup.10 × 20	0	None
Gagala	2014	20	m	MVA	V	Posterior	1 h	n.e.	n.e.	None	Superior	n.e.	None
Anthonissen	2016	20	m	MC	V	Anterior	1 h	One	Superior	None	Superior 20 × 15	0	None
Kong	2017	55	m	MVA	V	Anterior	1 h	None	Superior	None	None	n.e.	None
Coulomb	2017	16	f	MVA	V	Anterior	1 h	None	Ant.-sup.	None	Ant.-sup. 30 × 20	o	td
Passaplan	2023	21	m	n.e.	n.e.	n.e.	n.e.	n.e.	n.e.	n.e.	118 mm^2	n.e.	ABC
Passaplan	2023	39	m	n.e.	n.e.	n.e.	n.e.	n.e.	n.e.	n.e.	353 mm^2	n.e.	PW
Passaplan	2023	36	m	n.e.	n.e.	Posterior	n.e.	n.e.	n.e.	n.e.	346 mm^2	n.e.	None
Lee	2023	62	m	5 m fall	V	Anterior	8 h	Multiple	None	None	Sup.-lat. 35 × 27	0	0

MI mechanism of injury, *MVA* motor vehicle accident, *disl.* Dislocation, *i.a.* intra-articular/loose fragments, *OC #* osteochondral fracture, *FTCD* full-thickness cartilage defect, *Spw* small posterior wall avulsion

Table 14.7 Case descriptions of patients with FH impactions, treated with osteochondral autografts: surgical details and follow-up results

Author	Year	Age	Sex	Approach	Treatment	ips. GHL	After-treatment	f/u	Clinical result
Nam	2010	15 years	m	KL/SHD	CD, FOF (bPAp), 3 OCP (bPAs), MF	Knee	6w non-WB	12	VAS = 0, excellent
Krych	2012	15 years	m	KL/SHD	FOF (bPAp), 3 OCP (press-fit)	Knee	8w partial WB	50	Excellent, HO grade 1
Krych	2012	29	f	KL/SHD	FOF (screws), 2 OCP (press-fit)	Knee	8w partial WB	48	VAS = 0, excellent, HO grade 2
Gagala	2014	20	m	KL/SHD	FHFF (3 OCP (press-fit)), 1 OCP (press-fit)	Knee	n.e.	62	VAS = 0, excellent
Anthonissen	2016	20	m	KL/SHD	4 OCP (bPAp)	Knee	8w partial WB	24	VAS = mild, good, II° degeneration
Kong	2017	55	m	KL/SHD	4 OCP (press-fit)	Knee/FH	12w partial WB	19	VAS = 0, excellent
Coulomb	2017	16	f	Hueter/DAA	3 OCP (screws)	Knee	6w partial WB	12	VAS = 0, excellent

Passaplan	2023	21	m	KL/SHD	ORIF AC, 3 OPC (press-fit)	FH	6w partial WB	20y	
Passaplan	2023	39	m	KL/SHD	ORIF AC, 9 OPC (press-fit)	Knee	6w partial WB	17y	THR
Passaplan	2023	36	m	KL/SHD	3 OPC (press-fit)	FH	6w partial WB	15y	THR
Lee	2023	62	m	KL/SHD	6 OPC (press-fit)	FH	12w partial WB	24	Excellent

KL/SHD Kocher-Langenbeck+ surgical hip dislocation, *CD* cartilage debridement, *FOF* fixation osteochondral fracture, *OCP* osteochondral plugs, *bPAp* bioabsorbable polylactic acid pins, *bPAs* bioabsorbable polylactic acid screws, *MF* microfracture procedures, *sFR* small fragment removal, *FHFF* FH fracture fixation, *ORIF AC* open reduction internal fixation acetabular fracture, *GHL* graft harvesting location, *ips.* Ipsilateral, *WB* weight bearing, *f/u* follow-up, *VAS* Visual Analog Pain Scale, *HO* heterotopic bone formation

(ICRS) system—only one classification has been specifically developed to address cartilage lesions of the femoral head [58]. This system describes superficial lesion patterns including uniform thinning, cartilage softening, fibrillation, delamination, and exposed subchondral bone. In traumatic cases, treatment has largely been limited to excision of loose chondral fragments.

El Bitar et al. proposed a treatment algorithm for femoral head cartilage lesions based primarily on defect size, although it does not specifically address traumatic etiologies [14]:

- **< 2 cm²** → Microfracture or suture repair
- **2–6 cm²** → Microfracture or osteochondral allograft transplantation
- **6–8 cm²** → Total hip arthroplasty (THA) or possibly osteochondral allograft
- **> 8 cm²** → THA.

In 2017, the German Society of Orthopaedics and Trauma issued consensus guidelines for managing full-thickness cartilage defects of the hip joint [19]. These recommendations emphasized that age alone should not preclude joint-preserving procedures, although advanced degenerative changes of the hip remain a contraindication. Treatment strategies were outlined as follows:

- **Matrix-assisted autologous chondrocyte transplantation (MACT)** is preferred for full-thickness lesions >1.5–2 cm^2.
- **Minimally invasive MACT**, including injectable chondrocyte systems, is favored in the hip due to anatomical constraints.
- **Bone marrow-stimulating techniques combined with biomaterials** are recommended for lesions unsuitable for MACT.
- **Single-stage procedures** may be considered for smaller lesions (< 1.5–2 cm^2).

A recently proposed classification of femoral head fractures introduced a type V lesion, describing a superior collapse of the femoral head [11] (Fig. 14.1). This rare pattern was identified in 1 out of 32 cases (3.1%) in the context of combined acetabular fractures.

Several case reports have documented the use of mosaicplasty for managing severe and deep femoral head lesions, utilizing various surgical approaches such as the direct anterior approach or, more commonly, the posterior approach with surgical hip dislocation [1, 6, 12]. However, robust data regarding the optimal treatment strategy and long-term prognosis remain lacking.

One of the largest available case series included 12 patients—10 of whom had associated posterior acetabular fractures, predominantly involving the posterior wall—treated with osteochondral reconstruction and followed for a minimum of 5 years. The reported 5-year hip joint survivorship was 57.1% [26].

In a separate analysis of 128 patients with acetabular fractures, femoral head impaction injuries were identified in 5 patients (3.9%) via CT imaging at admission. An additional three patients (2.3%) were found to have femoral head impaction intraoperatively, bringing the total incidence to 6.25% [52].

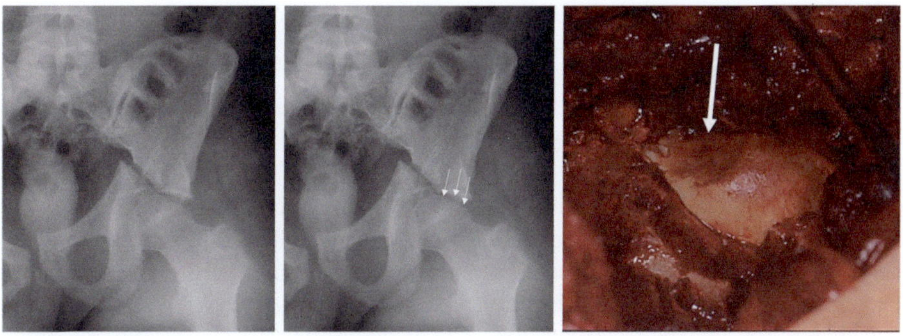

Fig. 14.1 Superior femoral head impaction in a patient with a transverse acetabular fracture. Typically, the femoral head is impacted by the medial edge of the iliac fragment

Given this unexpectedly low detection rate, a re-evaluation of the original CT scans was performed, which revealed a substantially higher true incidence—39.8% of patients exhibited femoral head lesions. Among these, 45% were classified as large and 55% as small. Concomitant hip dislocations were present in 19 of the 51 patients with femoral head injuries (37%).

Topographic analysis revealed that anterior-superior femoral head lesions were more commonly associated with isolated acetabular fractures, whereas lesions in the anterior-inferior quadrant were predominantly observed in cases with concurrent hip dislocation.

Importantly, the presence of femoral head impaction was associated with a significantly increased risk of secondary total hip arthroplasty (THA), with an odds ratio of 4.8.

> Femoral head impaction injuries are risk factors for secondary joint failure [56]. Thus, especially in younger patients, these concomitant injuries should possibly be addressed [24].

All surgical techniques for reconstructing femoral head (FH) cartilage defects reported in the literature remain experimental, and no universally accepted or gold-standard procedure has been established to date (overview in: [26]).

Reconstructive attempts for traumatic cartilage lesions in the context of femoral head fractures have a long history. Both osteochondral allografts and autografts have been utilized; however, the literature is limited to isolated case reports, without consistent protocols or long-term outcome data.

One of the earliest such cases was described by Meyers, who treated a Pipkin type II fracture-dislocation using a fresh osteochondral allograft. However, specific clinical and procedural details of the case were not provided [44].

In 2003, Hangody et al. reported on their broader experience with autologous osteochondral mosaicplasty for full-thickness cartilage defects in weight-bearing joints, yet their report did not detail any specific application or outcomes in femoral head injuries [25].

14.5 Autograft Reconstruction

Nam et al. were the first to provide a detailed account of autologous mosaicplasty for femoral head (FH) reconstruction in two young patients following posterior hip dislocation [45]. The first case involved a 15-year-old with a CT- and MRI-confirmed osteochondral fracture of the weight-bearing zone of the FH, featuring articular impaction and areas of full-thickness cartilage loss. The second case was a 21-year-old presenting with a Pipkin type II fracture. Both patients had intra-articular loose bodies.

Surgical intervention was carried out via the Kocher-Langenbeck approach, incorporating a surgical hip dislocation as described by Ganz. Defect reconstruction included cartilage fragment fixation using bioresorbable pins or screws, along with osteochondral autografts harvested from the ipsilateral knee in one case and from the inferior aspect of the femoral head in the other. Cartilage debridement was performed until stable margins were achieved, and bone perfusion was confirmed by subchondral bleeding.

Krych et al. reported on two additional patients with traumatic anterosuperior osteochondral FH defects following posterior hip dislocation [35]. Both underwent fixation of the impacted fragments, loose body removal, and osteochondral autograft transfer (OAT) from the ipsilateral knee using the surgical hip dislocation technique. At 4 years of follow-up, both had excellent clinical outcomes, although they developed grade I and II heterotopic ossification.

An alternative strategy was described by Gagala et al., who presented a small case series of three patients treated with osteochondral autologous transfer system (OATS) for fracture stabilization rather than classic defect filling [20]. In this approach, femoral head fracture fragments were first temporarily stabilized using K-wires. Subsequently, 4.5 mm drill holes were created and filled with press-fit osteochondral autografts, which acted as a biological fixation construct. Notably, these patients did not have discrete cartilage defects requiring resurfacing.

Anthonissen et al. described a case of anterior hip dislocation resulting in a posterosuperior cartilage lesion within the weight-bearing zone, managed with osteochondral autograft transfer system (OATS) [1]. Despite successful graft healing, the patient exhibited early degenerative changes and limited hip range of motion at 2 years postoperatively.

Won et al. reported a case involving a 31-year-old male who sustained a right posterior Pipkin type IV fracture-dislocation during a soccer match [69]. The femoral head fracture (Pipkin type II) was anatomically reduced and fixed using three 3.5 mm cannulated screws. Additional small osteochondral fragments were excised. A 2.5 × 1 cm superomedial cartilage defect was treated using a local OATS graft, secured with screws. At 1-year follow-up, the clinical outcome was rated as good (modified Harris Hip Score: 82), although the patient developed adhesive capsulitis and reduced flexion, necessitating hip arthroscopy.

Zelken later reported his own 13-year follow-up after undergoing hip preservation surgery for a Pipkin type II fracture with an associated osteochondral lesion—originally presented by Nam et al. in 2010 [45, 71]. Despite radiographic evidence of moderate joint degeneration (grades II–III) by the eighth postoperative year, the patient remained pain-free with a Harris Hip Score of 100 at 13 years, strongly advocating for joint-preserving techniques even in complex FH injuries.

Kong et al. presented a case of a 55-year-old male who sustained an anterior obturator hip dislocation with superolateral femoral head impaction after a motor vehicle accident [32]. Using the surgical hip dislocation (SHD) approach, OATS was performed with grafts harvested from the ipsilateral knee (one 10 mm and two 8 mm plugs) and an additional 9 mm graft from the inferior femoral head. At 1 year, second-look arthroscopy revealed well-integrated grafts with preserved cartilage morphology. The clinical result was excellent, with a Harris Hip Score of 96.

Coulomb et al. reported on a 16-year-old female who sustained an obturator hip dislocation with a 3 × 2 cm anterolateral femoral head defect and an associated teardrop acetabular fracture following a motor vehicle accident [12]. Through a direct anterior approach (Hueter), the lesion was accessed, debrided, and treated with OATS harvested from the ipsilateral knee. Residual voids were filled with cancellous autograft from the iliac crest, and definitive fixation was achieved using two headless compression screws. At 1-year follow-up, the patient demonstrated good functional recovery with no signs of degeneration.

Passaplan et al. reported a series of three patients with traumatic FH cartilage injuries treated via press-fit osteochondral autograft transfer [50]. Two of the three patients underwent successful hip preservation for 15–17 years before eventual conversion to total hip arthroplasty. The third patient, who sustained a both-column acetabular fracture, remained joint-preserved for nearly 21 years.

Lee et al. described a case of autologous osteochondral mosaicplasty in a 62-year-old male who sustained an anterior (obturator) hip dislocation following a 5-m fall [39]. Closed reduction was performed under general anesthesia approximately 8 h post-injury. Preoperative imaging with conventional radiographs and CT scans revealed a large superolateral cartilage defect of the femoral head, which was confirmed intraoperatively to measure 35 × 27 mm, along with multiple small intra-articular bony fragments.

Using the surgical hip dislocation (SHD) technique, the defect was debrided, and mosaicplasty was performed using six osteochondral plugs harvested from the inferior aspect of the femoral head. The grafts were inserted using a press-fit technique. At 2-year follow-up, the patient achieved an excellent clinical outcome, with no radiographic signs of joint degeneration, and a high modified Harris Hip Score.

14.5.1 Allograft Reconstruction

Nousiainen et al. were the first to provide a detailed account of osteochondral allograft reconstruction in 2010, involving an 18-year-old male who sustained a posterior-superior fracture-dislocation of the hip (Pipkin type IV) following a motor vehicle accident [46]. The injury included a small, peripheral posterior wall acetabular fracture and a large, medially displaced femoral head (FH) fragment, which appeared ischemic on MRI. A significant superior impaction injury of the weight-bearing surface of the FH was also identified.

Surgical management was performed via the Kocher-Langenbeck approach, incorporating surgical hip dislocation as described by Ganz. Due to the irreparability of the central third of the femoral head within the weight-bearing zone, a frozen osteochondral femoral head allograft was used to reconstruct the defect. The allograft was supported with autologous cancellous bone harvested from the greater trochanter, and fixation was achieved using bioabsorbable polylactic acid screws. Postoperative care included toe-touch weight bearing, restriction of hip flexion to a maximum of 60°, and avoidance of active hip abduction for 8 weeks.

In 2012, Kosashvili et al. reported another case involving a 22-year-old male treated with a fresh-stored osteochondral allograft for a femoral head defect following fracture [34]. At 54 months postoperatively, the patient achieved a Harris Hip Score of 84, reflecting a good functional outcome. The surgical approach utilized a modified trochanteric osteotomy in the lateral decubitus position. However, details regarding the initial injury, defect characteristics, and intraoperative findings were not provided.

14.5.2 Rotational Osteoplasty

Rotational osteoplasty has been introduced as a novel technique for reconstructing large femoral head (FH) defects when conventional fixation or grafting options are limited. Au et al. were the first to report its use in a patient with a Pipkin type II FH fracture following posterior hip dislocation [4]. Using the Hardinge approach, the Pipkin fragment was anatomically reduced, revealing a substantial superior FH defect. To restore the weight-bearing surface, the fragment was rotated until congruent articulation with the acetabulum was achieved and then fixed with three 3.5 mm cortical screws. The non-weight-bearing inferior defect was filled with corticocancellous bone harvested from the greater trochanter. At 18 months postoperatively, the patient had no functional limitations and radiographs confirmed joint preservation without signs of degeneration.

A similar approach was reported by Bartlett et al., who described a 40-year-old male with a Pipkin type IV injury following a high-energy pelvic crush trauma [5]. The injury included a small acetabular rim avulsion and a type II FH fracture with additional impaction and cartilage loss. Intraoperative findings using a Kocher-Langenbeck approach combined with surgical hip dislocation revealed a displaced medial FH fragment constituting 25–35% of the head, along with marginal impaction on the intact superior central FH accounting for 15–20% of the surface.

Following reduction, a large superior defect persisted that could not be reconstructed using the available osteochondral fragments. Consequently, the main Pipkin fragment was repositioned superiorly via rotational osteoplasty after wedge resection of the impacted cancellous bone. This reorientation resulted in an oval-shaped reconstructed FH, secured with three 3.5 mm screws. The acetabular rim avulsion was excised. Postoperative imaging showed a congruent joint. At 5-year follow-up, the patient reported mild subjective instability, but functional assessment showed a good Harris Hip Score, with only minimal signs of joint degeneration and no evidence of FH collapse.

14.5.3 Other Techniques

Lehmann et al. described a case of a Pipkin type II femoral head fracture associated with a significant cartilage defect [40]. Following fixation of the Pipkin fragment using screws, the residual femoral head defect was filled with cancellous bone harvested from the greater trochanter. A collagen membrane was applied over the graft to provide additional support, highlighting an early attempt at biological augmentation in joint-preserving surgery.

14.5.4 Arthroscopic-Assisted Treatment

Arthroscopic techniques have increasingly been explored as adjuncts or alternatives to open surgery in selected femoral head fractures. The literature distinguishes between true femoral head fractures and "clamshell-type" avulsion injuries.

Yamamoto et al. were the first to report arthroscopic management of hip trauma in 2003, including five Pipkin-type cases (three type I, one type II, one type III) [72]. Among them, only one patient with a Pipkin type I injury underwent arthroscopic osteosynthesis. The remainder were managed with debridement, lavage, or fragment excision.

Subsequent reports further detailed arthroscopic approaches:

- **Lansford et al.** treated two Pipkin type I fractures after posterior hip dislocation using an anterolateral and anterior portal [36]. Both cases involved fragment removal and debridement without fixation.
- **Park et al.** described a 45-year-old male with a posterior wall acetabular fracture treated by ORIF. Postoperative CT revealed intra-articular osteochondral fragments, which were arthroscopically removed, along with labral reconstruction [49]. No specific Pipkin-type fracture was reported, classifying this case under general hip trauma management.

A more definitive arthroscopic approach was described by **Park et al.** in a 50-year-old woman with a Pipkin type I fracture managed by arthroscopic-assisted percutaneous screw fixation [48].

Kekatpure et al. were the first to manage a Pipkin type IV injury arthroscopically, involving an infrafoveal Pipkin type I fragment and a small posterior wall fragment (<20%) displaced anteriorly [30]. The femoral head fragment was reduced arthroscopically, while the acetabular fragment was excised.

Hsu et al. published the first series with intermediate-term outcomes for arthroscopic fixation in seven femoral head fracture cases (five suprafoveal, two infrafoveal) [28]. Headless compression screws were used under arthroscopic control. At a mean follow-up of 18 months, patients had excellent clinical outcomes (mean Harris Hip Score: 90.8), with no signs of osteoarthritis, avascular necrosis, or heterotopic ossification. One patient experienced a transient sciatic nerve injury attributed to traction.

Aprato et al. later compared five arthroscopically treated Pipkin type I fractures with five ORIF cases performed via surgical hip dislocation [2]. Four of five arthroscopically treated cases achieved anatomic reduction, and functional outcomes were slightly better than the ORIF group (Harris Hip Score: 94 vs. 88). Arthroscopic management also resulted in lower morbidity. Their team has published a detailed technical description of the arthroscopic procedure [3].

Rojas-Sayol et al. contributed a case of a Pipkin type II fracture dislocation managed arthroscopically using anterolateral, midanterior, and posterolateral portals [55]. Fixation was performed via the posterolateral portal using headless compression screws. At 72-month follow-up, the patient maintained excellent hip function with no radiographic degeneration.

Finally, **Chen et al.** retrospectively compared 13 patients undergoing arthroscopic internal fixation and 8 patients treated with fragment excision for Pipkin type I and II fractures [9]. Fragment excision was associated with better functional outcomes (modified Harris Hip Score), although both groups demonstrated preserved joint structure radiographically. The authors recommended internal fixation for fragments larger than 2 cm.

14.6 Clamshell-Type Fractures

Clamshell-type femoral head fractures, first described by Matsuda, represent a specific subtype of osteochondral avulsion injuries involving the superior aspect of the femoral head [42, 43]. In 2009, Matsuda reported arthroscopic-assisted reduction and internal fixation of such a lesion in a 19-year-old woman who sustained a superior impaction injury with multiple small fracture fragments. Using an anterolateral portal and multiple accessory portals, the main osteochondral fragment was manipulated and fixed with two headless compression (Herbert) screws under fluoroscopic guidance. Additional arthroscopic debridement was performed to remove minor intra-articular debris. However, no long-term outcomes were provided.

In a subsequent 2012 report, Matsuda presented follow-up data from another patient with a similar lesion who returned to high-impact sports at 32 months postoperatively with excellent hip function and no radiographic signs of degeneration [43].

A comparable case was later reported by Sobczyk et al. in 2019, further supporting the feasibility of arthroscopic management for Clamshell-type femoral head injuries [61].

14.7 Current Concepts and State of the Art

Söylemez et al. conducted a systematic review on arthroscopic-assisted management of femoral head fractures, incorporating eight published studies [62]. The majority of reported cases involved Pipkin type I and II injuries, with surgery typically performed in the supine position on a traction table. Standard anterolateral and anterior portals were most commonly used, while additional portals were adapted according to fragment location, fracture configuration, and the surgical objectives (e.g., fixation vs. excision vs. debridement).

Complication rates across the reviewed studies were low, and clinical outcomes were generally favorable, suggesting that arthroscopic-assisted fixation is a safe and effective approach in select cases.

In addition to the conventional fixation technique using headless compression screws for larger fragments, a novel method known as the **"Letter V Technique"** was recently introduced for stabilization of infrafoveal femoral head fractures [70]. This technique combines screw and wire fixation in a V-shaped configuration to enhance fragment stability in anatomically challenging locations.

14.8 Conclusions

Pipkin fractures remain uncommon, and consequently, most surgeons have limited individual experience with their management. A subset of these injuries is associated with osteochondral defects (Fig. 14.2), either following initial trauma or during the course of surgical reconstruction, often accompanied by small osteochondral fragments.

Over the past two decades, increasing efforts have been directed toward reconstructing weight-bearing defects of the femoral head. These reconstructions have predominantly employed autografts harvested from the inferior femoral head or the ipsilateral knee, with promising mid-term results. In parallel, selective cases have demonstrated the utility of standard hip arthroscopy for fragment removal (Fig. 14.3) and even arthroscopic reconstruction in Pipkin type I and II fractures.

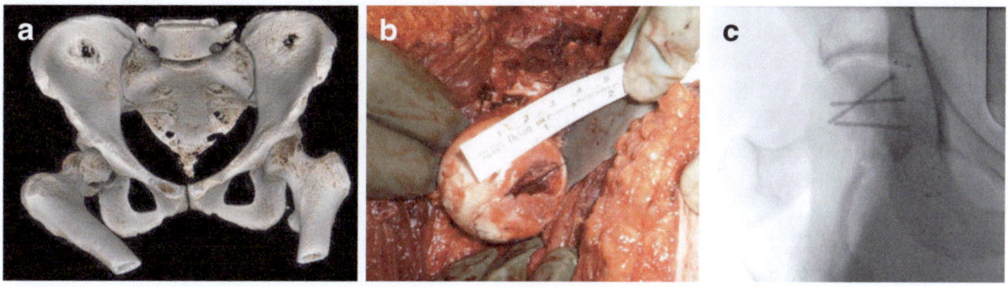

Fig. 14.2 Typical case of an anterior-inferior femoral head fracture with posterior hip dislocation (**a**). Using the Kocher-Langenbeck approach with surgical hip dislocation after open reduction, a typical defect anterior/medial/superior remains, which was not addressed but can optional be treated using a femoral head autograft (**b**). Intraoperative X-rays show a congruent joint (**c**)

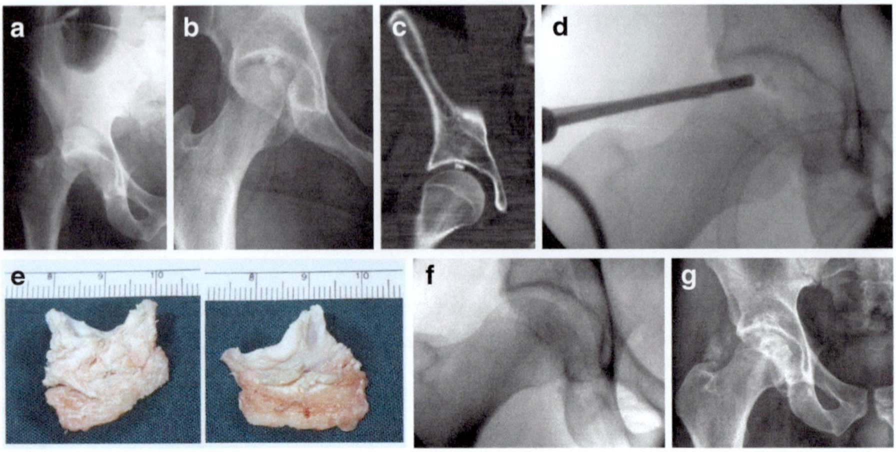

Fig. 14.3 Posterior-superior hip dislocation with an infrafoveal femoral head fracture fragment (**a**). After closed reduction, an acceptable fragment position was observed, but a superior intra-articular fragment was detected (**b**), which was confirmed during CT evaluation (**c**). Hip arthroscopy was used (**d**) to remove this fragment (**e**). Intraoperative imaging confirmed removal (**f**). The infrafoveal fragment was in an anatomic position and was not further addressed (**f**). At 6-month follow-up, some heterotopic ossifications developed, but no degenerative changes could be detected (**g**)

Although these minimally invasive and joint-preserving techniques show encouraging outcomes and may serve as valuable adjuncts, open reduction and internal fixation (ORIF) remains the current gold standard for the treatment of femoral head fractures.

Literature

1. Anthonissen J, Rommens P, Hofmann A. Mosaicplasty for the treatment of a large traumatic osteochondral femoral head lesion: a case report with 2 year follow-up and review of the literature. Arch Orthop Trauma Surg. 2016;136:41–6.
2. Aprato A, Buzzone M, Di Benedetto P, Masse A. Surgical hip dislocation vs arthroscopy for fixation of subfoveal femoral head fractures: a new technique for Pipkin type 1 fractures. Acta Biomed. 2021;92:e2021016. https://doi.org/10.23750/abm.v92iS3.11724.
3. Aprato A, Caruso R, Reboli M, Giachino M, Masse A. Arthroscopic reduction and fixation of a Pipkin type-I femoral head fracture. JBJS Essent Surg Tech. 2024;14
4. Au B, Jamieson M, Banerjee R. Rotational osteoplasty for femoral head fracture with cartilage loss. Orthopedics. 2013;36:e105–8.
5. Bartlett C, Birch C. Femoral head reduction osteoplasty for fracture dislocation: a surgical technique. Injury. 2015;46:1689–94.
6. Bastian J, Buchler L, Meyer D, Siebenrock K, Keel M. Surgical hip dislocation for osteochondral transplantation as a salvage procedure for a femoral head impaction fracture. J Orthop Trauma. 2010;24:e113–8.
7. Bettinelli G, Placella G, Moharamzadeh D, Belluati A, Salini V. Articular femoral head fracture management: a meta-analysis of literature. Ind J Orthop. 2021;55(Suppl 2):S304–13.

8. Böhler J. Experimentelle Untersuchungen über die Ursache der sog. Kopfnekrose nach Verrenkungen und Verrenkungsbrüchen des Hüftgelenkes. Chirurg. 1953;24:344–9.
9. Chen C, Hsu S, Hsu C, Liu H, Lu Y. Pipkin Type I and II femoral head fractures: internal fixation or excision?-from the hip arthroscopy perspective. J Hip Preserv Surg. 2023;10:31–6.
10. Chen Z, Lin B, Ding Z, Lian K, Kang L, Guo L, Zhai W. Treatment of Pipkin type I fracture of femoral head associated with posterior dislocation of the hip. Zhongguo Xiu Fu Chong Jian Wai Ke Za Zhi. 2011;25:521–5.
11. Chiron P, Lafontan V, Reina N. Fracture-dislocations of the femoral head. Orthop Traumatol Surg Res. 2013;99:S53–66.
12. Coulomb R, Alrubaie A, Haigniere V, Kouyoumdjian P. Femoral head mosaicplasty by direct anterior approach for an osteochondral impaction without performing surgical hip dislocation. SICOT J. 2021;7:22. https://doi.org/10.1051/sicotj/2021014.
13. Dallich A, Rath E, Atzmon R, Radparvar J, Fontana A, Sharfman Z, Amar E. Chondral lesions in the hip: a review of relevant anatomy, imaging and treatment modalities. J Hip Preserv Surg. 2019;6:3–15.
14. El Bitar Y, Lindner D, Jackson T, Domb B. Joint-preserving surgical options for management of chondral injuries of the hip. J Am Acad Orthop Surg. 2014;22:46–56.
15. Enocson A, Wolf O. Pipkin fractures: epidemiology and outcome. Eur J Trauma Emerg Surg. 2022;48:4113–8.
16. Epstein H. Posterior fracture-dislocation of the hip. J Bone Joint Surg. 1961;43-A:1079–98.
17. Epstein HC. Posterior fracture-dislocations of the hip; long-term follow-up. J Bone Joint Surg Am. 1974;56:1103–27.
18. Ferguson T, Patel R, Bhandari M, Matta J. Fractures of the acetabulum in patients aged 60 years and older: an epidemiological and radiological study. J Bone Joint Surg Br. 2010;92:250–7.
19. Fickert S, Aurich M, Albrecht D, Angele P, Buchler L, Dienst M, Erggelet C, Fritz J, Gebhart C, Gollwitzer H, Kindler M, Lampert C, et al. Biologic reconstruction of full sized cartilage defects of the hip: a guideline from the DGOU Group "clinical tissue regeneration" and the Hip Committee of the AGA. Z Orthop Unfall. 2017;155:670–82.
20. Gagala J, Tarczynska M, Gaweda K. Fixation of femoral head fractures with autologous osteochondral transfer (mosaicplasty). J Orthop Trauma. 2014;28:e226–30.
21. Gay B, Roman W, Arbogast R. Makroskopische und mikroskopische Veränderungen am Femurkopf nach Acetabulumfrakturen. Unfallheilkunde. 1984;164:663–9.
22. Gay B, Romen W. Makroskopische und mikroskopische Befunde am Femurkopf nach Acetabulumfraktur. Unfallheilkunde. 1983;86:201–4.
23. Giannoudis P, Kontakis G, Christoforakis Z, Akula M, Tosounidis T, Koutras C. Management complications and clinical results of femoral head fractures. Injury. 2009;40:1245–51.
24. Giordano V, Giordano M, Gloria R, de Souza F, di Tullio P, Lages M, Koch H. General principles for treatment of femoral head fractures. J Clin Orthop Trauma. 2019;10:155–60.
25. Hangody L, Fules P. Autologous osteochondral mosaicplasty for the treatment of full-thickness defects of weight-bearing joints: ten years of experimental and clinical experience. J Bone Joint Surg Am. 2003;85-A Suppl 2:25–32.
26. Hanke M, Keel M, Cullmann JL, Siebenrock K, Bastian J. Transfer of osteochondral shell autografts to salvage femoral head impaction injuries in hip trauma patients. Injury. 2020;51:711–8.
27. Hidden K, Yang J, Githens M, Firoozabadi R. Closed reduction technique for acetabular fractures with femoral head protrusion and concomitant superolateral impaction: a case report. JBJS Case Connect. 2023;13
28. Hsu S, Chen C, Ko J, Hsu C, Liu H, Lu Y. Hip arthroscopy-assisted reduction and fixation for femoral head fracture dislocations: clinical and radiographic short-term results of seven cases. J Orthop Surg (Hong Kong). 2019;27:2309499019881865. https://doi.org/10.1177/2309499019881865.
29. Hu H, Yang H, Wang G, Gan M, Li J, Cao Z, Wang Q. Analysis of influencing factors of hip functional recovery after Pipkin fracture surgery. Zhongguo Xiu Fu Chong Jian Wai Ke Za Zhi. 2012;26:433–6.

30. Kekatpure A, Ahn T, Lee SJ, Jeong M, Chang J, Yoon P. Arthroscopic reduction and internal fixation for Pipkin type I femoral head fracture: technical note. Arthrosc Tech. 2016;5:e997–e1000.
31. Kloen P, Siebenrock K, Raaymakers E, Marti R, Ganz R. Femoral head fractures revisited. Eur J Trauma. 2002;28:221–33.
32. Kong G. Osteochondral autograft transplants for femoral head impaction fracture: a case report with arthroscopic findings. J Clin Orthop Trauma. 2017;8:S29–31.
33. Konrath G, Hamel A, Guerin J, Olson SA, Bay B, Sharkey NA. Biomechanical evaluation of impaction fractures of the femoral head. J Orthop Trauma. 1999;13:407–13.
34. Kosashvili Y, Raz G, Backstein D, Lulu O, Gross A, Safir O. Fresh-stored osteochondral allografts for the treatment of femoral head defects: surgical technique and preliminary results. Int Orthop. 2013;37:1001–6.
35. Krych A, Lorich D, Kelly B. Osteochondral autograft transfer for a posttraumatic osteochondral defect of the femoral head. Am J Orthop (Belle Mead NJ). 2012;41:472–6.
36. Lansford T, Munns S. Arthroscopic treatment of Pipkin type I femoral head fractures: a report of 2 cases. J Orthop Trauma. 2012;26:e94–6.
37. Larson C. Fracture dislocations of the hip. Clin Orthop Relat Res. 1973:147–54.
38. Lederer S, Tauber M, Karpik S, Bogner R, Auffahrt A, Resch H. Hüftkopffrakturen – eine Mulicenterstudie. Unfallchirurg. 2007;110:513–20.
39. Lee H, Kim H, Jo S. Femoral head cartilage reconstruction using autologous osteochondral mosaicplasty: a case report. Medicine (Baltimore). 2023;102:e32913. https://doi.org/10.1097/MD.0000000000032913.
40. Lehmann W, Spering C. Pipkin-Frakturen. Unfallchirurg. 2022;125:313–23.
41. Letournel E, Judet R. Fractures of the acetabulum. 2nd ed. Berlin/Heidelberg: Springer; 1993.
42. Matsuda D. A rare fracture, an even rarer treatment: the arthroscopic reduction and internal fixation of an isolated femoral head fracture. Arthroscopy. 2009;25:408–12.
43. Matsuda D. The clamshell fracture and adjunctive acetabuloplasty in the arthroscopic osteosynthesis of femoral head fractures with femoroacetabular impingement. Arthrosc Tech. 2012;1:e5–e10.
44. Meyers M. Resurfacing of the femoral head with fresh osteochondral allografts. Long-term results. Clin Orthop Relat Res. 1985:111–4.
45. Nam D, Shindle M, Buly R, Kelly B, Lorich D. Traumatic osteochondral injury of the femoral head treated by mosaicplasty: a report of two cases. HSS J. 2010;6:228–34.
46. Nousiainen M, Sen M, Mintz D, Lorich D, Paul O, Buly R, Helfet D. The use osteochondral allograft in the treatment of a severe femoral head fracture. J Orthop Trauma. 2010;24:120–4.
47. Ordway C, Xeller C. Transverse computerized axial tomography of patients with posterior dislocation of the hip. J Trauma. 1984;24:76–9.
48. Park M, Her I, Cho H, Chung Y. Internal fixation of femoral head fractures (Pipkin I) using hip arthroscopy. Knee Surg Sports Traumatol Arthrosc. 2014;22:898–901.
49. Park M, Yoon S, Choi S. Hip arthroscopic management for femoral head fractures and posterior acetabular wall fractures (Pipkin Type IV). Arthrosc Tech. 2013;2:e221–5.
50. Passaplan C, Hanauer M, Gautier L, Stetzelberger V, Schwab J, Tannast M, Gautier E. Surface repair of the femoral head using press-osteochondral autograft transfer. Bone Jt Open. 2023;4:523–31.
51. Pipkin G. Treatment of grade IV fracture dislocation of the hip. J Bone Joint Surg. 1957;39A:1027–42.
52. Poletti P, Sahin M, Peter R, Boudabbous S, Herpe G, Rutschmann O, Platon A. Femoral head subchondral impaction on CT: what does it mean in patients with acetabular fracture? Skeletal Radiol. 2019;48:939–48.
53. Richardson P, Young J, Porter D. CT detection of cortical fracture of the femoral head associated with posterior hip dislocation. AJR Am J Roentgenol. 1990;155:93–4.
54. Riedel B. Längsfraktur von Schenkelkopf und –Hals. Bericht über die Verh Dtsch Ges Chir XIV. Congr Beilage Zbl Chir. 1885;12(24):92–3.

55. Rojas-Sayol R, De Caso J, Valera M. Arthroscopic-assisted percutaneous fixation of a femoral head fracture (Pipkin II): a case report. JBJS Case Connect. 2022;12
56. Rollmann M, Holstein J, Pohlemann T, Herath S, Histing T, Braun B, Schmal H, Putzeys G, Marintschev I, Aghayev E. Predictors for secondary hip osteoarthritis after acetabular fractures-a pelvic registry study. Int Orthop. 2019;43:2167–73.
57. Sahin V, Karakas E, Aksu S, Atlihan D, Turk C, Halici M. Traumatic dislocation and fracture-dislocation of the hip: a long-term follow-up study. J Trauma. 2003;54:520–9.
58. Sampson T. Arthroscopic treatment for chondral lesions of the hip. Clin Sports Med. 2011;30:331–48.
59. Scolaro J, Marecek G, Firoozabadi R, Krieg J, Routt M. Management and radiographic outcome of femoral head fractures. J Orthopaed Traumatol. 2017; https://doi.org/10.1007/s10195-017-0445-z.
60. Shakya S, Chen J, Sun J, Xiang Z. Management and outcome of patients with femoral head fractures: the mid-term follow-up with injuries and associated prognostic factors. BMC Musculoskelet Disord. 2023;24:311.
61. Sobczyk J, Drwiega M, Banasiewicz J, Laskowski J. Arthroscopic fixation of osteochondral fracture of head of femur. Case study. Ortop Traumatol Rehabil. 2019;21:219–26.
62. Soylemez M, Kemah B, Poyanli O. Arthroscopy-assisted reduction and fixation of femoral head and acetabulum fractures: a systematic review of the literature. Orthop Surg. 2022;14:652–62.
63. Stein H. Computerized tomography for ascertaining osteocartilagenous intraarticular (slice) fractures of the femoral head. Isr J Med Sci. 1983;19:180–4.
64. Stewart M, Milford L. Fracture-dislocation of the hip. An end-result study. J Bone Joint Surg. 1954;36-A:315–42.
65. Tannast M, Mack P, Klaeser B, Siebenrock K. Hip dislocation and femoral neck fracture: decision-making for head preservation. Injury. 2009;40:1118–24.
66. Tehranzadeh J, Vanarthos W, Pais M. Osteochondral impaction of the femoral head associated with hip dislocation: CT study in 35 patients. AJR Am J Roentgenol. 1990;155:1049–52.
67. Thompson V, Epstein H. Traumatic dislocation of the hip. J Bone Joint Surg. 1951;33A:746–78.
68. Tonetti J, Ruatti S, Lafontan V, Loubignac F, Chiron P, Sari-Ali H, Bonnevialle P. Is femoral head fracture-dislocation management improvable: a retrospective study in 110 cases. Orthop Traumatol Surg Res. 2010;96:623–31.
69. Won Y, Lee G, Kim S, Kim S, Yang K. Osteochondral autograft from the ipsilateral femoral head by surgical dislocation for treatment of femoral head fracture dislocation: a case report. Yonsei Med J. 2016;57:1527–30.
70. Yin X, Liu Y, Liu W, Yin Q. Arthroscopic fixation with absorbable suture anchors for Pipkin type I femoral head fractures-letter V technique. Arthrosc Tech. 2024;13:103090. https://doi.org/10.1016/j.eats.2024.103090.
71. Zelken J. First-person long-term follow-up using autologous mosaicplasty for osteochondral lesion accompanying femoral head fracture. J Orthop Trauma. 2016;30:e70–4.
72. Zotter K, Titze A. Femurkopffrakturen bei Verrenkungsbrüchen des Hüftgelenks – operative Versorgung mit Knochenschrauben. Hefte zur Unfallheilkunde Heft. 1974;124:85–7.

Outcome in Femoral Head Fractures

15

Srinivas Kasha and Ranjith Kumar Yalamanchili

Key Points

- The timing of intervention is crucial, as treatment that starts more than 6 h after injury increases the likelihood of ONFH and leads to worse functional outcomes.
- The surgeon's experience and fracture features are generally the deciding factors when selecting a surgical strategy, with anterior approaches yielding superior functional results.
- Optimizing results requires early closed reduction and anatomical fracture reconstruction in addition to a customized strategy depending on the type of fracture and patient-specific variables.
- Indentation injuries are often associated with poor outcomes, and among elderly patients, primary THA is strongly recommended for favorable outcomes.
- Although delayed and neglected cases have poor outcomes, considering patient-specific factors, a treatment algorithm appropriate for the fracture pattern should be selected, and THA in elderly patients can be considered an option for faster rehabilitation and good outcomes.

S. Kasha (✉)
Department of Orthopaedics, Krishna Institute of Medical Sciences, Secunderabad, Telangana, India

R. K. Yalamanchili
Department of Orthopaedics, All India Institute of Medical Sciences, Hyderabad, Telangana, India

R. K. Sen, S. K. Tripathy (eds.), *A Practical Guide to Management of Femoral Head Fracture-Dislocation*, https://doi.org/10.1007/978-981-96-9852-3_15

15.1 Introduction

Femoral head fractures are mostly associated with hip dislocation, with or without an acetabular fracture. Thus, many factors and complications related to hip dislocation and acetabular fractures also significantly influence the outcome of treatment for femoral head fractures. Injury to the proximal femur blood supply is also multifactorial and can occur either during injury or dislocation or at the time of surgical intervention to treat fractures, making the outcome of femoral head fracture alone more complex. Hence, these injuries must be seen as an entire perspective to the hip when assessing their outcome. Historically, femoral head fractures have been reported to have poor outcomes, as the mainstay of treatment has been mostly conservative management or excision of the fragments [1, 2]. In recent years, the extensive use of CT scans to understand fracture morphology, along with improved familiarity with surgical approaches and better orientation to surgical techniques, have changed the treatment protocols and improved the outcomes [3]. The poor outcomes following femoral head fracture are dictated by the major complications associated with these injuries, which include osteonecrosis of the femoral head (ONFH), posttraumatic osteoarthritis (PTOA), heterotopic ossification (HO), and peripheral nerve injury. Outcomes of the femoral head injuries are commonly assessed by Thompson and Epstein criteria [4], Merle d'Aubigne and Postel functional score [5] (based on pain, mobility, and walking ability), Stewart–Milford criteria [6] (combining roentgenographic and clinical findings), or Harris Hip Scores [7].

15.1.1 Outcome with Respect to Time to Intervention

Most studies have reported higher incidence of ONFH and posttraumatic osteoarthritis in patients with delayed treatment (>6 h after injury) of hip dislocation associated with femoral head fractures [8]. As most of the Pipkin fractures are associated with hip dislocation, emergency hip reduction within 6 h of injury minimizes the chances of ONFH and improves chances of outcome. The advantage of an emergency trauma operating room and experienced team in cases of irreducible hip dislocations is that the definitive procedure can be performed immediately if closed reduction fails, which will shorten the hospital stay and improve functional outcomes [9].

15.1.2 Outcome Trends in Conservative and Operative Management

The results of a randomized control trial (RCT) comparing conservative to surgical management of Pipkin type I fractures (where displacement of the fracture does not play a role in decision-making strategies) revealed that the outcome of the conservative group was worse than that of the fragment excision group [10]. A similar outcome was demonstrated in another RCT, in which Pipkin type II fractures were randomized to surgical and conservative groups [11].

15.1.3 Outcome vs. Surgical Approach Selection

Although the injury pattern itself amounts to damage to the femoral head cartilage and jeopardizes the blood supply of the femoral head, poor outcomes are also attributed to the difficulties encountered in obtaining adequate exposure for the reduction and fixation of these injuries [12].

The choice of surgical approach for treating femoral head fractures remains uncertain and is favored by surgeons' familiarity with the approach, keeping in view the fracture type and associated acetabular wall injuries. When the modified Hueter approach and the Kocher–Langenbeck approach for the treatment of Pipkin type I and II femoral head fractures were compared, differences were found only in surgical time and blood loss, whereas complication rates and functional outcomes were nearly similar [13]. Another study comparing the combination of the Kocher–Langenbeck approach with flip osteotomy performed through the Gibson interval and direct Kocher–Langenbeck approach alone revealed that the former was associated with a shorter operative time, less blood loss, and improved visualization, with no difference in the rates of complications or outcomes [14].

Kloub et al. used the Thompson and Epstein scoring systems and analyzed the functional outcome in relation to the surgical approach among 295 patients from 17 articles. They reported that the minimally invasive approach (57%) and flip osteotomy (54%) had higher rates of excellent results than did the medial (24%) or Kocher–Langenbeck approaches (28%) [15]. Type I and II injuries treated either by fragment excision or by open reduction and internal fixation (ORIF) had good to excellent results in both the fragment excision and ORIF groups, but the cases treated with anterior approaches had slightly better results [10, 13, 16].

Liu et al., in their study on the Pipkin type IV injury pattern, reported that the direct anterior approach combined with the posterior approach does not increase the operative time or intraoperative estimated blood loss but can promote favorable functional outcomes without increasing complications [17].

15.1.4 Outcomes for Specific Fracture Types (Pipkin Injury Classification)

15.1.4.1 Pipkin Type I

Nonoperative treatment is a good option in cases wherein the anatomic reduction is achieved with a stable hip joint as assessed in post-reduction CT scan. This may not be possible in type II injuries, wherein the fracture extends above the fovea into the weight-bearing region, given the inherent risk of displacement. Swiontkowski et al. demonstrated good outcome in their series with cases <1 mm displacement of fragments on CT scan and recommends serial radiographs to observe for chances of displacement [18]. Giannoudis et al. reported a favorable outcome of 87% (good to excellent) among their series of 71 patients who underwent excision of fractured fragments [19]. Most cases of this type of fracture involve anterior approaches, namely, the Hueter, Smith–Peterson, or medial Ludloff approaches.

Chen et al., in their randomized prospective study, reported better outcomes ($P = 0.032$) in the fragment excision group than in the closed reduction group among Pipkin type I femoral head fractures [10]. Park et al. evaluated the management of Pipkin I fractures with respect to fragment size and location and reported that large fracture fragments had excellent or good results with internal fixation (82.6%) [16].

Arthroscopic reduction and fixation of info-foveal fractures of the femoral head can be good minimally invasive options. The outcome following arthroscopic reduction was excellent in most cases, with patients returning to their previous occupation [20, 21]. Percutaneous osteosynthesis for nondisplaced large femoral head fractures helps in early rehabilitation and combines the advantages of conservative and surgical treatment, making it a good alternative choice for such nondisplaced congruent head fractures following hip dislocation [22].

15.1.4.2 Pipkin Type II

Pipkin type II fractures involve a larger area of the weight-bearing part of the femoral head and are more challenging injuries that are amenable to internal fixation [23]. Although these injuries can be approached with any of the surgical approaches to the hip joint, there has been an increasing tendency to use trochanteric flip osteotomy, which provides a 360° view of the femoral head. Early reduction of the hip and stable reduction with internal fixation following anatomical reduction are important factors in determining positive outcomes in these fracture patterns, whereas the development of ONFH and heterotrophic ossification lead to poor outcomes [24, 25] (Fig. 15.1).

Fracture comminution and displacement in general has poor outcomes in long-term follow-up but does not warrant excision. A trial of salvage with internal fixation using multiple headless screws to reconstruct the joint can yield mid-term good outcomes, although a longer follow-up evidence is required [26].

15.1.4.3 Pipkin Type III

These uncommon injuries are associated with increased rates of avascular necrosis in reconstructive procedures requiring secondary total hip arthroplasty. Fractures of the femoral neck and femoral head are dual insults to the blood supply of the head of the femur. Most such injuries have been reported to have poor outcomes, particularly when the neck of the femur is grossly displaced [27]. Patients with such injury patterns should be well informed about the poor outcome and need secondary THA following complications arising after primary internal fixation. Outcomes in series treated by internal fixation are poor, requiring revision to hip arthroplasty as early as 6 months [24, 27, 28]. As many as 50% of the patients treated by internal fixation methods reported poor outcomes following these injury patterns [29]. Younger age groups (<35 years) can be given a trial of reconstruction with hip salvage, but indications for internal fixation in middle-aged patients should be decided carefully.

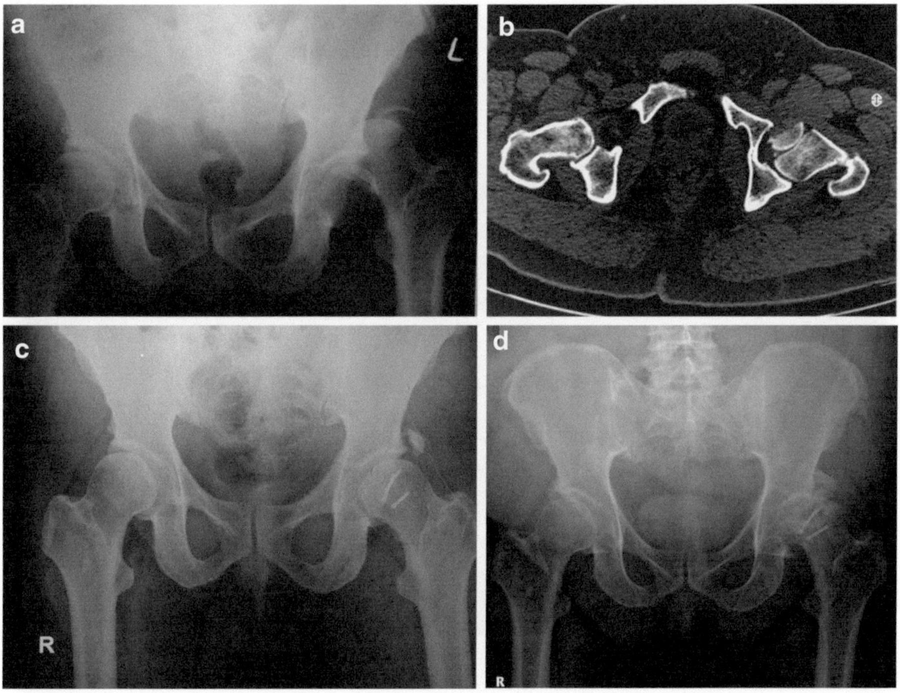

Fig. 15.1 A 48-year-old male patient who sustained a type II Pipkin fracture following a road traffic accident (RTA) and was treated with ORIF with headless compression screws via the Hueter approach. (**a**) Preoperative image showing posterior dislocation. (**b**) CT scan of the pelvis showing a femoral head fracture in a reduced hip dislocation. (**c**) Postoperative radiograph showing the femoral head fixed with Herbert screws. (**d**) Radiograph of the patient with ONFH at the 8-year follow-up

The use of the posterior approach should be discouraged to avoid poor outcomes due to vascular compromise of the femoral head [30].

15.1.4.4 Pipkin Type IV

Most of these injuries are treated with posterior approaches to the hip with or without trochanteric osteotomy. The combination of approaches (posterior and anterior) is another possibility, as the majority of head fractures are located on the anterior part of the femoral head and fixation can be demanding when a Kocher–Langenbeck or Gibson approach is used (Figs. 15.2 and 15.3).

15.1.5 Outcomes Following Fixation

Cichos et al. reported that Pipkin IV fractures managed surgically have a greater risk of secondary surgery (THA) within 1 year (28.5%), and the risk factors vary according to the fracture subtype [31]. Pipkin IV fractures are subclassified as OTA/

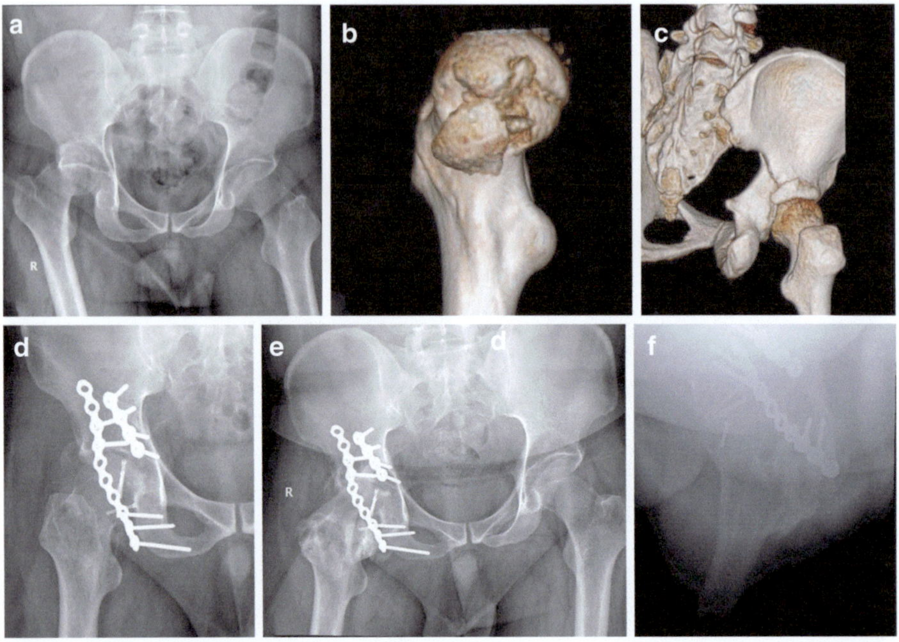

Fig. 15.2 (**a**) Preoperative radiograph of the pelvis of a 34-year-old male who underwent RTA with a type IV Pipkin fracture. (**b, c**) CT scan showing a posterior wall and posterior column fracture with an infra-foveal fracture of the femoral head. (**d**) Immediate postoperative radiograph showing column and wall fixation along with femoral head fixation. (**e, f**) Radiographs at follow-up showing heterotrophic ossification of the hip—Brooker grade IV ankylosis

AO 31C2 type fractures with supra-foveal and posterior head impaction, and older patients should be counselled on the need for a secondary procedure (THA) due to the poor outcomes of ORIF [31, 32]. The rate of conversion to THA ranges from 10% at 1 year [27] to 50% at long-term follow-up [33].

15.2 Outcomes in Fragment Excision

The biomechanical impact of removing fragments smaller than one-third of the femoral head is unclear; however, previous research recommended doing so [1, 2]. Previous studies indicate that internal fixation and fragment excision produce comparable results [11, 34]. Kokubo et al. recommended that larger fragments (>1 cm) should be salvaged, whereas those less than 1 cm should be removed [35]. Fragment size, comminution, and placement in relation to the weight-bearing area influence the outcome of femoral head fractures.

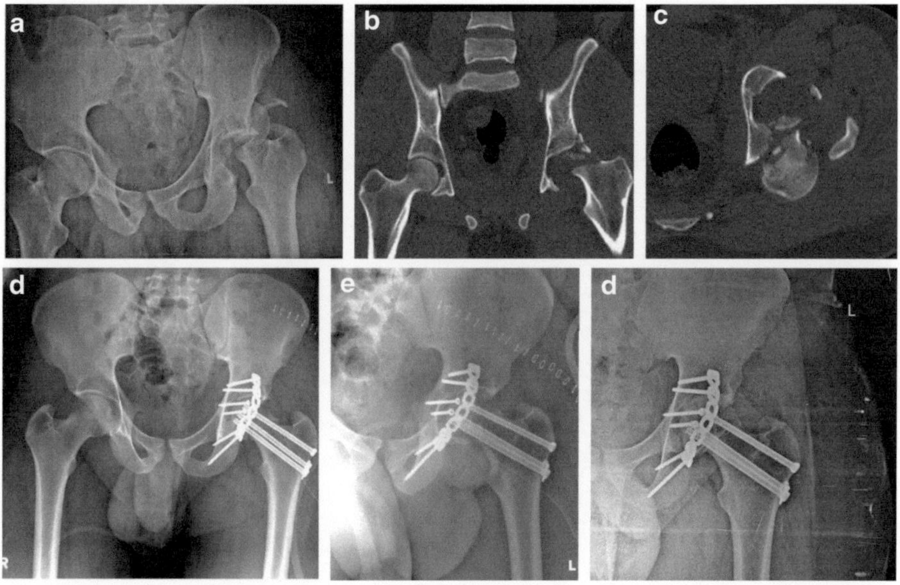

Fig. 15.3 (**a**) Preoperative radiograph of the pelvis of a 25-year-old male with femoral head fracture and neck of femur fracture associated with posterior wall injury. (**b, c**) CT scan showing marginal fracture of the femoral head with the neck of the femur fracture and posterior dislocation of the hip. (**d, e**) Immediate postoperative radiograph showing posterior acetabular wall fixation along with femoral neck fixation and excision of femoral head fragments. (**f**) Radiographs at the 6-year follow-up showing the healed neck of the femur fracture and posttraumatic osteoarthritis of the hip (PTOA)

15.2.1 Outcomes of Patients with Femoral Head Indentation Fractures

Femoral head indentation fractures and transchondral shear fractures of the femoral head are usually associated with anterior dislocations of the hip. DeLee et al. reported fair to poor outcomes in more than 50% of their series of such injuries [36]. These indentation fractures require elevation of the depressed part and sometimes bone grafting to prevent early collapse via a technique similar to the "trap-door" procedure performed for ONFH [30, 37]. In elderly patients with femoral head indentation injury, primary THA is strongly recommended for favorable outcomes [38, 39] (Fig. 15.4).

15.2.2 Outcome in Associated Acetabular Dome Impaction Fractures

Dome impaction fractures of the acetabulum can also be associated with femoral head injuries. Lai et al. reported that marginal impaction fractures of the acetabulum

Fig. 15.4 A case of an indentation fracture of the femoral head with a posterior wall fracture treated by primary THA. (**a, b**) CT scan showing an indentation fracture of the femoral head with a posterior wall fracture of the acetabulum. (**c**) Intraoperative image showing significant osteochondral loss of the femoral head. (**d**) Intraoperative image showing internal fixation of the posterior wall of the acetabulum and acetabular cup. (**e**) Follow-up X-ray image of the AP and (**f**) lateral view of the hip and proximal femur at 4 years after primary uncemented THA

had higher rates of ONFH than those without an impact injury and hypothesized that this was due to the greater forces on the femoral head during direct impact on the acetabulum [40]. Papachristos et al. suggested the need for posterior wall osteotomy along with surgical dislocation of the hip to treat such impaction injuries of the acetabulum and address concomitant osteochondral femoral head fractures [41]. Understanding such fracture morphology is necessary to plan a treatment strategy and select an approach to address femoral head fracture for favorable outcomes [42].

15.2.3 Outcomes of Associated Irreducible Hip Dislocation

While femoral head fractures are only rare injuries, irreducible hip dislocations are even less common. Apart from indentation injuries, button holing of the femoral head associated with capsulo-labral incarceration makes it challenging to reduce by closed means even under muscle relaxation. Such presentations require open reduction of the joint by freeing the tissues and subsequent congruent reduction of the joint followed by osteosynthesis of the fracture. These injuries require the use of an appropriate strategy for addressing the injuries of interest and are often associated with a high risk of ONFH and poor outcomes [43] (Fig. 15.5).

15.2.4 Outcomes in Children and Adolescents

These are very rare injuries and are mostly associated with dislocation following high-velocity injuries. The treatment perspective is very similar to that of adult injuries [44]. MRI plays a greater role in this age group for the assessment of labral damage and osteochondral defects following reduction of the hip joint to plan appropriate steps of definitive treatment [45]. MRI also has a role in evaluating the long-term complications associated with these injuries.

15.2.4.1 Outcomes in Delayed and Neglected Presentations

Sen et al. reported their series of 138 patients who presented delayed (where the hip was not reduced within 6 h of injury) and neglected (where the patients presented >6 weeks after injury) [46]. Late reduction of the hip (after more than 6 h of injury) had an adverse effect on the outcome, as most patients developed ONFH (14.5%). The incidence of avascular necrosis and the need for secondary procedures are greater in delayed and neglected femoral head fracture dislocations. In their series, Sen et al. reported that ONFH is commonly observed in Brumback type 2A injuries and posterior approaches and that all Brumback type 3B fractures should be treated with THA when presented late [46]. Osteosynthesis in other injury patterns among delayed presentations yields good outcomes. In their series, they reported good to excellent outcome results in 52.89% of patients and poor-to-fair results in 47.11% of patients and concluded that careful selection of a treatment plan can result in comparable functional outcomes even among patients with delayed presentations [46].

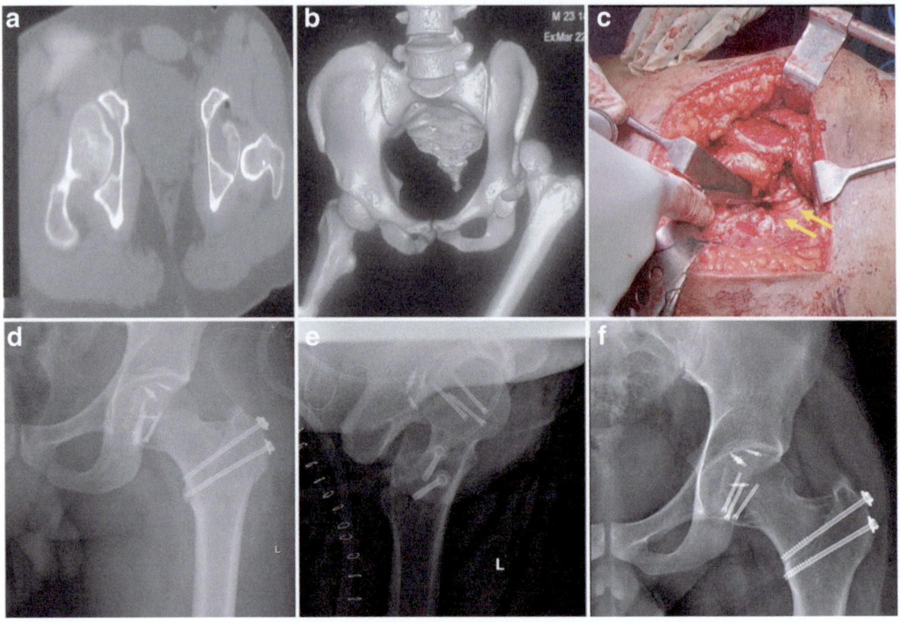

Fig. 15.5 A case of irreducible hip dislocation due to capsulo labral button holing of the femoral head treated by immediate open reduction and fixation with labral repair(**a, b**) CT scan showing a Pipkin type II fracture with irreducible hip dislocation. (**c**) Intraoperative image showing a labral tear (yellow arrow) that was repaired. (**d, e**) Immediate postoperative radiograph of the AP and lateral view showing reduction of the femoral head with suture anchors used for labral repair. (**f**) Radiograph at the 4-year follow-up showing no ONFH

In neglected presentations, particularly type IV injuries, stable cup insertion and acetabular bone conservation strategies are needed to improve the functional outcomes. Larger acetabular wall defects (>30%) caused by metal augments have better functions than those caused by structural femoral head grafts used to bridge the defects [47]. This is due to poor osteointegration of the acetabular component to the graft, which often results in the formation of a fibrous membrane in between, causing failure. However, there is no consensus for the recommendation of a reconstruction strategy in neglected presentations of type IV Pipkin with acetabular bone defects with respect to long-term (~10 years) survivorship.

15.2.5 Outcomes in Femoral Head Fractures Treated by THA

Although primary THA is reserved for elderly patients or those with complex injuries and relatively high chances of poor outcomes, THA is also the choice of treatment secondary to complications arising from femoral head fractures. The choice of bearing materials and fixation of components is the surgeon's preference, with the aim of increasing longevity and ease of revision if one fails. Elderly patients who undergo primary THA following the selected femoral head fractures discussed above have good to excellent outcomes. Hemiarthroplasty is reserved for patients with low functional demand and no associated arthritis or no associated acetabular injury [30].

15.3 Complications and Outcome

Since femoral head fractures are a part of high-velocity injuries, the outcome depends on associated injuries that can include head injury, pelvi-acetabular injury, genitourinary tract injury, spine injury, abdominal and chest injury, or combination of any of them. Poor outcomes in cases associated with systemic injuries are often due to delays in definitive treatment, as the severity of the systemic injuries may prevent timely surgery. Combined pelvi-acetabular injuries associated with femoral head fractures will have lower outcome than those associated with isolated acetabular injuries. Literature review attribute poor outcome in combined pelvi-acetabular injuries to the poor reduction of acetabulum and pelvic ring additional displacements than the isolated injury itself [48, 49].

The higher incidence of heterotopic ossification (HO) to about 35–40% is reported in western literature [19, 27]. Incidence of ONFH ranges from 8% to 14%, and higher rates of ONFH are found among delayed presentations, severe communition, and selection of posterior-based approach (posterior approach has 3.2 times increased risk) [3, 18]. Sen et al. observed osteolysis of the femoral head in follow-up among four patients, and this might be due to significant impact on articular cartilage that causes such focal osteolysis [46]. ONFH, focal osteolysis of the femoral head, and associated acetabular injuries on mid-term follow-up lead to osteoarthritis of the hip that have an impact on the outcome of the femoral head.

Sciatic injury is common with traumatic hip dislocations. The sciatic nerve, particularly its peroneal branch, is most often affected and can be injured through laceration, stretching, compression, or later encased in heterotopic ossification. While recovery occurs in 60–70% of cases, treatment outcomes remain controversial, and rehabilitation should focus on preventing foot deformities for better outcomes [50].

15.4 Summary

Complications following femoral head fractures play a pivotal role in determining the outcome. We believe that the functional outcome is not directly related to the treatment modality or approach but is attributed to many factors, such as the severity of the injury, general condition of the patient, morbidities, time to intervention from injury, associated cartilage injury, and level of comminution, along with the treatment modality adopted. Wide ranges in outcomes among each fracture type reported in the literature are possibly due to (a) a smaller sample size, (b) varied duration of follow-up reported, and (c) potential confounding effects of adoption of a treatment strategy along with expertise in its execution. For treatment, we should aim at early closed reduction of the joint and anatomic reduction of the fragments with minimum soft tissue injury by choosing the best approach for obtaining an excellent view of the fragments. Although delayed and neglected cases have poor outcomes, considering patient-specific factors, a treatment algorithm appropriate for the fracture pattern should be selected, and THA in elderly patients can be considered an option for faster rehabilitation and good outcomes.

References

1. Epstein HC. Posterior fracture-dislocations of the hip; long-term follow-up. J Bone Joint Surg Am. 1974;56(6):1103–27.
2. Epstein HC, Wiss DA, Cozen L. Posterior fracture dislocation of the hip with fractures of the femoral head. Clin Orthop. 1985;201:9–17.
3. Tripathy SK, Sethy SS, Sen RK. Femoral head fractures. In: Slullitel P, Rossi L, Camino-Willhuber G, editors. Orthopaedics and trauma: current concepts and best practices [Internet]. Cham: Springer;2024 [cited 2024 Sep 13]. p. 423–41. https://doi.org/10.1007/978-3-031-30518-4_34.
4. Thompson VP, Epstein HC. Traumatic dislocation of the hip; a survey of two hundred and four cases covering a period of twenty-one years. J Bone Joint Surg Am. 1951;33-A(3):746–78. passim
5. D'aubigne RM, Postel M. Functional results of hip arthroplasty with acrylic prosthesis. J Bone Joint Surg Am. 1954;36-A(3):451–75.
6. Stewart MJ, Milford LW. Fracture-dislocation of the hip; an end-result study. J Bone Joint Surg Am. 1954;36(A:2):315–42.
7. Chiron P, Lafontan V, Reina N. Fracture-dislocations of the femoral head. Orthop Traumatol Surg Res. 2013;99(1 Supplement):S53–66.
8. Wang S, Li B, Zhang Z, Yu X, Li Q, Liu L. Early versus delayed hip reduction in the surgical treatment of femoral head fracture combined with posterior hip dislocation: a comparative study. BMC Musculoskelet Disord. 2021;22(1):1057.
9. Lin D, Lian K, Chen Z, Wang L, Hao J, Zhang H. Emergent surgical reduction and fixation for Pipkin type I femoral fractures. Orthopedics. 2013;36(6):778–82.
10. Chen ZW, Lin B, Liang ZW, Min GZ, Liang Z, Zheng JP, et al. Conservative versus surgical management of Pipkin type I fractures associated with posterior dislocation of the hip: a randomised controlled trial. Int Orthop. 2011;35(7):1077–81.
11. Chen ZW, Liang ZW, Qi DZ, Jian LK, Qi KL, Xin GL, et al. Operative versus nonoperative management of Pipkin type-II fractures associated with posterior hip dislocation. Orthopedics. 2011;34(5):350.
12. Ozcan M, Copuroğlu C, Sarıdoğan K. Fractures of the femoral head: what are the reasons for poor outcome? Ulus Travma Ve Acil Cerrahi Derg Turk J Trauma Emerg Surg TJTES. 2011;17(1):51–6.
13. Wang S, Li B, Li J, Zhang Z, Yang H, Liu L. Comparison of the modified Heuter approach and the Kocher-Langenbeck approach in the treatment of Pipkin type I and type II femoral head fractures. Int Orthop. 2019;43(11):2613–20.
14. Mostafa MF, El-Adl W, El-Sayed MAE. Operative treatment of displaced Pipkin type I and II femoral head fractures. Arch Orthop Trauma Surg. 2014;134(5):637–44.
15. Kloub M, Látal P, Giannoudis P. Techniques and results of reconstruction of femoral head fractures: An Update. Injury. 2024;55(6):111473.
16. Park KS, Lee KB, Na BR, Yoon TR. Clinical and radiographic outcomes of femoral head fractures: excision vs. fixation of fragment in Pipkin type I: what is the optimal choice for femoral head fracture? J Orthop Sci. 2015;20(4):702–7.

17. Liu B, Zhao B, Zhang Q. Efficacy of direct anterior approach combined with direct posterior approach in Pipkin IV femoral head fractures. J Orthop Surg. 2022;17(1):160.
18. Swiontkowski MF, Thorpe M, Seiler JG, Hansen ST. Operative management of displaced femoral head fractures: case-matched comparison of anterior versus posterior approaches for Pipkin I and Pipkin II fractures. J Orthop Trauma. 1992;6(4):437–42.
19. Giannoudis PV, Kontakis G, Christoforakis Z, Akula M, Tosounidis T, Koutras C. Management, complications and clinical results of femoral head fractures. Injury. 2009;40(12):1245–51.
20. Chen CY, Hsu SL, Hsu CH, Liu HC, Lu YD. Pipkin Type I and II femoral head fractures: internal fixation or excision? – from the hip arthroscopy perspective. J Hip Preserv Surg. 2023;10(1):31–6.
21. Hsu SL, Chen CY, Ko JY, Hsu CH, Liu HC, Lu YD. Hip arthroscopy-assisted reduction and fixation for femoral head fracture dislocations: Clinical and radiographic short-term results of seven cases. J Orthop Surg Hong Kong. 2019;27(3):2309499019881865.
22. Kloub M, Holub K, Peml M, Urban J, Latal P. Closed reduction and minimally invasive screw osteosynthesis of Pipkin femoral head fractures. J Appl Biomed. 2023;21(1):1–6.
23. Shakya S, Chen J, Sun J, Xiang Z. Management and outcome of patients with femoral head fractures: the mid-term follow-up with injuries and associated prognostic factors. BMC Musculoskelet Disord. 2023;24(1):311.
24. Yoon TR, Rowe SM, Chung JY, Song EK, Jung ST, Anwar IB. Clinical and radiographic outcome of femoral head fractures: 30 patients followed for 3-10 years. Acta Orthop Scand. 2001;72(4):348–53.
25. Butler JE. Pipkin Type-II fractures of the femoral head. J Bone Joint Surg Am. 1981;63(8):1292–6.
26. Hafez MA, Hamza H. Is fixation an option for comminuted femoral head fracture? Ann Transl Med. 2015;3(14):203.
27. Scolaro JA, Marecek G, Firoozabadi R, Krieg JC, Routt ML. "Chip." Management and radiographic outcomes of femoral head fractures. J Orthop Traumatol. 2017;18(3):235–41.
28. Tonetti J, Ruatti S, Lafontan V, Loubignac F, Chiron P, Sari-Ali H, et al. Is femoral head fracture-dislocation management improvable: a retrospective study in 110 cases. Orthop Traumatol Surg Res. 2010;96(6):623–31.
29. Wang S, Yu X, Li B, Ding Q, Wang T, Li Q, et al. Pipkin type III femoral head fracture: which treatment strategy can be recommended? J Orthop Traumatol. 2023;24(1):28.
30. Giordano V, Giordano M, Glória RC, de Souza FS, di Tullio P, Lages MM, et al. General principles for treatment of femoral head fractures. J Clin Orthop Trauma. 2019;10(1):155–60.
31. Cichos KH, White PA, Bergin PF, Ghanem ES, McGwin G, Hawkins J, et al. Risk factors for early conversion total hip arthroplasty after Pipkin IV femoral head fracture. J Orthop Trauma. 2023;37(4):181–8.
32. Ullmark G. Femoral head fractures: hemiarthroplasty or total hip arthroplasty? Hip Int J Clin Exp Res Hip Pathol Ther. 2014;24(Suppl 10):e12–4.
33. Engel JL, Johnsen P, Patel NK, Satpathy J, Mounasamy V. Pipkin type IV femoral head fractures: a case series and review of literature. Eur J Orthop Surg Traumatol Orthop Traumatol. 2021;31(4):791–5.
34. Droll KP, Broekhuyse H, O'Brien P. Fracture of the femoral head. J Am Acad Orthop Surg. 2007;15(12):716–27.
35. Kokubo Y, Uchida K, Takeno K, Yayama T, Miyazaki T, Negoro K, et al. Dislocated intra-articular femoral head fracture associated with fracture-dislocation of the hip and acetabulum: report of 12 cases and technical notes on surgical intervention. Eur J Orthop Surg Traumatol Orthop Traumatol. 2013;23(5):557–64.
36. DeLee JC, Evans JA, Thomas J. Anterior dislocation of the hip and associated femoral-head fractures. J Bone Joint Surg Am. 1980;62(6):960–4.
37. Church DJ, Merrill HM, Kotwal S, Dubin JR. Novel technique for femoral head reconstruction using allograft following obturator hip dislocation. J Orthop Case Rep. 2016;6(1):48–51.
38. Stannard JP, Harris HW, Volgas DA, Alonso JE. Functional outcome of patients with femoral head fractures associated with hip dislocations. Clin Orthop. 2000;377:44–56.

39. Henle P, Kloen P, Siebenrock KA. Femoral head injuries: Which treatment strategy can be recommended? Injury. 2007;38(4):478–88.
40. Lai PJ, Lai CY, Tseng IC, Su CY, Yu YH. Influence of associated femoral head fractures on surgical outcomes following osteosynthesis in posterior wall acetabular fractures. BMC Musculoskelet Disord. 2022;23(1):830.
41. Papachristos IV, Johnson JP, Giannoudis PV. Treatment of incarcerated impaction of acetabular fractures with concomitant osteochondral femoral head fractures by the use of a posterior wall osteotomy and surgical hip dislocation: a novel technique. J Am Acad Orthop Surg. 2019;27(24):e1086–92.
42. Kasha S, Yalamanchili RK. Articular disimpaction in acetabular fractures. J Clin Orthop Trauma. 2020;11(6):1025–30.
43. Menger MM, Braun BJ, Herath SC, Küper MA, Rollmann MF, Histing T. Fractures of the femoral head: a narrative review. EFORT Open Rev. 2021;6(11):1122–31.
44. Mehlman CT, Hubbard GW, Crawford AH, Roy DR, Wall EJ. Traumatic hip dislocation in children. Long-term followup of 42 patients. Clin Orthop. 2000;376:68–79.
45. Strüwind CM, von Rüden C, Thannheimer A, Bühren V, Schneidmueller D. Relevance of MRI after closed reduction of traumatic hip dislocation in children. Z Orthopadie Unfallchirurgie. 2018;156(5):586–91.
46. Sen RK, Tripathy SK, Goyal T, Aggarwal S, Kashyap S, Purudappa PP, et al. Complications and functional outcome of femoral head fracture-dislocation in delayed and neglected cases. Indian J Orthop. 2021;55(3):595–605.
47. Singh A, Telagareddy K, Kumar P, Singh S, Singh RN, Singh PK. THA in patients with neglected acetabular fractures. SICOT-J. 2022;8:37.
48. Vaidya R, Blue K, Oliphant B, Tonnos F. Combined pelvic ring disruption and acetabular fracture: outcomes using a sequential reduction protocol and an anterior subcutaneous pelvic fixator (INFIX). J Orthop Trauma. 2019;33(Suppl 2):S66–71.
49. Hess AE, Johal HS, O'Toole RV, Nascone JW. Early postoperative displacement of combined pelvic ring injury with acetabular fracture. Orthopedics. 2017;40(3):163–8.
50. Cornwall R, Radomisli TE. Nerve injury in traumatic dislocation of the hip. Clin Orthop [Internet]. 2000 [cited 2024 Nov 27];377. Available from: https://pubmed.ncbi.nlm.nih.gov/10943188/

MIX
Papier aus verantwortungsvollen Quellen
Paper from responsible sources
FSC® C105338

If you have any concerns about our products,
you can contact us on
ProductSafety@springernature.com

In case Publisher is established outside the EU,
the EU authorized representative is:
Springer Nature Customer Service Center GmbH
Europaplatz 3, 69115 Heidelberg, Germany

Printed by Libri Plureos GmbH
in Hamburg, Germany